The World of Girolamo Donzellini

Girolamo Donzellini was born in 1513. He was a religious dissenter, a physician, and a bibliophile involved in the Medical Republic of Letters. He was put to death by the Venetian Inquisition in 1587, after being tried five times in his lifetime.

Extending beyond an individual case study to a granular and probing account of the many connections between Venetian physicians and heterodox religious movements in the wake of the Protestant Reformation, this innovative monograph reveals the heretical networks of physicians in sixteenth-century Venice. In addition to Donzellini himself, the web of actors includes printers, scholars, women, and alchemists who were all committed to fighting against religious dogma and violence in a time and place when both were the order of the day.

This book will appeal to researchers and students alike interested in the History of Medicine, the History of religious heterodoxy and tolerance, as well as the History of the Catholic Inquisition in Venice.

Alessandra Celati has been a Marie Curie Global Fellow between Stanford University and the University of Verona. She works as a researcher in collaboration with the University of Verona.

Routledge Studies in Early Modern Religious Dissents and Radicalism

Series editors: Federico Barbierato, Hannah Marcus, Stefano Villani, and Xenia von Tippelskirch

Titles in this series address the discursive constructions of religious dissent and the practices of radical movements in the early modern world. The series transcends traditional national and confessional historiographies to examine early modern religious culture as a dynamic system that was essential in forging complex identities and encouraging dialogue among them. The editors seek manuscripts that consider questions of dissent, radicalism, dissidence, libertinism, heresy, and heterodoxy, and that examine these themes historically as socio-cultural constructions.

British Protestant Missions and the Conversion of Europe, 1600–1900
Edited By Simone Maghenzani, Stefano Villani

Bodies in Early Modern Religious Dissent
Naked, Veiled, Vilified, Worshiped
Edited By Elisabeth Fischer, Xenia von Tippelskirch

Early Modern Diasporas
A European History
Mathilde Monge and Natalia Muchnik

The History of the Jews in Early Modern Italy
From the Renaissance to the Restoration
Marina Caffiero

Apocalypse Now
Connected Histories of Eschatological Movements from Moscow to Cusco, 15th–18th Centuries
Edited by Damien Tricoire and Lionel Laborie

The World of Girolamo Donzellini
A Network of Heterodox Physicians in Sixteenth-Century Venice
Alessandra Celati

The World of Girolamo Donzellini

A Network of Heterodox Physicians in Sixteenth-Century Venice

Alessandra Celati

Routledge
Taylor & Francis Group
LONDON AND NEW YORK

First published 2023
by Routledge
4 Park Square, Milton Park, Abingdon, Oxon OX14 4RN

and by Routledge
605 Third Avenue, New York, NY 10158

Routledge is an imprint of the Taylor & Francis Group, an informa business

British Library Cataloguing-in-Publication Data
A catalogue record for this book is available from the British Library

Library of Congress Cataloguing-in-Publication Data
Names: Celati, Alessandra, author.
Title: The world of Girolamo Donzellini : a network of heterodox physicians in sixteenth-century Venice / Alessandra Celati.
Description: Milton Park, Abingdon, Oxon ; New York, NY : Routledge, [2023] | Series: Routledge studies in early modern religious dissents and radicalism | Includes bibliographical references and index. |
Identifiers: LCCN 2022020149 (print) | LCCN 2022020150 (ebook) | ISBN 9781032112046 (hardback) | ISBN 9781032112060 (paperback) | ISBN 9781003218852 (ebook)
Subjects: LCSH: Donzellini, Girolamo, -1588. | Physicians--Italy--Venice--16th century. | Medicine--Italy--Venice--History--16th century. | Medicine--Religious aspects--Italy--Venice--History--16th century.
Classification: LCC R147.D66 C45 2023 (print) | LCC R147.D66 (ebook) | DDC 610.945/311--dc23/eng/20220727
LC record available at https://lccn.loc.gov/2022020149
LC ebook record available at https://lccn.loc.gov/2022020150

ISBN: 978-1-032-11204-6 (hbk)
ISBN: 978-1-032-11206-0 (pbk)
ISBN: 978-1-003-21885-2 (ebk)

DOI: 10.4324/9781003218852

Typeset in Times New Roman
by MPS Limited, Dehradun

To my family.

Contents

Acknowledgements

I have been lucky enough to discuss the content and methodology of this book with many scholars, some of whom are also friends. They have all made a fundamental contribution to the finished product.

My thanks go to Federico Barbierato, under whose supervision I conducted the project *Marie Skłodowska-Curie (Netdis 748645), Horizon 2020*. This book was conceived during and as a result of this experience. My personal development was enhanced by his kindness and intellectual generosity, as well as our regular cultural discussions about Venice and the religious context during the early modern period. Our shared thinking on different methodological and historiographical approaches and on the layout of this book also proved valuable for writing the text. I also thank him for reading various drafts of this text.

Equally heartfelt thanks go to Professor Massimo Firpo, whose lectures and books first led me to nurture a passion for the world of sixteenth-century Italian religious dissent. Even after many years, this enthusiasm has never faded. I also thank him for teaching me the discipline required for research, for generously providing me with books and unpublished sources, for the many hours of discussions about my work, and his countless suggestions and advice, to which this book owes much. He also read the first drafts with great patience and attention.

The outgoing phase of my Marie Curie project at the University of Stanford made a fundamental contribution to the development of my research. My thanks go first to Paula Findlen, the host supervisor of my project, who involved me in the academic environment at Stanford and made some valuable suggestions for circulating and discussing the results of my work in the USA. I also thank her above all for sharing her immense knowledge of the history of medicine and science in the early modern period and for offering guidance when this book first started to take shape and structure. Many people at Stanford contributed to an enriching and productive experience. I thank Elaine Treharne and Giovanna Ceserani for welcoming me to CESTA, the Centre for Space and Textual Analysis at Stanford, and giving me access to a wide range of resources, techniques, and tools. Thanks also to Katherine McDonough, Rachel Midura, Nicole Coleman, Luca Scholz, and Zuyi Zhao for the indispensable support they provided for the digital processing of my data. My stay in the USA opened up fresh perspectives and opportunities for my work, and I am indebted to many people to this end. I thank Hannah Marcus in particular for reading the first version of my text, as well as the productive time we spent working together at the Venetian State Archives. The ongoing stimulating dialogue with her, Mackenzie Cooley, and Brian Brege about our respective research interests, which are complementary in many ways, was fundamental in allowing me to bring into focus the problems and methods of my work.

Alessandro Arcangeli read the draft of my book with precision and attention to detail. I also thank him, along with Luca Ciancio and Federica Favino, for following the progress of my work with interest and inspiring me to reflect on content and methodology with a critical eye.

I would also like to express my heartfelt gratitude to Eleonora Belligni for her interest in my work over the past ten years, for discussing its direction and results, and for reading the draft of this text. Lucia Felici also read the manuscript of my book and gave me significant suggestions, for which I am very grateful. Sincere thanks also go to Luca Addante for the numerous occasions on which he listened to the latest developments in my research and gave me the benefit of his profound knowledge of sixteenth-century Italian religious history.

Thanks to Franco Angiolini and Giovanni Salmeri at the PhD School of History at the University of Pisa, as well as John Henderson, Simonetta Adorni Braccesi, Michaela Valente, Giorgio Caravale, Nicholas Terpstra, Stefano Villani, Xenia Von Tippelskirch, Diego Pirillo, Pietro Adamo, Enrico Pasini, and Monica Azzolini, for providing me with precious inspiration and stimuli. For the same reasons I thank Michele Camaioni, Simone Maghenzani, Stefano Colavecchia, Helena Wangefelt Ström, Fabrizio Baldassarri, and Tommaso Scaramella.

Francis Gordon translated this book with precision and diligence, and I thank him for his professionalism. Thanks also to the team at the research office at Verona University, especially Cecilia Negri and Alessio Lorenzi, as well as the staff at the archives and libraries that I used over the years while conducting this research, in particular the Venetian State Archive.

Profound thanks also to my family: my mother Margherita, my sister Marta, a fellow humanist aficionado, and my father Nedo, who now lies at rest among pine trees, caressed by the sea breeze and salty air. Without him, even now, nothing of what I have achieved would have been possible. I am extremely grateful to Andrea Benino, my life partner, who is also a philosopher in a sense that Girolamo Donzellini would certainly have appreciated. He has supported me with love, care, and intelligence at every stage of the development and writing of this book, offering me the reassuring perspective of a refined and restless mind. This book came into being at the same time as my baby boy, Giuliano. I thank him for his sweetness and for the strength I derive just from knowing he is there, also during the time spent away from him while working on this book.

Introduction

Orzi Nuovi, a little town near Brescia in the Venetian Republic, was afflicted by the deadliest plague in its history in 1513. Historical sources chronicle the spread of the disease in apocalyptic terms, describing houses packed with sick and maimed people, corpses thrown out of windows, and terrifying screams of fear and grief echoing throughout the streets. As the armies fighting the so-called Italian Wars raged across the landscape and terrorised the population, the town was increasingly beset by plague and famine. Even an angel was seen flying through the pestilential air wielding a bleeding sword. In their desperation, the population opened the gates and surrendered to anyone who wanted to take control. The town council then pledged a vow to Saint Vincent and, as legend has it, the epidemic vanished as suddenly as it had broken out.[1]

Against this backdrop, Buonamonte Donzellini arrived in Orzi Nuovi to escape the war between the Venetian Republic and the League of Cambrai, which had devastated his home city of Verona, and married a wealthy Brescian woman. Buonamonte's son Girolamo – the main character of this book – was born soon afterwards amid these tragic events. Against all the odds, he survived. Considering the difficulties he faced in his adult life, and yet how many times he managed to escape death, it is tempting to imagine that all the dying and sorrow surrounding him in the early months of his life somehow made him invulnerable to various perils – all but one that is. After enduring the plagues of 1513 and 1575, torture, and religious exile, at the age of seventy-four Donzellini was drowned by the Inquisition in the Venetian lagoon on a spring night in 1587.

In order to reconstruct the events which led to this tragic denouement, we need to start from the beginning and expand the scope of the story. This will demonstrate that the case of Donzellini is representative of a wider phenomenon encompassing the exposure of Italian physicians to the ideas of the Reformation, their involvement in the heretical movement, the general relationship between late Renaissance medicine, knowledge and heterodoxy, and the specific characteristics of the 'Reformation of physicians' as an intellectual and social movement.

DOI: 10.4324/9781003218852-1

I.1 Girolamo Donzellini and his world

Aside from being a 'heretic,' as he was defined by the Inquisition, Girolamo Donzellini was a medical doctor, a bibliophile, and a philosopher. He was fascinated by Hermetic discourse and the attempt to study secret correspondences in nature; he was open to ideas for change in the medical world, and his rational nature gradually led him to reject any kind of medical or religious dogma. With his intellectual vitality, he was the epitome of Cinquecento humanist medical culture in the Italian peninsula.

Girolamo was born into a family of men of culture (who were to become religious dissenters) at the height of the Renaissance in 1513, four years before the start of the Reformation. The surrounding world was still animated by the values of humanism: the 'cult of the ancients,' the practice of philology, the passion for authentic, restored, reliable knowledge, and the merit of intellectual curiosity. After 1517, the storm of the Reformation raged against this realm of refined culture and intellectual research, triggering various forms of religious conflict and violence in numerous places. Launched by Luther in Germany, Reformation ideas soon crossed the Alps to Italy, where they were embraced by long-term campaigners for reform of the Roman Church. Donzellini's father was one such individual. Religious non-conformism thus played a major role in Girolamo's upbringing, remaining one of his main traits throughout his life along with tenacious opposition to dogmatism and genuine fervour for humanist culture. After graduating from Padua, the most advanced Italian university for medicine and philosophy, Donzellini worked as personal physician to two cardinals in Rome. He was welcomed by a community of thinkers who embraced spiritual pluralism. It was here in 1546 that he encountered Inquisition repression for the first time.

The reaction of the Roman Church to the Reformation was slow and late, but by the 1540s the Catholic 'intransigent party' led by Cardinal Gian Pietro Carafa had started to recognise the great danger presented by the movement.[2] Pressure from this party led to the foundation of the 'Sant'Uffizio dell'Inquisizione' (Holy Office of the Inquisition) in 1542 to repel the Reformed doctrines now circulating widely among the Italian population. All pre-existing Italian Inquisition courts were then unified under this institution, which became increasingly pervasive and powerful.[3] One exception to this rule was the Venetian Inquisition, where three lay patricians – the *Savi Sopra l'Eresia* – worked alongside the ecclesiastical judges. While these figures made a vital contribution to the repression of religious dissent, they also played a monitoring role that limited the influence of the Roman Inquisition.[4] The religious policy of La Serenissima was one of the reasons that prompted Girolamo to move to Venice in the mid-1540s, his home for the next seven years.

He was in his element there. As well as being the European capital of the printing industry, Venice had a reputation as a land of tolerance and cosmopolitanism with lively cultural, scientific, philosophical, and religious debate, and humanists gathering from all over Italy (and indeed Europe). While in Venice, Donzellini became part of a dense network of heterodox thinkers; he disseminated heterodox ideas and liberally undertook religious and scientific research. However, when the Counter-Reformation started to take effect in the 1550s, he was one of those targeted.[5] After a trial was set against him in 1553, he was forced like many others to leave the peninsula to escape religious persecution.

The experience of exile marked a significant change in his intellectual and religious approach. He travelled across Germanic lands and probably reached Basel in around 1559. Here he associated with the radical group of humanists fighting for religious tolerance and made a personal contribution to this campaign. It was thanks to his experience in exile that Girolamo met Theodor Zwinger, the humanist from Basel who was a crucial figure for the reception and spread of innovative ideas in medicine and philosophy at a European level, as well as an active defender of religious and intellectual freedom.[6] Along with other German physicians, Zwinger remained part of Girolamo's epistolary network in the years to come. Over the time he spent abroad, Donzellini consolidated the Neoplatonic and Hermetic influences that had inspired his Venetian circles and moved towards 'more inclusive' spiritual beliefs.

Returning to Italy in the 1560s, he settled his debt with the religious legal system and became an upright citizen in Verona, working as a reputable doctor. Nonetheless, he was subjected to three further Inquisition trials, in the last of which he was sentenced to death. For the preceding thirty years or so, Donzellini exploited his connections with humanists and exiles abroad to collaborate on editing and publishing texts which could not be printed in Italy, also smuggling forbidden books into the Republic of Venice (his fate was probably sealed by the possession and distribution of such books). Religious repression had escalated when he died in 1587, and he was one of the few 'heretics' executed in Venice in the sixteenth century (significantly, as we shall see, the others were members of his network). As the following pages will show, however, even at the height of the Counter-Reformation the values of tolerance and mutual understanding were sought and sometimes found, along with the channels to express them, through tenacious networks of dissent that operated at the intersection between religion, medicine, and philosophy.

In examining the life, work, and world of Girolamo Donzellini, this book aims to enrich our understanding of the history of medicine and religious heterodoxy in sixteenth-century Italy. As Donzellini's life is documented in a wealth of sources, it can be used to reflect on burgeoning spiritual beliefs and to understand key developments in medical culture, underlining and contextualising the link between the evolution of medicine on the eve of the scientific revolution and the religious upheaval that affected the whole continent in the sixteenth century. However, as his chosen path was by no means an isolated case, these pages will explore the connection between sixteenth-century medicine and heterodoxy by outlining the experiences of many other heterodox physicians, thereby unveiling a dense network of dissent. I argue in this book that the aims of this network went far beyond the Protestant Reformation and eventually took a radically different direction. Indeed, their aspirations for deep-rooted reform of knowledge and the sacred realm were as irreconcilable with Scholastic philosophy as they were with both the old and new religious institutions.

The chapters document the history of this network in the Republic of Venice and explore its branches elsewhere in the Italian peninsula (especially the Kingdom of Naples) and on foreign soil against a backdrop of changing historical contexts. The period of reference almost completely spans the century of the Reformation and the Counter-Reformation. This was a time of momentous change, ranging from opportunities for real religious reform in Italy to the gradual segmentation of Europe into incompatible confessional areas and the progressive regulation of behaviour through the intensification and standardisation of mechanisms of control. The activities undertaken by the network between the 1540s and the 1580s took shape in different forms and objectives. At the turn of the century, free eclectic religious experimentation and concerted efforts to spread heterodox doctrines gave way to intellectual positions that no longer aimed to revolutionise the established historical frameworks. Nevertheless, rather than hiding in an ivory tower, this community mounted resistance that opposed any form of fanaticism and dogmatism.

This book is interdisciplinary both in its content and methodology. Through a chronological biography of Girolamo Donzellini and analysis of the circles he moved in, it explores numerous issues: religious reform, spiritual heterodoxy, attempts at repression by the Inquisition and strategies of opposition from religious dissidents; social, religious, and intellectual networks and the process of knowledge creation and transfer; developments in medical theory and practice; and continuity, ruptures and interplay in philosophical, scientific, and religious culture. Methodologically speaking, the book sits at the junction between different historiographical genres, offering a blend of religious history and history of medicine. With regard to the biographical aspect, a myriad of other figures is included alongside Donzellini with reconstructions of their relational networks and descriptions of their experiences. The book is underpinned by the laborious mining of an extraordinary cache of archival trial records which I used to recreate the lives, thought, and world of Donzellini and his cohorts. This research draws significantly on the microhistorical tradition, which is closely intertwined with the interpretative approach of the history of ideas.[7] On the one hand, the microhistorical narration of the story of Donzellini and those who shared his attitudes, practices, and contacts captures fragments of heterodox daily life in sixteenth-century Venice. On the other hand, it contributes to the history of ideas by shedding light on the link between heterodoxy, medicine, and philosophy in the Italian Cinquecento.

The following sections provide an overview of the theoretical, historiographical, and methodological notions at the core of this book. The overlap between medicine and religion in the sixteenth century has been well established, along with the points of intersection between their respective crises.[8] The book will not analyse the theoretical and epistemological links between these two fields or describe either critical situation in any great detail. Nevertheless, as its interdisciplinary research is aimed equally at scholars in the fields of the history of religion and the history of medicine, this introduction will offer a brief outline.

I.2 Medicine, Reformation, and heterodoxy in the sixteenth century

The Inquisition sources (both published and unpublished) demonstrate that physicians were heavily involved in religious dissent in the peninsula at a time when the fundamental crisis in the medical world led to major modifications to theory and practice, with Italian universities playing a central role. While care of the body and care of the soul continued to be considered as one and the same, the changes in the medical world – with healing practices gradually moving into the experimental realm – became intertwined with a distinctive approach to the Christian faith. Against the backdrop of widespread religious disquiet triggered by the explosion of Reformed ideas and the theological debate, the experimentalism now favoured by many physicians offered fertile ground for unconventional solutions resisting the dogmatism and rigidity imposed by the authorities, also in the religious field. While schoolmasters, notaries, jewellers, booksellers, and jurists, who had often received a humanist education, were all highly exposed to heretical ideas because they were culturally and socially proactive and involved in intellectual exchange, there was also a markedly professional aspect to the 'Reformation of physicians.'[9] Playing key roles in developing knowledge and claiming greater margins of freedom in the religious debate, Donzellini and his colleagues deserve to be studied as a historical phenomenon in their own right.

With its return to Hippocrates and Galen, medical humanism had conservative premises but eventually revolutionised the approach to the body and to nature. In their desire to imitate the ancients, physicians rediscovered the value of experience and started to perceive medicine as a 'rational practice' with its own speculative logic that gradually became more inductive.[10] While striving to connect the teachings of the ancients to the reality of the natural world, they also focused on new fields of research, perceiving the rift between the theoretical and practical realms of medicine, first established in the Middle Ages, to be increasingly specious and unproductive. Humanist physicians could now undertake more boldly empirical research without jeopardising their social and intellectual status as scholars and 'philosophers,' embracing rational knowledge for practical purposes when addressing the intrinsically unstable subject of the body with its states of health and disease. During this phase they became involved in new fields of knowledge ranging from pharmaceutical preparation, which sometimes strayed into esoteric interests and alchemical practices, to the study of anatomical structures, which often took shape in dissections of corpses of varying legality. This methodological and epistemological change eventually affected not only the work of Italian physicians but also the purpose of their profession, their social role, and the way in which they related to the different disciplines associated with medical practice.

In Galenic and humanist thinking, body and soul formed a unified whole that the philosopher physician had to focus on in its entirety; rooted in Scripture, this concept had been underlined extensively during the Middle Ages.[11] As a result, medical intervention was deemed necessary in every aspect of human life: while medicine was the philosophy of the body, philosophy was the medicine of the soul. The philosopher physician was thus responsible for providing all-round care to the individual – the synolon of flesh and spirit[12] – and seeking 'truth' in whatever form it took. By virtue of their training and vocation, some humanist physicians saw philosophical study and philological practice as conceptual and methodological platforms for increasingly unconventional research into nature, humankind, and God. In this way, they began to discuss the individual destiny of the soul after death, along with moral questions, the reliability of the holy texts transmitted through the ecclesiastical tradition, and the truthfulness of the dogma and principles of the faith. Although not unprecedented, the overlap between philosophy (moral as much as natural) and theology became a remarkably common occurrence on Italian soil in the sixteenth century.

The profound religious crisis in the peninsula at the time stemmed from exasperation with the abuses of the clergy – considered corrupt, greedy, and ignorant – and exploded with the spread of the Protestant Reformation. Italy provided fertile ground for the burgeoning of Reformed doctrines for a number of reasons: the influence of humanist and philological culture; a high number of prestigious universities; a network of densely populated cities, especially in the north; and the fact that the noble political class was interested in religious issues, partly driven by competition with papal power and the desire to reduce its jurisdiction.[13] The doctrines of Luther, Zwingli and, especially from the 1550s onwards, Calvin, became crucial for the heterodox Italian communities.[14] However, the multiple roots of the Italian Reformation combined the teaching of the German Reformers with prophetism, radicalism (such as the Anabaptist and Antitrinitarian movements), popular culture, and the influence of philology, humanism and Neoplatonism (which were especially important for physicians). The heterodox circles in the peninsula also deeply absorbed the influence of

Erasmus of Rotterdam and Juan de Valdés and many heterodox thinkers would not have received the seal of approval from the leading lights of the Reformation.[15] The so-called Italian Reformation highlighted the moral aspects of Christianity. From a doctrinal point of view, it developed a flexible, undogmatic concept of the cornerstones of the religion, while in ecclesiological terms it tended to favour compromise and mediation. This led to the flourishing of spiritual and radical positions, which were often interconnected, as recent studies on Valdesianism have shown.[16] Due to the lack of solid theological guidance at an institutional level, religiosity became an increasingly internal, personal matter and Nicodemism (the justification of religious simulation and dissimulation grounded in the primacy of inner faith) was adopted both for practical and theoretical reasons.[17] In-depth analysis of the Christian religion – unrestricted in terms of both scriptural-philological research and doctrinal experimentation – generated theological formulae that questioned the Catholic system to the point of rejecting the very foundations of Christianity (the divine nature of Christ, the virginity of Mary, the immortality of the soul, and so on).

Physicians played a leading role in this context because of their cultural background, their experimental approach, and their penchant for addressing the health of both body and soul. The Inquisition documents give the impression that there were physicians in almost every heretical group in the peninsula between the 1530s and the 1560s, with many acting as intellectual leaders. Private houses, hospitals, convents, military barracks, and stately palaces provided them with a broad margin of freedom – they were generally undisturbed because of their social prestige and indispensable professional role – and numerous opportunities for digesting and spreading unconventional religious ideas. The exposure of physicians to heterodox discourse was also acknowledged by the Catholic authorities. Indeed, during the Counter-Reformation they made several attempts to place the medical profession under control and to exploit medical practices to discipline society.[18]

Medical and religious reforms also developed in tandem at a European level, including the countries where the Reformation took hold. In his *Reformation der Apotecken* (*Reform of Pharmacies*, Strasbourg, 1536), the German physician, botanist, and radical theologian Otto Brunfels set out his hopes for a comprehensive overhaul of medical and pharmaceutical knowledge in line with the profound religious reform underway at the time.[19] At around the same time, Philip Melanchthon made medicine one of the most prominent fields of study when he reorganised the curricula at the University of Wittenberg, a project subsequently embraced by other German universities. He placed particular importance on anatomy, which, on the basis of the link between body and soul, offered insight into the development of spiritual activities involving thinking, imagination, and will. According to Melanchthon's plan, every true believer had to undertake anatomical study under the constant supervision of Lutheran theologians and acquire new knowledge, starting from Vesalius's *De humani corporis fabrica* (*On the Fabric of the Human Body*, Basel, 1543).[20]

The key figure illustrating the influence of religious ideas on the development of medical knowledge is Michael Servetus. This Spanish physician, astrologer, theologian, and heretic, who was convinced of the unity of all philosophical and religious systems, was burned in effigy by the Roman Inquisition and burned at the stake along with his books by Calvin in 1553. Starting from the issue of individual salvation and the desire to understand the human relationship with the Eternal, Servetus devised a solution that blended Renaissance thinking, imbued with Hermetic influences, with Reformed ideas.[21] His most significant contribution to medical science was his main theological text, the *Christianismi restitutio* (*Restoration of Christianity,* Vienne, 1553), which he published anonymously. In his attempt to explain how the divine spirit came into contact with humankind, he posited the theory of the pulmonary circulation of blood, grounded as much in anatomical observation as in scriptural knowledge. From its title onwards, the whole work took shape as a bid to restore Christianity to its authentic form. Its polemical target was the Trinitarian conception of divinity established at the Council of Nicaea in 325 but never mentioned in the Bible. Servetus claimed that it had led to the corruption of the Christian message and the growth of papal temporal power. He believed, by contrast, that everyone could ascend to God and partake of his essence because of the human nature of Christ and the 'spark of divinity' – the soul – in every human being. The vehicle for this 'transmission of divinity' was the Holy Spirit, who was thought to make every individual vital and divine by entering the body through breathing and circulating in the blood.

Servetus's ethical, spiritual, and radical take on Christianity was influenced by Spanish *alumbradismo*, Erasmianism, and the evangelical groups he frequented in Basel and Strasbourg in the 1530s. Neoplatonism also had a great impact on Servetus's thought (as it already did on the teacher of Servetus, Symphorien Champier). As we will see, similar influences, concepts, and social circles feature in the thought and experiences of Girolamo Donzellini. This similarity demonstrates that at the time of the sixteenth-century theological unrest, a common cultural and religious background could lead to the development of specific positions with the same intricate blend of philosophical and theological questions.

The relationship between medicine and religious dissent, if not out-and-out unbelief, even became a topos in the seventeenth century. The Gomarist theologian Gisbertus Voetius (Gijsbert Voet) wrote a disputation *De atheismo* (*On Atheism,* Utrecht, 1639), in which he attacked the Dutch physician Henricus Regius (Henri le Roy) in order to target his mentor, Descartes; among other things, the medical profession was described as a repository of atheists.[22] Focusing on the Italian context, he argued that the study of ancient literature during the Renaissance had led, on one hand, to the rediscovery of the thinking of Lucian, Epicurus and Lucretius, and, on the other hand, to the overhaul of the mathematical sciences and the revival of Galenic medicine. These developments had in turn prompted the emergence of irreligious thinking dissimulated under the cult of *bonae litterae* (literally 'good letters,' or classical literature). Voetius explained that physicians had been particularly exposed to a highly potent blend of harmful influences: Aristotelian empiricism, Averroistic mortalism and the doctrine of the eternity of the world, Galen's psychological agnosticism, and Avicenna's concept of natural prophecy.[23] Even from his partisan position he identified certain fundamental aspects of medical 'atheism' but failed to grasp the prominent role of physicians in spirited religious unrest before such subversion came to fruition. Indeed, in addition to the influence of the Renaissance philosophical tradition and Galen's medical theory, it must be stressed that the sixteenth-century religious crisis offered speculative opportunities and that a large proportion of the medical profession was involved in the Reformed movement for almost a century.

In analysing the connection between medical science and religious reform, historians first focused on Michael Servetus, the 'total heretic.'[24] Attention then shifted to the ties between medicine and religious dissent with studies on some of the most significant heterodox physicians. Aldo Stella's research on Niccolò Buccella, a Paduan medical practitioner, outlined that 'Christological problems' were often solved at Padua University in the second half of the sixteenth century through physiology and medicine rather than philosophical and theological speculation.[25] From a more general perspective, Antonio Rotondò analysed the works published by Pietro Perna – a radical Basel-based printer who is a major figure in this book – and the most culturally advanced groups in the city, observing that their basic intellectual outlook derived from a combination of changes in the philosophical-scientific paradigm (moving beyond the Scholastic Aristotelian framework) and a spiritual and irenic religious approach.[26] Although Stella and Rotondò suggested some intriguing lines of research, they did not explore the matter further by analysing methodology, contexts, or medical practices. Only more recently did Alessandro Pastore return to the common ground between medical and religious history by focusing, among other things, on the link between religious discipline and the increasing rigidity of medical institutions in the confessional age (2006).[27] A few years afterwards, the section on Scipione Capece in Luca Addante's 2010 work reiterated the importance of the relationship between naturalistic investigation, Renaissance philosophy, and ideas of religious renewal.[28] Finally, Silvia Ferretto's writings (2009, 2011) on Pomponio Algieri, Bassiano Lando, and more generally the relationship between Padua University, freedom of research, and religious discipline helped to explore the connections between religious feeling, philosophical investigation, and medicine in the Republic of Venice in the sixteenth century.[29]

Some of these studies draw on previous insights made by Alexandre Koyré (1955)[30] and Walter Pagel (1958),[31] who highlighted the overlap between spiritualism and alchemy by analysing Paracelsus and other 'spiritual mystics.' These works prompted Gary Waite to reflect on the link between radical spiritualism and medicine by analysing the social circle of the Anabaptist David Joris in a 2002 article.[32] Charles Webster (2008) confirmed the connection between Paracelsus's thinking and medical work, stressing the prevalent spiritual climate among the protagonists of the Radical Reformation.[33] In the field of Anglo-Saxon historiography, which has made a particularly vibrant contribution to research on the history of medicine, special mention should go to the innovative volume *Medicine and the Reformation* edited by Andrew Cunningham and Ole Peter Grell (1993). It includes an essay by Richard Palmer on the relationship between heterodox physicians and the Venetian Inquisition in the sixteenth century; focusing on Donzellini, it is of great interest for identifying both sources and further research prospects.[34] The volume edited by John Brooke and Ian Maclean (2005) should also be cited: even though it does not strictly address the medical field, it offers key ideas for exploring the relationship between religious heterodoxy and the genesis of modern science, stressing the intertwining of discourses on nature and God in sixteenth- and seventeenth-century Europe in a context where scientific and religious heterodoxy were intrinsically linked.[35]

Palmer's work did not lead to any systematic research on Italian heretical physicians or on the association between medicine and religion until a flurry of studies at the beginning of this century. One of the main themes in these works was the role of Italian physicians in the *Respublica medica*, an international and interconfessional medical 'republic.' Nancy Siraisi and Alessandra Quaranta investigated the matter from this perspective.[36] The latter focused on the frequent heterodox proclivities of medical practitioners, stressing that the experience of exile for religious reasons (*religionis causa*) was a key factor for Italian heretical physicians in creating lasting relationships in the fields of religion and science. Quaranta presented three case studies of heretical physicians (including Donzellini) and examined their correspondence to reconstruct their ties with the German-speaking world and pinpoint potential links (which are sometimes somewhat forced) between medical and religious reform in their life stories. Johanna Kostylo pursued a similar path, underlining that physicians in exile established connections between Venice and Poland; her research developed studies on Italian heretics in Poland, Moravia, and Transylvania first undertaken by Domenico Caccamo and Massimo Firpo in the late 1970s.[37] Finally, Riccarda Suitner examined connections between the Republic of Venice – above all Padua University – and the broader context of sixteenth-century religious and scientific reform in a 2016 essay that drew on the work of Stella and Cantimori.[38]

This book fits into this historiographical context by advancing the hypothesis that there was a close relationship between religious and philosophical spiritualism. My inferences focus in particular on the connections between a conception of the cosmos as animated by secret correspondences and occult forces, an emanationist and pantheist philosophical framework, and a propensity for religious tolerance aimed at defending freedom of thought. Yet, the study does not only examine philosophical, medical, and religious works. The conclusions are the partly unexpected result of extensive archival research, mainly using Inquisition sources, which reconstructs a comprehensive and systematic overview of the flesh-and-blood protagonists of the phenomenon: Italian heterodox physicians, above all in the Republic of Venice, along with their operative framework and networks of relationships.

I.3 A network of dissident physicians

Starting from the case of Donzellini, this book explores the ideas, relationships, and practices in a *community of dissent* in which heterodox physicians featured prominently, examining its formation, development, and results. As is often the case, the preliminary research for this book was lengthy and tortuous. I first adopted a quantitative perspective to confirm the significance of the relationship between medicine and heterodoxy. My sample of around two hundred cases was assembled from archival research in the files of the *Savi Sopra l'Eresia* in Venice and documents held in the archives of Milan, Modena, Pisa, Belluno, and Trent. I supplemented these archive-based studies with an examination of published trial records and the historiography on the Italian Reformation.[39] In this phase, I analysed all the trial dossiers in the Venetian archive for the years 1541–75, indexing not only the physicians directly accused of heresy but also those accused but never traced by the magistrates, those mentioned as accomplices, and those named as active members of heretical groups with no further information provided. My idea was to investigate the intersection between the medical profession and the reform movement without taking shortcuts (such as considering trials as the only source of inquiry), in the knowledge that the heretical movement in Venice and throughout the Italian peninsula lacked a fixed doctrinal framework. The group could encompass both strong affiliations and fleeting affinities, and religious ideas could derive from social and cultural causes. My comprehensive analysis of hundreds of dossiers produced a clear picture of the relationship between medicine and heterodoxy, with an estimate that around 25% of physicians in Venice displayed heterodox tendencies between the 1540s and 1570s.[40]

However, this initial survey, which forms the conceptual and contextual framework of the present research, did not take into account the concrete experiences of the main protagonists. As a result, there was a danger of offering a somewhat clichéd picture of their professional values, philosophical visions, and religious ideals. While the examination of individual trials clearly showed that physicians encountered all walks of life, an aspect that they exploited to absorb and endorse nonconformist ideas, very little was known about these relationships and the way in which they influenced their intellectual and religious lives. Several questions remained unanswered. What role did physicians play in the contestations that shook the foundations of the Catholic Church for at least half a century? By focusing excessively on theoretical connections such as the link between body and soul, have we lost sight of the practical objectives that prompted many physicians to (sometimes literally) dedicate their lives to this ideal of reform? And what kind of reform are we talking about? Was heresy just a consequence of the mindset (*forma mentis*) of the humanist philologist? And what was the *heretical* element of their *heresy*? Was it merely a category devised by their accusers? Or, besides their mental restlessness, might their lifestyle have become irreconcilable with the growing inflexibility in the early modern period? In order to address these questions, I made a comprehensive reconstruction of the networks of heterodox physicians to include their mutual contacts, societal relations, ties with others involved in the same field of action, and intellectual output. This approach helped to reveal the *world* of medical religious dissent with its intricate blend of characters, ideas, and circumstances. Donzellini and his community shared ideas and practices which became more and more irreconcilable with Catholic and even Protestant orthodoxy, raising the urgent need for freedom of research in the fields of medicine, philosophy, and religion.

I felt that the ambitious nature of the project would be best served by starting from an individual case study in a specific context. This book is mainly set in the Republic of Venice, not only because it was home to many heterodox physicians but also due to its distinctive nature in the sixteenth century. As an important European commercial and publishing centre, it was seen as the 'gateway' ('porta') of the Reformation in Italy in the 1540s.[41] The Republic boasted the most prestigious university in Europe – in Padua – and its geographical position bordering Germanic, Slavic, and Turkish lands guaranteed presence and authority in the Mediterranean and Northern Europe as a pivotal hub for trading goods, books, and cultural and religious information. There was also an extremely strong German presence through the 'Germanic nation' ('nazione germanica') at Padua University – the largest contingent of foreign students – and the Fondaco dei Tedeschi in Venice, which was the headquarters of the city's German merchants and an important distribution centre for Reformed ideas and books from Northern Europe. Furthermore, the Republic's aversion to papal interference, which made it fiercely possessive of its own religious jurisdiction, limited the influence of the Roman Inquisition.[42] Such factors made the Republic (above all Padua and Venice) a particularly attractive place for physicians. Not only were they men of culture looking for job opportunities and news of the latest publications, but they also often sympathised with heterodox ideas. For them, the Republic stood out as a major European cultural hub that could provide shelter from the Inquisition as far as possible and, in the event of arrest, offered a legal system complete with guarantees.

The city of Venice is a protagonist in its own right in the narrative: its streets, bridges, shops, and houses are all key elements in the life of the movement, while the waters of its lagoon were used to do away with unrepentant heretics. My idea was to outline the experiences of heterodox physicians by systematically examining the ways that their lives interacted with historical contexts (including spatial and environmental variables). Such a perspective required a main character. Among the many candidates, Donzellini seemed to stand out as the most representative heterodox physician.[43] First of all, as his life spans the majority of the sixteenth century (1513–87), it can be used to gauge the significance of the experiences of a heterodox physician in the long term and through changing contexts. Donzellini regularly appeared on the Inquisition's radar for over thirty years (1553–87) against a backdrop of volatile political scenarios: while the international stage assumed different characteristics, the religious environment gradually became stricter through inflexible confessionalism and consolidated repressive strategies. The surviving records of four of Donzellini's five trials for heresy, held at the State Archive in Venice, offer a wealth of information in this respect.[44] Furthermore, notwithstanding ecclesiastical censorship, Donzellini acted as an intermediary between the Republic and German-speaking lands in the clandestine circulation of scientific, philosophical, and religious books for a similar length of time, paying no heed to confessional barriers. This role can be reconstructed through his correspondence with humanists and physicians like Theodor Zwinger in Basel and Joachim Camerarius in Nuremberg; such documentation allows us to follow the heretical-medical networks beyond limited geographical contexts.[45] Finally, an analysis of Donzellini's contribution to the medical debate and his epistemological conception of medical science offers significant elements for understanding the relationship between medicine and religious dissent. His philosophical works of 1559 and 1586 reveal the way in which heterodoxy and medical humanist culture fed off each other in the second half of the sixteenth century.

While the number and variety of available sources on Donzellini cast light on the historical issue, my objectives would not be met by writing a biography, however quintessential it may be. Donzellini's comprehensive network included colleagues who, like him, shared alternative religious ideas to Catholicism, were victims of repression, or were forced into religious exile. More generally, it also consisted of friends, acquaintances, relatives, and accomplices who made up the social body in which and through which the interplay between medicine, religious dissent, and philosophy took shape. I have therefore extended my analysis to include other emblematic heterodox physicians with extensive social networks and/or singular experiences in the heretical movement about whom information was available. I have provided a complete picture of the events they were involved in by using Inquisition trial records as my main sources as well as notarial documents, proceedings of colleges of physicians, private correspondence, documentation of involvement in academies, and intellectual output (medical and philosophical texts).

The concept of heretic/heresy has a rich and controversial historiographical tradition and I have employed it with full awareness of its complexity. The term 'heterodox' has generally been preferred – to avoid using 'heretic,' a label employed by the Inquisition – to denote the behaviours, attitudes, and ideas that were incompatible with Roman orthodoxy and condemned by the Church authorities.[46] As the theological fluidity of Italian religious dissent prevents us from applying rigid confessional labels to the spiritual sensibilities of Donzellini and the other protagonists, their religious development is described in the terms they used themselves, documented in the sources. Nevertheless, problematising the concept of heresy does not mean reducing the magnitude of the Italian religious crisis or the resulting dissent that spread most notably in Venice. Indeed, the historical importance of this phenomenon is one of the premises of this book. At least until the 1550s, the heterodox movement in Venice and throughout the Italian peninsula was driven by many different groups (including Lutherans, Calvinists, Anabaptists, and Valdesians). On their journeys through the movement and in their encounters with these groups, though, Donzellini and other men of culture adopted a flexible approach that was open to contradictions and developments. Yet, as some of their dramatic fates illustrate, this fluidity did not compromise their active commitment to dissident action. Their involvement must therefore be framed in a perspective that excludes clear doctrinal affiliations and rigid dichotomies (Catholic/Lutheran; orthodox/heretic).

The same level of circumspection needs to be applied to the decision to use inquisitorial documents. These sources reveal the 'dynamic' aspects of intellectual and religious life by capturing the everyday life of members of the heterodox movement and highlighting their network (which I reconstructed by systematically cataloguing witnesses, accusers, relatives, and other contacts mentioned during trials).[47] As the events outlined in these documents are retrospective depictions partly influenced by the repressive circumstances, I decided to proceed with caution (supplementing them with other documentation where available such as letters, wills, and published works). Nevertheless, if trial records are read thoroughly with attention to the specific nature of individuals, contexts, and roles, they remain an essential resource for studying sixteenth-century religious history, above all in this type of research.

The abundance of sources means that the case study can be viewed through a lens that broadens the perspective of the experiences of Donzellini and his peers and reflects the numerous links between people, ideas, and places. In accordance with the assumption that historical phenomena can only be understood if *all* those involved are studied, this research features both men and women with different social and intellectual profiles.[48] By adopting an 'intensive technique for reconstructing [the] biographies,' relationships, and environments in which these individuals were involved, I have analysed complex cultural trends and events from a micro-historical perspective that complements the macro-historical viewpoint.[49] Indeed, the relationship between microhistory and general historical questions is the organising principle of this book. The narrative combines a focus on individual stories and specific local contexts with philological analysis of books and ideas, offering a comprehensive examination of historical processes (the spread of certain religious movements, the emergence of a specific medical culture, the onset of Counter-Reformation repression, the dynamic of religious migration, and so on).[50]

Sociologists use the term 'social movements' to refer to 'groups that focus on specific issues, and aim to produce, resist, or undo, by means of a collective effort, certain historical change.'[51] The sociological concept of a movement is adopted here to describe the dimension of active militancy in which Donzellini and his cohorts were involved. This does not mean, though, that their actions were driven by fixed objectives. At a time of radical change in the intellectual and religious spheres, countered through discipline and repression, every decision regarding religion, work, relationship building, and lifestyle was the result of compromise, ambiguity, uncertainty, and sometimes even chance (see for example the epilogue to the story of Girolamo Donzellini). One of the objectives of this book is to restore the ambivalence of the precarious circumstances that led some members of the network to their deaths at the hands of the Inquisition. As the case of Donzellini successfully illustrates, although it was impractical to prevent all forms of domination of minds and bodies employed at the time, it was possible to temper them and broaden the scope of action. This was done by exploiting the inconsistencies between the religious regulations and the application of penalties in Venice in the sixteenth century, and by combining respectable public profiles with clandestine practices.[52]

The opportunity to establish 'a politics of everyday life' ('una politica della vita quotidiana') and escape from situations with no apparent way out (see the episode involving Donzellini at the time of the plague in Chapter 5) owed much to the construction of networks: social, intellectual, and political connections stemming from a knowing strategy or contingent circumstances.[53] The network is one of the key concepts of this book. The term refers to groups of individuals providing mutual material support, exchanging items or knowledge, and making a collective effort to circulate ideas and information through letters, conversations, and other forms of interaction. Networks played a fundamental role in early modern society, especially in high-density environments like Venice where they became essential for movements opposing the predominant norms. The construction of networks was also sometimes the result of shared spaces and forms of knowledge (such as studying medicine at Italian universities) and could contribute to a successful professional career.

The concept of networks thus provides a useful perspective for examining the history of heterodox physicians. We can definitely think of them as a community clustered into informal groups or more formal aggregations (such as affiliation to Colleges, universities, or editorial projects). They shared the same education and mental framework, which led them to develop common ways of looking at nature and the body. They also performed their medical duties in similar places (hospitals, pharmacies, and private houses) and adopted the same vocational practices, professional values, and ambitions. As my research shows, many also tended to question religious orthodoxy and elaborated personal theological (or a-theological) constructs. By systematically exploring physicians' social connections, we can highlight the mechanisms underpinning their intellectual and religious output such as trust, competition, mutual support, the exchange of goods, and so on. In this book, such dynamics are highlighted by examining the relationship between Donzellini and the members of his network (friends, relatives, colleagues, patients, cohorts involved in the Italian heterodox movement – Chapters 1 and 2 – and humanists active in the Republic of Letters – Chapter 5) and investigating the wider network of dissent made up of physicians in exile (Chapter 3) and local physicians in their heterodox associations and practices (Chapters 4 and 7). Moreover, by focusing on these networks, the book recreates the everyday life of Donzellini and the other protagonists as far as possible, with elements such as secret reading, book smuggling, personal recommendations, shared living and working spaces, imprisonment, 'ephemeral' distribution of ideas and texts in city streets, and medical practices.[54] Such a historiographical methodology based on the reconstruction of historical networks can therefore unearth, illustrate, and clarify the social and intellectual dynamics alluded to in the sources. In this way, the focus shifts from the abstract level of ideas to the concrete dimension of the people who received, shared, and reformulated these ideas in their daily lives. Attention is thus also placed on the *process*: the sequence of actions and interactions that led to what is now called the heterodox movement.[55] This movement was the result of a specific historical, social, and cultural context and the action of all those involved.

When examining archival documents, historians have always sought connections between the different individuals involved. By and large, scholars of the Reformation and the Counter-Reformation have adopted a historiographical perspective associated with the history of ideas. In this approach, the reconstruction of networks is not undertaken systematically (with figures seemingly uninvolved in intellectual output thereby ignored) and is related to the study of the development of religious doctrines and movements.[56] By contrast, although this book draws on and develops the excellent results of historiography on the Italian Reformation and early modern medicine, it embraces the idea that the concept of network and the methodical reconstruction of relational systems are useful both for social history and intellectual history, seen as the history of those who facilitated the development of ideas and the relationship between texts, contexts, and individuals.[57] In reconstructing Donzellini's relational system, the aim is not only to contextualise the events in which he was involved but also to shift the spotlight onto the network itself and identify its structure, complexity, and interactive levels wherever possible. Focusing on a relational network rather than just an individual can cast new light on the constituent relations and the choices they involve.

In theoretical terms, the starting point of this research is the idea that reality is both *procedural* and *relational*.[58] This means that the subjectivities driving the dynamics of history are the result of a continual process of transformation, contamination, and evolution. This process stems from concrete individual action, which is in turn the result of various evolving forms of interaction (personal, familial, professional, social, intellectual, and spatial). In this respect, historical actors are no longer the monolithic ontological basis for certain religious or intellectual categories (such as 'heretic,' 'humanist,' 'Lutheran,' and 'philosopher'). In philosophical terms, it could be said that 'existence precedes essence.'[59]

The definition of the reach of a network is naturally somewhat arbitrary (after all, any two people can be connected with 'six degrees of separation'); in the case of historical networks, the sources place limits on the reconstruction. During my research, I followed the traces left by the different protagonists and by their social relations, examining all the available sources about those with ties to the heterodox physicians: individuals who supported their work like humanists, apothecaries (*speziali*), and booksellers, as well as their friends and relatives, unrelated to the medical context, and figures from the lower social ranks such as alchemists, empirical physicians, and servants. The analysis of these additional processes has highlighted how intellectual convergences could even be developed without direct contact, revealing the existence of a close-knit network uniting everyone involved.

In some chapters it was more straightforward to interweave personal and collective questions with aspects of doctrinal history, while in others it was necessary to address contexts, practices, and ideas separately. The first chapter examines Donzellini's religious and professional formation by comparing his story with the experiences of other heterodox physicians in Orzi Nuovi, Padua, and Rome. The second chapter focuses on Venice. It starts by reconstructing the heretical circles in the city between the 1540s and 1560s, taking into consideration social, spatial, and religious aspects. It then analyses Donzellini's female contacts: women often acted as intermediaries between different networks, assuming specific roles in the heterodox movement and fostering special relations with physicians in their capacity as patients. Finally, the focus shifts to the texts read in Donzellini's Venetian network, along with the doctrines and practices that were embraced.

Chapter 3 examines the religious exile that Donzellini and other heterodox physicians experienced in the 1550s, describing the paths they took and their medical and religious output. It then focuses specifically on Donzellini, outlining the different phases of his exile, his career, and his abandonment of Protestant doctrines in favour of a more inclusive form of religiosity. This aspect emerges above all from an analysis of his text *De successione doctrinae ab origine mundi* (*On the Continuity of Doctrine since the Origin of the World*), steeped in Hermetic influences.

The fourth chapter returns to Venice for a close-up view of the impact of repressive policies on physicians in the city and the response of the movement. Donzellini does not appear in this chapter because he was in Verona rather than Venice during the period in question (between 1560 and the early 1570s). After describing how the medical world was affected by the consolidation of the Counter-Reformation, the chapter examines two case studies. Firstly, the story of Teofilo Panarelli shows the growth and defeat of the heretical movement that had developed over the preceding decades in Venice. Secondly, the events involving two rivals, Decio Bellebuono and the empirical healer Antonino Volpe, prompt considerations on the link between heterodoxy, medicine, alchemy, and social aspects in Counter-Reformation Venice.

Chapter 5 charts Donzellini's return to the Republic of Venice. After examining his years in Verona (1560–73), focusing on his professional experience and the development of his network, it explores his legal troubles between 1560 and 1587, and analyses his correspondence and role in the *Respublica medica*. The final section of the chapter focuses on the book smuggling network that Donzellini was involved in and the denouement of his life.

While Chapters 1–5 are structured around a combination of the history of ideas and microhistory/network reconstruction, the final two chapters (6 and 7) address these issues separately. Chapter 6 explores Donzellini's intellectual output by considering various constituent elements: his involvement in the spread of Paracelsianism in Italy, the influence of Hermeticism on his philosophical thinking, his possible penchant for radical religious doctrines, and his medical proclivities. The final chapter ties up all the loose ends. Specifically, by examining the connections between Donzellini, Panarelli, and Bellebuono, I reconstruct an even broader network (a network of networks) and demonstrate that they were part of a 'social movement.' This community of dissent was varied from a social perspective but uniform in terms of cultural values, theological and philosophical approaches, and religious and scientific practices. This group rejected religious dogmatism and intolerance and opposed the disciplinary measures of the Catholic Church by actively reworking the characteristic spiritualism of the Italian Reformation into a functional, rational, and militant approach imbued with irenicism, Hermeticism, and natural inquiry.

What emerges today from the experiences of Donzellini, Panarelli, and the other protagonists is a tangle of fragmentary threads and traces. It will be possible to verify or consolidate my hypotheses, thereby broadening our knowledge, by using the same methodology to conduct further research through additional case studies on Venice, the city's ties with other territories (by adopting the approach suggested, for example, in the concluding pages of this book), or other areas of the Italian peninsula.

Note: I used the methodology and tools of the Digital Humanities in my research on heterodox-medical networks as an exploratory resource. In this book I employ it, to a limited extent, for illustrative purposes Figures I.1 and I.2.[60]

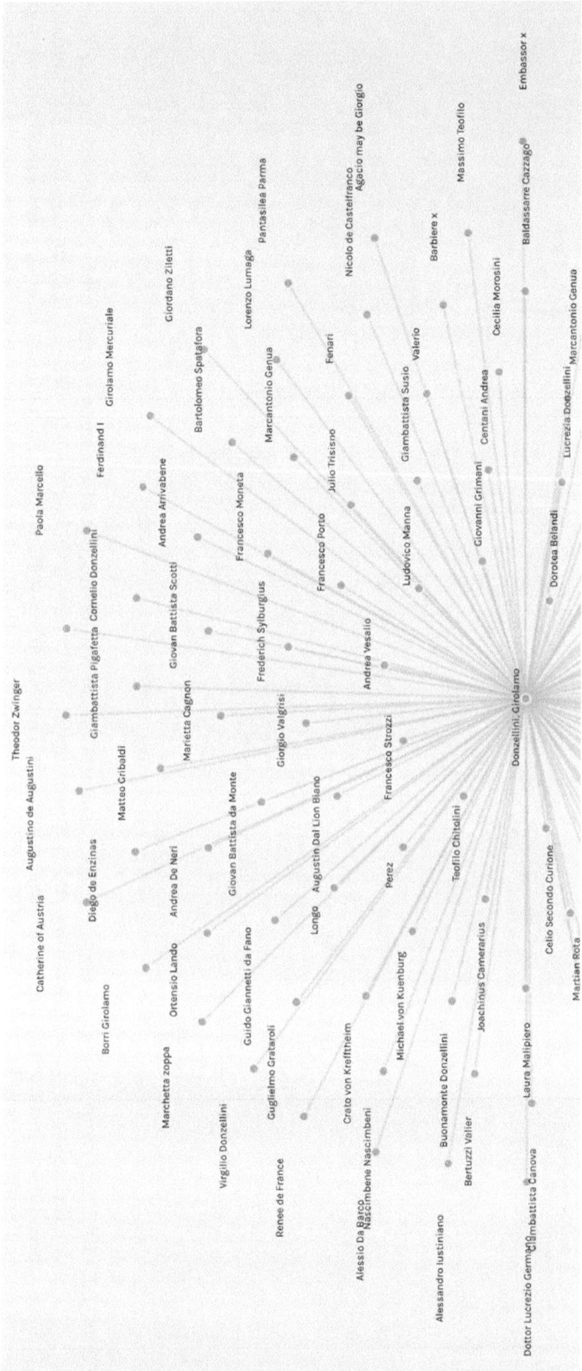

Figure I.1 Girolamo Donzellini's ego-network.

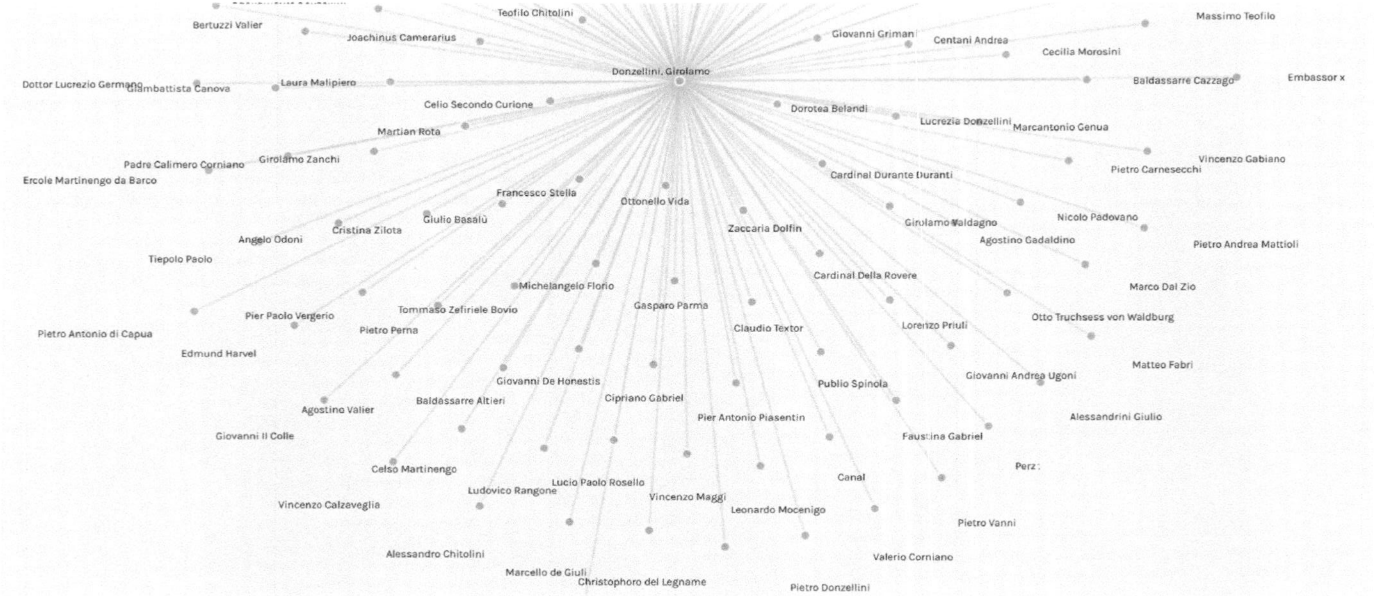

Figure I.2 Girolamo Donzellini's ego-network. The visualisation shows the breadth of the network that a heretical physician like Donzellini could develop in sixteenth-century Italy (approximately 150 nodes populate his network - as they emerge from the sources). Such breadth suggests a rather eclectic social strategy in Donzellini's experience: he could initiate relationships with the most important political figures of his time (even with the Emperor Ferdinand I), but he was also in touch with clergymen, quacks, printers, and an alleged witch (Laura Malipiero), whom he healed in prison. The connections that Donzellini established with these people derived from a mutual exchange of books; from a familiar relationship or a relationship of patronage; from university education; or from sharing the same profession, the same humanistic culture, and, of course, similar heterodox ideas. A heretical relationship, however, could develop on different bases and overlap with other forms of connection (for instance from the practice of medicine, both with colleagues and patients).[61]

Notes

1 Domenico Codagli, *Historia Orceana* (Orzinuovi: Borella, 1592), 130–31.
2 Massimo Firpo, *La presa di potere dell'inquisizione romana (1550–1553)* (Rome – Bari: Laterza, 2014).
3 Andrea Del Col, *L'Inquisizione in Italia dal XII al XXI secolo* (Milan: Mondadori, 2006), 342–94; Christopher Black, *The Italian Inquisition* (New Haven: Yale University Press, 2009).
4 Paul F. Grendler, 'The Tre Savi Sopra l'Eresia 1547–1605: a Prosopographical Study,' *Studi Veneziani*, 3, (1979), 283–340; Del Col, *L'Inquisizione*, 342–94.
5 The concept of Counter-Reformation has a controversial historiographical tradition. On this concept and the related historiographical debate see Massimo Firpo, 'Rethinking 'Catholic Reform' and 'Counter-Reformation': What Happened in Early Modern Catholicism—A View from Italy,' *Journal of Early Modern History*, 20, no. 3 (2016), 293–312; see also Simon Ditchfield, 'Decentering the Catholic Reformation: Papacy and Peoples in the Early Modern World,' *Archiv für Reformationsgeschichte*, 101 (2010), 186–208; Alexandra Bamji, Geert Janssen, Mary Laven, *The Ashgate Research Companion to the Counter-Reformation* (London – New York: Routledge, 2013); Elena Bonora, 'Il ritorno della Controriforma (e la Vergine del Rosario di Guápulo),' *Studi Storici,* 57 (2016), 267–95.
6 On Theodor Zwinger see Carlos Gilly, *Theodor Zwinger e la crisi culturale della seconda metà del Cinquecento*, provisional draft, 2012, available online at https://www.saavedrafajardo.org/Archivos/LIBROS/Libro0844.pdf (5 December 2020). Additional bibliography on Zwinger and the Basel context will be provided in the following chapters.
7 For the microhistorical approach see as a starting point Carlo Ginzburg, *Il formaggio e i vermi. Il cosmo di un mugnaio del 500* (Turin: Einaudi, 1976); Natalie Zemon Devis, *The return of Martin Guerre* (Cambridge, Harvard University Press, 1983); Robert Darnton, *The Great Cat Massacre and Other Episodes in French Cultural History* (New York: Basic Books, 1984); Giovanni Levi, *L'eredità immateriale. Carriera di un esorcista nel Piemonte del Seicento* (Milan: Il saggiatore, 2020, first edition 1985), 21; Ginzburg, *Microhistory, Two or Three Things That I Know about It*, in *Threads and Traces. True, False, Fictive*, translated by Anne C. Tedeschi and John Tedeschi (Berkeley – Los Angeles – London: University of California Press, 2012 – first Italian edition, 2006), 193–214. The tradition of history of ideas with which my book aligns is the one opened by Cantimori: Delio Cantimori, *Eretici italiani del Cinquecento e Prospettive di storia ereticale*, Adriano Prosperi (ed.), (Turin: Einaudi, 2009, first edition 1939). The works of Antonio Rotondò, Massimo Firpo, Adriano Prosperi, Domenico Caccamo, Lucia Felici, Luca Addante, to mention but a few, which will be quoted in this book, refer to this tradition.
8 There is a vast bibliography on the general relationship between medicine and religion between the Middle Ages and the early modern period. See as a starting point the collection of essays, Maria Pia Donato, Luc Berlivet (eds.), *Médecine et religion: compétitions, collaborations, conflits (XIIe-XXe siècles)* (Paris – Rome: Editions de l'Ecole française de Rome, 2013); on the relationship between early modern Catholicism and medicine see also two valuable recent volumes, and their copious bibliographies: Bradford A. Bouley, *Pious Postmortems: Anatomy, Sanctity, and the Catholic Church in Early Modern Europe* (Philadelphia: University of Pennsylvania Press, 2017); Hannah Marcus, *Forbidden Knowledge. Medicine, Science and Censorship in Early Modern Italy* (Chicago: University of Chicago Press, 2020).

9 On the leading role played by notaries in Italian religious dissent, see Silvana Seidel Menchi, *Erasmo in Italia, 1520–1580* (Turin: Bollati Boringhieri, 1987), 322–37; on the role of jewellers, see Massimo Firpo, *Artisti, gioiellieri, eretici. Il mondo di Lorenzo Lotto tra Riforma e Controriforma* (Rome – Bari: Laterza, 2001).

10 Simone Mammola, *La ragione e l'incertezza, Filosofia e medicina nella prima età moderna* (Milan: Franco Angeli, 2012).

11 There is a verse in Ecclesiasticus (38:1) which states: 'Honour a physician with the honour due unto him for the uses which ye may have of him: for the Lord hath created him.' For an effective summary of the relationship between medicine and Christianity in the Middle Ages, see Jole Agrimi, Chiara Crisciani, 'Carità e assistenza nella civiltà medievale,' in Mirko Grmek (ed.), *Storia del pensiero medico occidentale*, vol. I: *Antichità e Medioevo* (Rome – Bari: Laterza: 1993), 217–59.

12 The Scholastics summarised this as 'where the philosopher ends, there begins the physician' ('*ubi desinit physicus ibi incipit medicus*') on the basis of Aristotle's considerations on the relationship between philosophy and medicine in *Sense and Sensibilia*, 436a17–b1. On the interpretation and uses of Aristotle's passage in the field of disputes between the arts and sciences ('dispute delle arti'), see Charles B. Schmitt, 'Aristotle among the Physicians,' in Andrew Wear, Roger French, Iain M. Lonie (eds.), *The medical Renaissance of the Sixteenth Century* (Cambridge: Cambridge University Press, 1985), 1–16.

13 On the Italian Reformation, see as a starting point the seminal works by Cantimori, *Eretici italiani*; Massimo Firpo, *Riforma protestante ed eresie nell'Italia del '500: un profilo* storico (Rome – Bari: Laterza, 1993); Salvatore Caponetto, *La Riforma protestante nell'Italia del Cinquecento* (Turin: Claudiana, 1997); and Antonio Rotondò, *Studi di storia ereticale del Cinqucento* (Florence: Olschki, 2008). Additional bibliography will be found in the next pages.

14 On the spread of Calvinism in Italy see Susanna Peyronel Rambaldi, *Dai Paesi Bassi all'Italia. «Il Sommario della Sacra Scrittura». Un libro proibito nella società italiana del Cinquecento* (Florence: Olschki, 1997); Lucia Felici, *Calvino e l'Italia* (Turin: Claudiana, 2010).

15 On the spread of Erasmus's thought in Italy, see Seidel Menchi, *Erasmo in Italia*; on Valdés, see Massimo Firpo, *Juan de Valdés and The Italian Reformation* (Farnham: Ashgate, 2016).

16 Luca Addante, *Eretici e libertini nel Cinquecento italiano* (Rome – Bari: Laterza, 2010).

17 On the concept of Nicodemism, which has been widely debated in historiography, see at least Delio Cantimori, *Spigolature per la storia del Nicodemismo italiano*, in Delio Cantimori, Giorgio Spini, Franco Venturi, Valdo Vinay (eds.), *Ginevra e l'Italia. Raccolta di studi promossa dalla facoltà Valdese di teologia di Roma* (Florence: Sansoni, 1959); Antonio Rotondò, 'Atteggiamenti della vita morale italiana del Cinquecento. La pratica nicodemitica,' *Rivista storica italiana*, 59 (1967), 991–1030; Ginzburg, *Il nicodemismo*; Albano Biondi, 'La giustificazione della simulazione nel Cinquecento,' in Antonio Rotondò (ed.), *Eresia e Riforma nell'Italia del Cinquecento*, Miscellanea 1 (Chicago – Florence: The Newberry Library – Sansoni, 1974), 9–68; Paolo Simoncelli, *Evangelismo italiano del '500: questione religiosa e nicodemismo politico* (Rome: Istituto Storico Italiano, 1979). For a historical and historiographical overview of the concept, see Adriano Prosperi, 'Confessione e dissimulazione' in *Dissidence et Dissimulation*, Jean Pierre Cavaillé and Antony Molho (eds.), 2009, available online at https://journals.openedition.org/dossiersgrihl/3671 (1 May 2021); Eleonora Belligni, *Renata di Francia (1510–1575). Un'eresia di corte* (Turin: Utet, 2011), 193–200. On the subject of religious simulation and dissimulation in urban contexts see also *Dis/simulazione e tolleranza religiosa*

nello spazio urbano dell'Europa moderna, Élise Boillet, Lucia Felici (eds.) (Turin: Claudiana, 2020).

18 About this issue see infra Chapter 4 – in particular see the case of the *Contra Medicos* Inquisition trial held in Venice in 1571, Archivio di Stato di Venezia (ASV), Sant'Uffizio, *Processi, Contra Medicos*, Bu. 35.

19 William Eamon, *Science and the Secrets of Nature. Books of Secrets in Medieval and Early Modern Culture* (Princeton: Princeton University Press, 1994), 98. On Otto Brunfels, considered the key figure in the development of Nicodemism (the defensive strategy of religious [dis]simulation) as a theological doctrine, see Carlo Ginzburg, *Il nicodemismo. Simulazione e dissimulazione nell'Europa del '500* (Turin: Einaudi, 1970).

20 See Jürgen Helm, 'Religion and Medicine: Anatomical Education at Wittenberg and Ingolstadt,' in idem, Annette Winkelmann (eds.), *Religious Confessions and the Sciences in the Sixteenth Century* (Leiden – Boston: Brill, 2001); Andrew Cunningham, 'Protestant Anatomy,' ivi, 44–50; Vivian Nutton, 'Wittenberg Anatomy,' in Ole Peter Grell, Andrew Cunningham (eds.), *Medicine and the Reformation* (New York: Routledge, 1993), 11–32.

21 Angel Alcalá, 'What Remains as the Servetus' Heritage, Conclusions from my Life in Touch with his Writings,' in Marian Hillar, Juan Naja (eds.), *Michael Servetus, Heartfelt: Proceedings of the International Servetus Congress 20–21 October 2006* (New York: City University of New York, 2011), 166.

22 On Regius see Theo Verbeek, 'From "Learned Ignorance" to Scepticism. Descartes and Calvinist Orthodoxy,' in Richard Popkin, Arie Johan Vanderjagt (eds.), *Scepticism and Irreligion in the Seventeenth and Eighteenth Centuries,* (Leiden – Boston: Brill, 1993), 31–45; idem, 'The Invention of Nature: Descartes and Regius,' in Stephen Gaukroger, John Schuster, John Sutton (eds.), *Descartes' Natural Philosophy* (New York: Routledge, 2000), 149–67.

23 Gijsbert Voet, *De atheismo, pars quarta, resp. Gualtero de Bruyn Amisfurt, Ad diem 13 Iulii 1639*, in idem, *Selectarum Disputationum Theologicarum, pars prima* (Utrecht: Johannes van Waesbergen, 1639), 217.

24 Cantimori, *Eretici italiani*, ad indicem (especially 49–62); Roland Bainton, *Vita e morte di Michele Serveto,* Adriano Prosperi (ed.), (Rome: Fazi, 2012); Giuseppe Ongaro, 'La scoperta della circolazione polmonare e la diffusione della *Christianismi restitutio* di Michele Serveto nel XVI secolo in Italia e nel Veneto,' *Episteme,* 5 (1971), 3–44; Claudio Manzoni, *Umanesimo ed eresia: Michele Serveto* (Naples: Guida, 1974). Servetus's works are published in Miguel Servet, *Obras completas*, Ángel Alcalá (ed.) (Zaragoza: Prensas Universitarias De Zaragoza, 2003).

25 Aldo Stella, 'Intorno al medico padovano Niccolò Buccella anabattista del '500,' *Atti e Memorie dell'Accademia Patavina di Scienze, Lettere ed Arti,* 74 (1961–1962), 333–61; idem, *Dall'anabattismo al socinianesimo nel Cinquecento veneto: ricerche storiche* (Liviana: Padua, 1967), 121–43. On Buccella, see also Domenico Caccamo, *Eretici italiani in Moravia, Polonia, Transilvania* (Florence – Chicago: Sansoni – The Newberry Library, 1970), ad indicem and especially 51–60.

26 Antonio Rotondò, 'Pietro Perna e la vita culturale e religiosa di Basilea fra il 1570 e il 1580,' 273–91, in idem, *Studi di storia ereticale*; See also idem, 'L'uso non dogmatico della ragione,' ivi, 635–702, which focuses on the radical naturalism, influenced by Bernardino Telesio, put forward by the heterodox physician Agostino Doni.

27 Alessandro Pastore, *Le regole dei corpi. Medicina e disciplina nell'Italia moderna* (Bologna: Il Mulino, 2006).

28 Addante, *Eretici e libertini*, 61–76.

29 Silvia Ferretto, 'Il "caso" Pomponio Algieri. Appunti di una ricerca in corso,' *Bruniana & Campanelliana,* 16, no. 1, (2009), 65–79; eadem, *La cultura medica all'Università di Padova tra istanze di rinnovamento culturale e poteri politici nel Cinquecento* (Padua: Cleup, 2011).
30 Alexandre Koiré, *Mystiques, spirituels, alchimistes du XVIe siècle allemand* (Paris: Armand Colin, 1955).
31 Walter Pagel, *An Introduction to Philosophical Medicine in the Era of the Renaissance* (Basel: Kerger, 1958).
32 Gary Waite, 'Radical Religion and the Medical Profession: The Spiritualist David Joris and the Brothers Weyer (Wier),' in Hans-Jürgen Goertz, James M. Stayer (eds.), *Radikalität und Dissent im 16. Jahrhundert/Radicalism and Dissent in the Sixteenth Century*, special edition of the *Zeitschrift für historische Forschung*, (Berlin: Duncker & Humblot, 2002) 167–85.
33 Charles Webster, *Paracelsus. Medicine, Magic and the Mission at the End of Time* (New Haven: Yale University Press, 2008).
34 Richard Palmer, 'Physicians and the Inquisition in Sixteenth-Century Venice,' in Grell, Cunningham, *Medicine and The Reformation*, 118–33.
35 John Brooke, Ian Maclean (eds.), *Heterodoxy in Early Modern Science and Religion* (Oxford: Oxford University Press, 2005).
36 Nancy G. Siraisi, *Communities of Learned Experience. Epistolary Medicine in the Renaissance* (Baltimora: Johns Hopkins University Press, 2013); Alessandra Quaranta, *Medici italiani eretici nella seconda metà del Cinquecento, Esperienze d'esilio e rapporti culturali e scientifici con il mondo di lingua tedesca* (Palermo: New Digital Frontiers, 2019).
37 Johana Kostylo, 'Commonwealth of all faiths. Republica Myth and The Italian Diaspora in Sixteenth-Century Poland-Lithuania,' in Karen Friedrich, Barbara M. Pendzich (eds.), *Citizenship and Identity in a Multinational Commonwealth: Poland-Lithuania in Context, 1550–1772* (Leiden-Boston: Brill, 2008), 184–85; eadem, 'Pharmacy as a centre for Protestant reform in Renaissance Venice,' *Renaissance Studies*, 30, no. 2 (2015), 236–53; Caccamo, *Eretici Italiani*; Massimo Firpo, *Antitrinitari nell'Europa Orientale del '500, Nuovi testi di Szymon Budny, Niccolò Paruta e Iacopo Paleologo* (Florence: La Nuova Italia, 1977).
38 Riccarda Suitner, 'Reformation, Medicine, and Religious Dissent in the Late Renaissance: The Case of the University of Padua,' *Nuncius. Journal of the Material and Visual History of Science*, 31 (2016), 11–31.
39 Archivio di Stato di Milano, *Carteggio delle cancellerie dello Stato*, bb. 78, 88, 93, 164; ivi, Fondo *Culto,* bb, 2107, 2104 (where there is also information about Pietro Bresciani, Callisto Villani, Girolamo Maccagno, Bernardo Appiano, and Cristoforo Canale); Archivio di Stato di Trento, Archivio del Principato Vescovile, *sezione latina*, capsa 4, *Contro Ascanio Schrattenberg*; Archivio vescovile di Belluno, sez. 1, rep. IV, *Processo Venzo* (sic) *1579–1580,* Bu. 11; Archivio Arcivescovile di Pisa, *Contro Girolamo Borri*, Bu. 1; Archivio della curia patriarcale di Venezia, *Archivio Segreto, Inquisizione*, *Contro Francesco Severi*, Bu. 2; Archivio di Stato di Modena, *Inquisizione*, Bu. 2, 5, 6 (including information about the heterodox physicians Giovanni Grillenzoni, Antonio De Bendeis, and Paolo Roccacciolo). For the published trial records, see Carlo Ginzburg, *I costituti di Don Pietro Manelfi* (Florence-Chicago: Sansoni – The Newberry Library, 1970); Massimo Firpo, Dario Marcatto (eds.), *I processi inquisitoriali di Pietro Carnesecchi, 1557–1567. Edizione critica*, vols. I–II (Vatican city: Archivio Segreto Vaticano, 1998–2000); Massimo Firpo, Sergio Pagano (eds.), *I processi inquisitoriali di Vittore Soranzo (1550–1558), Edizione critica*, vols. I-II (Vatican city: Archivio Segreto Vaticano, 2004); Massimo Firpo, Dario Marcatto (eds.), *Il processo inquisitoriale del Cardinal Giovanni Morone. Nuova*

edizione critica, vols. I-III (Vatican City: Libreria Editrice Vaticana, 2011–15). The historiography on the Italian Reformation is extensive and will be abundantly quoted in the following pages and chapters.

40 Alessandra Celati, *Medici ed Eresie nel Cinquecento italiano* (PhD diss., University of Pisa, 2016).

41 'Christ has already started to seep into Italy, but I would like him to enter there gloriously and openly, and I believe that Venice will be the gateway' ('Già Christo ha incominciato penetrare in Italia, ma vorrei che v'intrasse glorioso, a la scoperta e che credo che Venezia sarà la porta'); see the letter written by Bernardino Ochino on 7 December 1542, cited in Firpo, *Riforma protestante ed eresie*, 17. On the history of the Protestant Reformation and the spread of heresies in Venice in the sixteenth century, see John Martin, *Venice's Hidden Enemies. Italian Heretics in A Renaissance City*, (Berkeley-Los Angeles: University of California Press, 1993).

42 Paul F. Grendler, 'The Tre Savi Sopra l'Eresia 1547–1605: a Prosopographical Study,' *Studi Veneziani*, 3, (1979), 283–340; Andrea Del Col, *L'Inquisizione in Italia dal XII al XXI secolo* (Milan: Mondadori, 2006), 342–94.

43 On Donzellini, see Ann Jacob Schutte, entry 'Donzellini, Girolamo,' in *Dizionario biografico degli Italiani,* 41 (Rome: Treccani, 1992); Alessandro Pastore, 'L'onore della corporazione. Il collegio medico di Verona fra tardo Quattrocento e gli inizi del Seicento,' in *Studi di storia per Luigi Ambrosoli* (Verona: Cierre edizioni, 1993), pp. 7–28; Alessandra Celati, 'Medicine, Heresy and Paracelsianism in Sixteenth-century Italy: The Case of Girolamo Donzellini (1513–1587),' *Gesnerus, Swiss Journal of the History of Medicine and Sciences*, 71, no.1 (2014): 5–37, Quaranta, *Medici italiani.*

44 ASV, Sant'Uffizio, *Processi, Contro Girolamo Donzellini*, Bu. 39.

45 For the correspondence between Girolamo Donzellini and Theodor Zwinger, see the collection of letters held in Basel at the Universitätsbibliothek, Abteilung Frey-Gryn Mscr I and II, and in Erlangen at the Universitätsbibliothek, Briefsammlung Trew. The latter archive also contains Donzellini's letters to Joaquim Camerarius the Younger.

46 The same holds true for the term 'sect,' used in this book to describe the experience of Giorgio Siculo and his followers. It was taken from sources and historiography that outline the group's initiatory dimension and characteristics of secrecy and exclusivity.

47 Seidel Menchi, *Erasmo in Italia*, 14.

48 Ginzburg, *Microhistory*, 205.

49 The expression 'intensive technique for reconstructing biographies' ('tecnica intensiva di ricostruzione delle biografie') is taken from Levi, *L'eredità immateriale*, 21.

50 This approach is inspired by the assertions made by Ginzburg in *Microhistory*, 207, 213: 'Marc Bloch offered the best solution in his *Feudal Society:* a constant back-and-forth between micro- and macrohistory, between close-ups and extreme long shots, so as to continually thrust back into discussion the comprehensive vision of the historical process through apparent exceptions and cases of brief duration. […] reality is fundamentally discontinuous and heterogeneous. […] any social structure is the result of interaction and of numerous individual strategies, a fabric that can be reconstituted only from close observation. […] the relationship between this microscopic dimension and the larger contextual dimension became […] the organizing principle in the narration.'

51 For a thorough examination of the concept of social movement see Donatella Della Porta, Mario Diani (eds.), *Social Movements. An Introduction* (Malden: Blackwell Publishing, 2006, first edition 1997).

52 On the 'inconsistency between systems of rules and penalties' ('incoerenza tra sistemi di regole e sanzioni') and the chance to use 'the ambiguity of rules' ('l'ambiguità delle regole') and compromises between 'subjectively desired behaviours and socially required behaviours' ('comportamenti soggettivamente desiderati e comportamenti socialmente richiesti') as an interpretative category, see Levi, *L'eredità immateriale,* 21–22.
53 'Una politica della vita quotidiana'; ibidem.
54 This expression is inspired by Rosa Salzberg, *Ephemeral City. Cheap Print and Urban Culture in Renaissance Venice* (Manchester, Manchester University Press, 2014).
55 This approach is useful for avoiding the 'anthological bias': that is to say focusing on those who occupied a prominent position in the history of religious dissent. I have drawn this expression from Christian Jacob, 'Lieux de savoir. A comparative approach to the tools and techniques of scholarly work. (Conférence donnée à la Bibliothèque royale, Copenhague, 24 september 2009),' available at https://www.academia.edu/2581140/Lieux_de_savoir_A_comparative_approach_to_the_tools_and_techniques_of_scholarly_work, January 2022.
56 See for instance Cantimori, *Eretici italiani*; Rotondò, *Pietro Perna*; Firpo, *Riforma protestante ed eresie*; Addante, *Eretici e libertini.*
57 Manuela Albertone, Enrico Pasini, 'Editorial,' *History of European Ideas* 40, no. 4 (2014), 452, available at https://www.tandfonline.com/doi/abs/10.1080/01916599.2013.826433 (22 February 2021). For an introduction to the application of network research to intellectual history and its value, see Rachel Midura, 'Conceptualizing Knowledge Networks: Agents and Patterns of 'Flow,' in *Empires of Knowledge*, ed. Paula Findlen (New York: Routledge, 2018), 373–77.
58 Between the 1950s and the 1960s, a group of British social anthropologists from the School of Cambridge rejected the structural paradigm (and its interpretation of society as essentially static) as inappropriate for describing complex communities and started to experiment with the concept of 'network.' In their approach, they emphasised themes like change, discontinuity, and conflict, suggesting that reality is fluid and unstable. In particular, history is the result of the set of connections that took place in the past. See Fortunata Piselli, 'Il network sociale nell'analisi del potere e dei processi politici,' *Stato e Mercato* 50, no. 2 (1997), 288–89; Federica Ruspio, 'Network analysis e microstoria: il caso della nazione portoghese,' in *Microstoria. A venticinque anni dall'eredità immateriale*, Paola Lanaro (ed.), (Milan: Franco Angeli, 2011), 133; Claire Lemercier, 'Formal network methods in history: why and how?,' in *Social Networks, Political Institutions, and Rural Societies*, Brepols (2015), 281–310. I will not attempt to provide a complete overview of works grounded in a networked approach and will just mention some of the most significant studies: Alan Macfarlane, Sarah Harrison and Charles Jardine, *Reconstructing Historical Communities* (Cambridge: Cambridge University Press, 1977); Natalie Zemon Davis, 'The Sacred and the Social Body in Sixteenth-Century Lyon,' *Past & Present* 90, no. 1 (1981), 40–70; John F. Padgett and Christopher K. Ansell, 'Robust Action and the Rise of the Medici, 1400–1434,' *American Journal of Sociology* 98, no. 6 (1993), 1259–1319; Francesca Trivellato, *The Familiarity of Strangers: The Sephardic Diaspora, Livorno, and Cross-Cultural Trade in the Early Modern Period* (New Haven and London: Yale University Press, 2009); Simone Testa, *Italian Academies and their Networks, 1525–1700. From Local to Global* (New York: Palgrave Macmillan, 2015); Tijl Vanneste, *Global Trade and Commercial Networks: Eighteenth-Century Diamond Merchants* (New York, Routledge, 2011); Georg Fertig (ed.), *Social Networks, Political Institutions, and Rural Societies* (Turnhout: Brepols, 2015). With regard to the history of the

Reformation, see Ole Peter Grell, *Brethren in Christ. A Calvinist Network in Reformation Europe* (Cambridge: Cambridge University Press, 2011); Vivienne Larminie (ed.), *Huguenots networks 1560 1780: The Interactions and Impact of a Protestant Minority in Europe*, (New York: Routledge, 2018); Ruth Ahnert, Sebastian E. Ahnert, Nicole Coleman, and Scott Weingart, The Network Turn. Changing Perspectives in The Humanities (Cambridge: Cambridge University Press, 2020).

59 'What do we mean by saying that existence precedes essence? We mean that man first of all exists, encounters himself, surges up in the world—and defines himself afterwards. If man as the existentialist sees him is not definable, it is because to begin with he is nothing. He will not be anything until later, and then he will be what he makes of himself. [...] Man simply is. [...] But what do we mean to say by this, but that man is of a greater dignity than a stone or a table? For we mean to say that man primarily exists—that man is, before all else, something which propels itself towards a future and is aware that it is doing so. Man is, indeed, a project which possesses a subjective life, instead of being a kind of moss, or a fungus or a cauliflower. Before that projection of the self nothing exists; not even in the heaven of intelligence: man will only attain existence when he is what he purposes to be. Not, however, what he may wish to be. For what we usually understand by wishing or willing is a conscious decision taken—much more often than not—after we have made ourselves what we are'; Jean Paul Sartre, *L'existentialisme est un humanisme (Existentialism Is A Humanism)* (first French edition 1946), English translation available online at https://warwick.ac.uk/fac/cross_fac/complexity/people/students/dtc/students2011/maitland/philosophy/sartre-eih.pdf (2 September 2021).

60 The Digital Humanities research has heuristic value. It is useful for showing the density and extent of relational phenomena, outlining any interruptions and anomalies, and identifying individuals worthy of further research (with the corresponding sources). Furthermore, by using data modelling and visualisation in digital networks, a concrete quantitative relational perspective can be added to the qualitative context, thereby fine-tuning the research hypothesis, overcoming interpretative bias, and confirming or refuting the insights offered over time by historiography. Notwithstanding these considerations, Digital Humanities findings should not be taken as definitive and must be combined with qualitative research. I explained the way in which I processed the sources and transformed them into digital imaging, as well as the contribution of the digital humanities to my research (with their potential and problems) in: Alessandra Celati, 'A Digital Exploration of 16th-Century Heretical Networks in the Italian Medical Context: Methodological Challenges and Research Perspectives,' *Journal of Interdisciplinary History of Ideas*, 7, no. 14 (2018), 4–47. This article includes several network visualisations of the individuals who feature in this book. For an introduction to the methodology of the digital humanities and the benefits of using them in the reconstruction of historical networks, see Giovanna Ceserani, Caroline Winterer, Dan Edelstein, Paula Findlen, Nicole Coleman, 'Historical Research in a Digital Age: Reflections from the Mapping the Republic of Letters Project,' *The American Historical Review* 122, no. 2 (Apr. 2017), 400–24.

61 See Celati, 'A Digital Exploration,' 18–19.

1 Becoming a heretic. Medical studies and religious dissent, 1513–1545

Girolamo Donzellini was born during a raging pestilence under the influence of an earth zodiac sign, which supposedly determined his 'melancholy' ('maninconico') nature.[1] He was around four years old when the religious crisis exploded in Germany, before it spread throughout Europe and reached the north of Italy in the early 1520s. *Lutheranism* was defined as a heretical plague (*peste ereticale*) by the Roman authorities, seen as perhaps even more dangerous than the physical disease since it affected the souls of believers rather than their bodies.

Located near the foot of the Adige valley at the junction of several routes between the Alps and Veneto, Brescia favoured contact with the German-speaking world. Many German traders worked in the city, allowing the circulation of Lutheran books and ideas. The first evidence of an official Catholic stance against Lutheranism in Brescia is an order given by Clement VII on 25 January 1524, in which the nuncio was instructed to seek out all 'Lutheran' books in the city and burn them. Two years later, Peter Martyr Vermigli preached in the church of Sant'Afra, having already been exposed to Lutheran ideas in Padua and Bologna.

Religious dissent was far from a new phenomenon in Brescia. Indeed, various forms had taken shape in the city and the surrounding area since the Middle Ages, highlighting the risk of conducting theological and spiritual research outside the Catholic precepts. One of the main episodes centred on Arnold of Brescia, who was condemned as a heretic in 1115 as a result of his appeal for purity and poverty in Christianity. The following decades saw the persecution of Cathars and Waldenses, while in the early sixteenth century the Val Camonica witch trials sentenced hundreds of women to burn at the stake. Such events did not curb the religious unrest, however, and the Brescia area became one of the main entry points for the penetration and spread of Lutheran thinking throughout northern Italy.[2] This was the backdrop against which Girolamo grew up. Although he went on to develop his heterodox ideas in Padua and Rome, his first influences of this kind were absorbed in his birthplace and, as in the case of many of his colleagues, in his domestic environment. This chapter examines the growth of Donzellini's

DOI: 10.4324/9781003218852-2

heterodox mind by considering his family, the Paduan university context, and the first stages of his professional career.

1.1 A family of dissidents, 1513–35

Buonamonte Donzellini, Girolamo's father, established a theological discussion group in his house in Orzi Nuovi in the early 1520s. He used his contact network of booksellers and printers in Brescia, which included Giordano Ziletti (who will reappear in later chapters) and Piertantonio Piasentin, to procure various, unfortunately unspecified Reformed texts to share with his three sons. In this way, from a tender age Girolamo, Cornelio, and Pietro Donzellini were educated in Lutheran principles such as individual reading and interpretation of the holy texts, a direct relationship with God, and justification by faith alone.[3] Girolamo was also introduced to Protestant thinking through his logic tutor, Michelangelo Florio, personally selected by Buonamonte. As the Holy Office judges later underlined during Girolamo's trial in 1560, Florio was 'a former conventual friar minor, now a heretical apostate' ('già frate minore conventuale ora apostata heretico'). The teacher-pupil relationship that they developed must have been significant for Donzellini, who in fact remained in contact with Florio over the years. They met up again in Venice in the 1540s, with Florio 'dressed as a layman' ('vestito da layco'), and Girolamo shared with him the advantages of belonging to a rich network of heterodox men of culture. Florio came bearing his translation of St Augustine's treatise *De gratia et libero arbitrio* (*On Grace and Free Will*) and asked Girolamo to deliver it to the Calvinist Duchess of Ferrara, Renée of France, knowing that his former pupil was friends with people who worked at the duchess' court, such as the Greek scholar Francesco Porto.[4]

The three Donzellini brothers followed a path of dissent that led first to an Inquisition trial and then to either recantation (Pietro) or prison and death (Cornelio and Girolamo). The sources reveal that Buonamonte also had a daughter, Maria, but little is known about her except that she was confined to a nunnery.[5] In this respect, she shared the fate of many Italian girls offloaded by their families to avoid paying dowries and to preserve property. However, this choice cannot be interpreted as a sign of the family's loyalty to the Catholic Church. Indeed, as Girolamo confessed to the Inquisitors in 1574 that both his parents shared his non-conformist religious thinking, it seems that Buonamonte's wife 'inclined towards heresy' too.[6] Furthermore, since Cornelio, the most radical brother, was also initially intent on an ecclesiastical career, it is perfectly feasible that Maria's entry into the nunnery was equally unrelated to Catholic devotion.

While sources provide scant details about Pietro, a 'doctor of law' ('dottor di legge'), they are more revealing about Cornelio. The former played an active role in Girolamo's defence when he was still at liberty in the 1550s but subsequently fell afoul of the Holy Office and recanted in Brescia a few years before Girolamo's trial in 1560, although the exact date is unknown.[7] As for Cornelio, whereas his brothers pursued an academic education, he joined the Dominican Order as a young man. He never felt at ease in his religious habit, though, and soon became an apostate. He then moved to Istria, where Lutheran ideas had already spread widely through the preaching of the heterodox bishop Pier Paolo Vergerio. Here, he tutored the latter's nephew Aurelio and gave sermons which were attended, among others, by Vergerio's niece Antonia and her entourage.[8] Cornelio duly became so active in the heterodox movement that the inquisitors referred to him as a 'heresiarch' in 1549.[9] The repressive atmosphere imposed by the Roman authorities soon prompted him to flee to Venice, where he worked with Protestant humanists Giovanni degli Onesti and Lucio Paolo Rosello on the vernacular version of three sacred texts: Calvin's *Petit traicté de la saincte céne* (*Short Treatise on the Lord's Supper*), a collection of ten sermons *De divina providentia* (*On Divine Providence*) by Theodoret of Cyrus, and a *Testamento novo* (*New Testament*) translated from the Greek and Latin versions. During his Inquisition trial, Rosello suggested that the latter text reflected Cornelio's views more than orthodox Catholicism.[10] After raising the suspicions of the Inquisition once more, Cornelio moved to Ferrara, where he joined the circle of Renée of France. He probably first introduced the Calvinist duchess and her entourage to Girolamo, who later temporarily fled to Ferrara to escape his first Venetian trial in 1553. By 1550, however, Cornelio had already moved to Florence. This was no coincidence, as the Tuscan capital was widely perceived at the time as a city where the Reformation could triumph, almost to the same extent as in Venice.[11] While working as a teacher at the Medici Court in Florence, he dedicated a Greek grammar to Giovanni and Francesco de Medici, making the book a covert vehicle to disseminate his heretical religious views. In 1552, he was arrested as part of Duke Cosimo's crackdown on Lutherans and Anabaptists.[12] He was forced to recant and sentenced to row on the galleys for the rest of his life, one of the harshest punishments in early modern legislation. He was unable to survive such a regime and died in the Stinche prison in Florence after only a year.[13]

The existence of an entire family of religious dissidents attracted the interest of the Inquisition, as shown by the records of the legal proceedings against Girolamo Donzellini. In his first trial in 1560, Girolamo exploited his deceased brother's case to prove his innocence, claiming that he had been led astray.[14] In the second process in 1574, the judges investigated Girolamo's heretical background. Although he initially refused to cooperate to protect his family's reputation, he was eventually forced to admit their involvement.[15] Both the letters he wrote to his father during his religious exile and his brothers' recantations clearly show that Reformed principles were firmly established in the Buonamonte home.

There are various instances – at least fifteen other cases – of a culture of heterodoxy flourishing in the households of physicians.[16] Although the subject of family heterodoxy has never been approached as a separate historical issue, scholars have touched on the matter while outlining the lives of certain leading figures in the landscape of the Italian Reformation.[17] The fact that religious dissent circulated in heterodox physicians' homes in a significant number of cases, however, suggests that family heresy should be considered as a specific historical phenomenon. The climate of free theological debate typically found in the domestic environments of these dissidents must be seen in relation to their developing critical attitude towards religious discourse and subsequent intellectual growth. While the medical profession admittedly offered excellent guarantees in terms of earnings and social prestige, it is also plausible that some aspiring young physicians were inspired by home-nurtured religious feelings. Indeed, a parental focus on theological debate almost certainly influenced the decision to enter the medical field. In the first place, in-depth knowledge of the human body was strongly associated with spiritual salvation at the time. Furthermore, the everyday practice of the profession was sometimes compared to works of mercy (*operae misericordiae*).

Among the many cases of physicians whose upbringing involved an education in dissent, one notable example is Teofilo Panarelli, who we will return to in the following chapters. Parallels can certainly be drawn between his family and the Donzellinis, with the addition of a female protagonist. Besides forcing his offspring into a peripatetic lifestyle with a rich range of cultural stimuli, Teofilo's father, Nicola Antonio Panarelli, a district physician (*medico condotto*), steered his children towards unorthodox religious choices. While he sent Teofilo to Bartolomeo Fonzio to further his heterodox education during the family's stay in Istria,[18] he was personally involved in instructing his daughter, Virginia, who later developed an unusual cultural awareness for a woman of her time. At his behest, she would read out passages from Ochino's sermons to her brothers.[19] Nicola Antonio also encouraged his other son, Agostino, to move to German soil, where he pursued a university education with clear Protestant leanings, encountering Matthias Flacius Illyricus and Philip Melanchthon along the way.[20] Instead, Virginia settled in Venice, where she married the polygraph Girolamo Ruscelli.[21] The couple maintained close relations with Teofilo, now a physician, who treated Ruscelli for the illness that eventually killed him in 1566.[22] A few years later, when Teofilo attracted the interest of the Inquisition, mutual accusations levelled by the two siblings brought to light the religious dissent in the Panarelli family. On this occasion, Virginia claimed that her brother had been alone in tainting their parents' orthodoxy due to his rebellious nature.[23] This did not save her from a trial for heresy, though, while the physician was sentenced to death in 1571.

After receiving his early education in Orzi Nuovi, the young Girolamo Donzellini forged relationships with members of the Reformed movement in Brescia and Lombardy, many of whom proved to be long-standing acquaintances. Most notably, he shared heterodox opinions with friends like

Celso Martinengo da Barco, Ippolito Chizzola, Andrea Ugoni, and Publio Francesco Spinola, known as *il Milanese*, who were all tried for heresy in Venice or became religious exiles between the 1540s and 1560s. In the early 1530s, Brescia saw the flourishing of an Erasmian circle centred around Vincenzo Maggi, who had left the priesthood under the influence of Francesco Negri and was to become one of Girolamo's best friends in Venice in the late 1540s. In this context, Emilio Emigli produced the first Italian translation of Erasmus's *Enchiridion militis christiani* (*Manual for a Christian Soldier*). Donzellini was an adolescent at the time, and it is not known whether he was already in contact with Vincenzo Maggi. However, his mature philosophical works show the impact of the Christian humanism of Erasmus on his thought. This was the backdrop against which the heterodox influences he later absorbed managed to thrive.

1.2 *Patavina libertas*

In the mid-1530s Donzellini moved to Padua, which had the most advanced university in Europe in terms of philosophical debate and medical research. He studied medical theory and practice during his eight years there, immersing himself in a dynamic scientific and philosophical environment.[24] The title of Doctor in arts and medicine was awarded at Italian universities after at least seven years of study. After focusing on the basics of medicine in the second part of the course, the training period ended with a working apprenticeship alongside an expert physician. The local medical authorities then administered an exam before finally granting a licence to practise. The medieval structure of the curriculum of studies had not changed over the centuries, but the emerging influence of humanistic culture in Italian universities led to content-based changes in research and teaching. This benefitted previously neglected disciplines like anatomy, botany, and clinical medicine.[25] At this juncture, with Padua at the helm, universities became places of experimentation, debate, and direct observation of the human body and pathological phenomena. The research conducted in the field of anatomy was arguably the main medical innovation of the century. The key player in these developments was Andreas Vesalius, one of Donzellini's masters, who taught in Padua in the late 1530s and in the 1540s.[26] His efforts led to the acceptance of physiological and anatomical studies as an essential discipline. Even before the construction of anatomical theatres (the first of which was designed by Hieronymus Fabricius in 1594), students and professors at Padua expected the civil authorities to provide them with a regular supply of cadavers to dissect.[27] Private dissections were even organised to meet this demand (sometimes at the house of the heterodox surgeon Nicholas Buccella in the 1560s and 1570s).[28]

Another of Donzellini's masters in Padua was Giovan Battista da Monte, a great innovator in the field of humanistic medicine who moved teaching at the university from the lecture theatre to the sickbed. This overcame the artificial distinction between the practical and theoretical components of medicine, generating interest in the previously unknown clinical aspect. Furthermore, Padua was at the forefront in the study of simples (medicinal plants): aspiring doctors could use the botanical garden, created in 1545, to learn about the properties of plants cultivated for their medical value. Donzellini had already graduated by then, but his adult interest in medicinal remedies and simples might well have originated at university. Finally, he studied philosophy with the Alexandrist Marcantonio Passeri, known as *il Genua*; when they met up again years later in Venice, they engaged in theological discussions with a heterodox flavour.

Donzellini was awarded the 'extraordinary second chair' in medical theory straight after graduating on 28 April 1541.[29] It is also known that he obtained a lectureship from the Reformers of the University of Padua while practising in Venice in 1552. He was aided in this by the mediation skills of his friend and fellow believer Gasparo Parma, who persuaded the nobleman Vincenzo Molino to recommend the appointment to the academic authorities.[30]

Although few details about his experience in Padua are available, the years he spent there undoubtedly further developed his profile as a dissident physician. Padua was the most important university city in sixteenth-century Italy with the largest community of German students (followed by Bologna and Siena).[31] Seething religious unrest flourished in this context, as the sources show. We do not know who Donzellini associated with in his student days, but the example of the aforementioned Teofilo Panarelli, who studied medicine there in the 1550s, illustrates the city's role in engendering heterodox doctrines and 'contaminating' young Italians. After his initial heterodox education from his father, it was in Padua that he first came into contact with unorthodox texts: the *Institutio christianae religionis* (*Institution of the Christian Religion*) and a 'Bible from Germany' ('Bibbia di Alemagna').[32] We also know that he shared a strong interest in theological debate with his fellow Italian and Northern European students. Indeed, they even visited an active preacher in the city, Fra' Franceschino, to express their doubts on various important matters of faith. The main issues raised by Panarelli were the interpretation of the passage 'this is my body' ('hoc est enim corpus meum') and the value of confession, which he did not perceive in the 'Papist way' ('modo papista').[33] The preacher responded by strongly discouraging him from addressing certain delicate questions or sharing opinions that contradicted Catholic orthodoxy. Panarelli did not heed the friar's warning, though, and continued his theological research. In this way, the doubts he harboured on the main truths of Catholic faith were transformed into pronounced heterodox sensibilities. He embraced the opportunity to read Reformed texts and explore sensitive doctrinal questions by exchanging opinions with peers and less orthodox preachers than Fra' Franceschino. When he expressed his views on Calvin's doctrine to one such preacher in 1556, he received confirmation that Calvinism contained reliable truths. However, he was recommended not to expound such ideas in public 'because it was something extremely dangerous' ('perché era cosa molto pericolosa').[34]

The lectures attended by Panarelli included those given by Matteo Gribaldi, a well-known heterodox jurist.[35] The aspiring physician was presumably attracted by the lecturer's humanistic knowledge and references to Reformed doctrines as the course was totally unrelated to his university specialisation. These lectures were also extremely well attended by German students, a fundamental vehicle of heterodox 'contagion' both inside and outside the university.[36] In Padua, young people were introduced to heretical opinions in shared accommodation, in printing houses where students bought books, and during their leisure time, learning from German students or Italian peers that had already converted to Reformed doctrines. Panarelli, for example, stated that he had debated religious questions at the Paduan printing house owned by Grazioso Percacino, who later became part of his Venetian network. Another medical student, Manusso Maran, a native of Crete, which was under Venetian rule at the time, was exposed to Protestant ideas by reading Reformed books left behind by the former tenant of his room when he returned to Flanders.[37] The Cretan then attempted to convert his new co-tenants to the same beliefs, raising their suspicions in the process.[38]

Alarmed by the proliferation of Reformed doctrines in the university environment, the Catholic authorities implemented a series of measures to curb the spread of heresy, most notably by placing checks on foreign students. The bull *In sacrosanta beati Petri* of 1564 established that a doctorate could only be obtained if the candidate professed the Catholic faith. While Northern European students were naturally hostile to this sudden change, the secular authorities – at least in Padua – often turned a blind eye if German scholars failed to swear the relevant oath (one should not forget that Protestants, Jews, and Orthodox Christians that refused to swear the oath could still be awarded a degree by counts palatine, which the governments tolerated). The secular authorities were particularly keen not to alienate the German rulers with whom the Venetian Republic had major trade links but also had a clear interest in maintaining the high number of foreign students living in the city. As well as bringing international prestige to the university, the latter provided a significant user base for related money-spinning activities. Rich earnings were guaranteed through the real estate market and the revenue generated by students from all over Europe, not to mention the university enrolment fees.

At the doctoral examination, the aspiring physician also had to be presented by an older colleague who vouched for his orthodoxy. Here too, the sources show that loopholes were available to those that were reluctant to renounce their heterodox religious faith. Such students could benefit from the solidarity network of Italian heterodox dissenters, which was especially close-knit among physicians who shared unorthodox religious tendencies and the same cultural and professional background. Manusso Maran, for example, used the physician Agostino Gadaldino to obtain the reference he required for a doctoral place.[39] This was duly granted by an Augustinian friar, Agostino Sostegni, a relative of Cardinal Fregoso with the title of cavalier and count palatine who 'had an understanding with schismatics and heretics' (si intendeva con schiesmatici e heretici').[40] As Gadaldino had been an active member of heretical circles in the Venetian Republic until at least ten years before, he was probably willing to lend his support out of solidarity for the young Cretan. It is significant that the inquisitors scrutinised every detail of Maran's university experience when he was apprehended. This involved investigating the relationships he had forged and reconstructing the dynamics that had allowed a young man seriously tainted by heretical dissent to obtain a doctorate – a frequent occurrence at Padua and other Italian universities.

Student heterodoxy was not only the result of friendships with Protestant peers, though. Lectures could also open up perspectives that were incompatible with Catholic orthodoxy. This is not the place to revisit the complex and heated philosophical debate triggered by the materialistic reading of Aristotelian precepts which, above all in Padua, led the most daring philosophers to claim that it was impossible to use rational means to demonstrate the immortality of the human soul, drawing on commentaries by Averroes and Alexander of Aphrodisias.[41] What should be underlined, however, is that the combination of passionate philological inquiry into sources and empirical observation of natural phenomena created the conditions for unrestricted study of natural philosophy. This sometimes generated intellectual views that were considered dangerous by the ecclesiastical authorities. It is said that medical students in Pisa – including the future heretical physician Matteo Gentili – shouted out 'soul, soul!' ('anima, anima!') when the well-known philosopher Simone Porzio, a disciple of Pomponazzi, entered the lecture theatre on 6 November 1546.[42] Similarly, students in Padua objected 'we want the soul!' ('vogliamo l'anima') in 1550 when it was suggested that the focus of the natural philosophy course would shift from Aristotle's *De anima* (*On the Soul*) to his treatise *Meteorologica* (*On Meteorology*).[43] Clearly, the efforts made by the fathers of the Fifth Council of the Lateran in 1513 to curb the 'cockle' and the 'extremely pernicious errors' scattered 'in the Lord's field' by philosophy professors had been fruitless.[44] The bull *Apostolici regiminis* had promulgated the decree of the eighth session of the Council, re-establishing the immortal soul as the only possible truth, but this did not silence the debate. Student physicians never missed an opportunity to quibble over the most delicate philosophical questions and leapt at the chance to practise theological debate, which often took a heretical turn whenever medical studies assumed spiritual connotations. The lack of faculties of theology in the Italian peninsula presumably contributed to the formulation of non-conformist religious notions among medicine and philosophy students. It was easy to overstep the boundaries of orthodoxy in a context where the intellectual verve of students was not corrected or regulated by scholastic theological teaching. In this way, natural philosophy lectures ended up addressing questions such as the destiny and origin of the individual soul. Although the ecclesiastical authorities claimed a monopoly on such matters, the humanistic interpretation of Aristotelian precepts and the development of the discourse on the biological origins of human life provided a natural scope for atheological inquiry. At the end of the century, Padua continued to be the major centre of diffusion for philosophical theories denying the immortality of the soul. The Aristotelian Cesare Cremonini, who had taught at Padua since 1592, was 'one of the most, if not the most, thoroughly investigated thinkers in the early modern Catholic world.'[45]

The impact of radical Aristotelianism did not wane in Padua after the death of Pomponazzi and developed independently in heretical conventicles. Extremist ideas were also sometimes acquired outside the university environment. For example, radical heretics Giulio Basalù and Girolamo Busale, former members of radical coteries in Naples, influenced the young future theologian Lelio Sozzini in Padua with their heterodox preaching.[46] Donzellini encountered Basalù in Venice in the 1550s; as we shall see, the latter cited the former as a heretical acquaintance during his trial in 1555.

In the meantime, the heretical thinking of Michael Servetus had reached the Venetian Republic in the mid-1530s. Imparted through two works, the *De Trinitatis erroribus* (*On the Errors of the Trinity*, Hagenau, 1531) and the *Christianismi restitutio* (*The Restitution of Christianity*), his ideas were promoted by professors at the university, above all Matteo Gribaldi, and physicians working in the Republic. The Paduan milieu proved particularly receptive to a religious discourse that blended scientific speculation with theological issues. Moreover, physicians were more likely to be attracted to the Spaniard's ideas on physiology, anatomy, religion, and philosophy as they shared his cultural background. They therefore probably supported and spread Servetian thinking by word of mouth, as well as through his printed works. We know that the *Christianismi restitutio* was available in Padua and throughout the Venetian Republic through Pietro Perna, a printer from Lucca living in exile in Basel whose contact network featured many heterodox physicians (including Girolamo Donzellini). Perna was a key player in the distribution of the works of Servetus[47] and was said to be responsible for the many copies in circulation in Italy. Heinrich Bullinger, the Reformer of Zurich, was informed of Perna's involvement by the Calvinist physician Guglielmo Grataroli, a native of Bergamo who fled to Basel in 1551. The texts were apparently distributed throughout the north of the peninsula after being sent to Matteo Gribaldi and Giorgio Filalete, alias *Turchetto*, a figure also identified as Ortensio Lando, an apostate friar with an interest in medicine who was part of Donzellini's network.[48] In Reformed Europe too, physicians like Girolamo Massari and Giorgio Biandrata were involved in distributing Servetus's works.

Padua was not only a meeting place for students from the Venetian Republic. The young aspiring physicians (and future heretics) who gathered there from all over the peninsula included Simone Simoni[49] and Leonardo Marchio[50] from Lucca, Fabio Nifo[51] from Sessa in Campania, and Jacomo (whose surname is unknown), the 'physician of the Kingdom' of Naples ('medico del Regno'). The latter's heretical feelings seem to have blossomed in the lecture theatres, almost mirroring the experiences of Manusso Maran[52] and Teofilo Panarelli. Jacomo became a member of a radical heterodox group in Padua that also included Pomponio Algieri from Nola in Campania, another medical student who later became a martyr.[53]

Although Padua was a unique hub for bringing together scientific experimentalism, radical theological and philosophical research, and Protestant ideas, all Italian universities served as a breeding ground for humanists with 'free-thinking' tendencies. For example, the physician Agostino Vanzo, who was tried by the Inquisition of Vicenza in Belluno in 1579, stated that he had acquired the basics of Protestant discourse at Ferrara University between 1553 and 1557.[54] His fellow students had taught him the value of examining the holy texts freely, above all the New Testament, which he started to read and study by himself.[55] When he noted a stark discrepancy between his personal findings and the teachings of the ecclesiastical authorities, he developed his own heterodox sensibilities. These would cost him dearly, though, and he was burned at the stake in 1580.

More generally, many Italian university graduates created intellectual networks spanning great distances, often featuring a strong element of religious dissent. The final chapter will highlight such connections established between Venice and the Kingdom of Naples. For now, we will focus on the example of Lelio Sozzini, son of the Sienese jurist Mariano, who worked in Padua from 1525 to 1542. After prudence forced him to take flight, Lelio followed his father to Bologna and joined the heretical group that also included the future physician Ulisse Aldrovandi. The latter had first become involved with heterodox groups influenced by Camillo Renato's spiritual thinking as a young man, embracing radical opinions on the definition of the sacraments and the destiny of the soul after death. Humanists and men of culture who sympathised with demands for reform were united throughout the peninsula by their academic education and a questioning mindset that favoured critical investigation. Physicians played an essential role in this community.[56]

Finally, a significant number of heterodox physicians attended the Medical College in Venice. As the institution benefitted from university privileges such as granting doctorates, it took shape as an alternative for those who wanted to study in Padua but could not afford the final exam. Girolamo Mercuriale was one of the leading sixteenth-century physicians that graduated from here, completing his studies in 1555.[57] Various members of the heretical movement in Venice and elsewhere also received their doctorate from the College, including Vincenzo Negroni, who was investigated in the late 1560s in Venice; Guglielmo Grataroli from Bergamo, who was tried on several occasions in the 1540s and 1550s before becoming a religious exile; and Pietro Giudici from Rivoltella, who was executed as a follower of Giorgio Siculo in 1568.[58]

As far as Girolamo Donzellini is concerned, there is no concrete evidence of elements of religious dissent in his medical studies. However, this brief overview of the religious crisis affecting Italian university life in the sixteenth century strongly suggests that his student days influenced his cultural and heterodox development.

1.3 Medical career and the growth of a heretical mind: Rome

University education played an essential role in forming the intellectual and professional identity of philosopher-physicians in the sixteenth century. For many, including Donzellini, their common academic experiences laid the foundations for dense correspondence-based networks spanning regional and international borders.[59]

After leaving the university lecture theatres, however, the newly qualified physicians undertook different career paths. One particularly enticing option was a return to the halls of academia to take up a chair in theoretical medicine, practical medicine, surgery, or simples. Another highly coveted position was that of archiater at the court of an Italian lord, a European prince, the Holy Roman Emperor, or the Pope. Indeed, a brilliant courtly career was a recurring element in the biographies of many heterodox physicians who were forced to flee Italy to avoid persecution. As Chapter 3 will highlight, the area encompassing Poland and Transylvania held a special attraction for Italian heterodox medical practitioners. To name but a few, Giorgio Biandrata, Niccolò Buccella, and Simone Simoni all enjoyed successful careers in these lands, each specialising in different branches of scientific experimentation: gynaecology, anatomy, theoretical and philosophical research, and the observation of nature according to its own principles.[60]

For those who prioritised job stability over career prospects and earnings, one viable solution was to practise as a district physician in small rural communities or villages.[61] Contracts were usually awarded on an annual basis but could be renewed after a satisfactory first year. The position made it possible to proselytise, spreading heterodox doctrines with greater ease and less risk than in the city because of the closer ties between physicians and patients. One pertinent example is Antonio Massimo, who moved from Venice to Oderzo (a small village close to Treviso), precisely for this purpose although he was then forced to flee to Geneva when the Inquisition authorities caught up with him.[62] Another is Gian Battista Goineo, the district physician in Pirano (a coastal town in present-day Slovenia), who was held responsible for converting the whole village to heresy with the complicity of his family and a schoolmaster. In a similar case in Gardone, on Lake Garda, the Anabaptist Stefano de Giusti managed to combine medical practice, heterodox propaganda, and works of mercy before being arrested and forced to abjure.[63]

This was not the life for Donzellini, though, as he clearly harboured higher professional ambitions. After working in Padua for two years, he moved to Rome in 1543 and became the personal physician to two cardinals: Durante Duranti, a native of Brescia, and Giulio Della Rovere. The fact that a heterodox physician decided to work in the papal city should come as no surprise. Firstly, the system of control and repression in the early 1540s still left ample scope for dissidents. Furthermore, as heresy had permeated the upper echelons of the Roman authorities, members of the clergy and various types of heterodox dissenters were guaranteed an unprecedented level of collusion. In his years in Rome, Donzellini was a member of a heterodox circle that revolved around Pietro Antonio Di Capua, Archbishop of Otranto, who in turn was influenced by the thinking of the most important theologian of the Italian Reformation, the Spaniard Juan de Valdés.

After making the acquaintance of Valdés between 1534 and 1541, Di Capua forged relations with his followers, read his books, and shared his theological insights. After the Spaniard died, Di Capua settled in Rome, where he associated with Valdesians like Cardinal Reginald Pole and the humanist Marcantonio Flaminio. He even welcomed the heterodox group that included Donzellini into his home. In this way, against the backdrop of the papal city, pervaded by spiritual anxieties and Reformed tendencies, Girolamo absorbed a form of religiosity that advocated complete inner freedom. This aspect offered potential for greater religious subjectivism and left room for Nicodemite overtones. The main spiritual message of Valdesianism was based on the supremacy of illumination of the spirit and the centrality of the internal forum, combining justification by faith with elements of Spanish Alumbradism and the Erasmian ethical concept of Christianity. With Valdesian teachings focusing on the necessary unity of the Christian community, there was no room for new orthodoxies, exclusive confessional affiliation, or indeed polemicists and controversialists. Preaching potentially radical ideas disguised in moderate tones, Valdesians reassured the faithful through a message of salvation within everyone's reach, made possible by the sacrifice of the cross.[64]

As we shall see, there is evidence of Donzellini's affinity with doctrines, texts, and individuals with Valdesian associations throughout his life. Valdesianism remained a constant in his religious anti-conformism, developing into a candidly ethical and spiritual notion of Christianity devoid of sectarian emphasis and open to radical perspectives. However, Valdesian ideas were only part of a more complex religious profile. This derived from an intricate interplay of influences and experiences, which all collimated with Donzellini's humanist religious orientation. This syncretism was the key feature of his intellectual and spiritual thought.

For now, however, we will focus on his heterodox circle in Rome. Some idea of their meetings can be constructed from the testimony of Pietro Carnesecchi, an apostolic protonotary convicted by the Holy Office, although it is somewhat short on detail.[65] It seems that the Averroist Girolamo Borri, a philosopher and physician from Arezzo, generally read out 'the epistles of St Paul or other epistles of Scripture' ('le epistole di san Paolo o altre epistole della Scrittura'), while Archbishop Di Capua and his secretary, Guido Giannetti from Fano, procured prohibited books. Although Donzellini's role in the group is unknown, it is certain that the time he spent with these figures significantly broadened his religious outlook. His intellectual aspirations and restless anti-Roman feelings were probably stoked by Giannetti's politically revolutionary Lutheranism and by Borri's radical Averroism, whose basics Donzellini was already familiar with from his university days in Padua. Borri was described as a man converted 'to modern heretical opinions' ('alle opinioni heretiche moderne'), most notably the Sacramentarian doctrine, and Carnesecchi testified 'that he said at almost every word: blessed be God, or the name of Jesus Christ' ('che quasi a ogni parola diceva: sia benedetto Dio, overo il nome di Iesu Cristo').[66] It is perhaps no coincidence that both Borri and Donzellini, who shared this experience and a spiritual-style religious education, used the same terms in their mature writings to describe their concept of the divine. As we shall see, these expressions, which refer to negative theology and the lexicon of Ficino, are indicators of a form of radicalism that should not be pigeonholed using the dichotomous terms 'Aristotelianism' and 'Platonism.'[67]

Donzellini's heretical experience in Rome came to an end in 1545, no more than two years after he had arrived in the city. In the same year, at Christmas, a letter to Luther was confiscated from the Spanish copyist Diego de Enzinas, a member of Donzellini's circle. The epistle asked for clarification on the thorny issue of the real presence of the body of Christ in the Eucharist. Enzinas, who had written on behalf of the 'very few believers' ('perpauci fideles') gathered in the papal city, was arrested and tortured. A few days later, he revealed the names of his companions, leading the inquisitors onto the trail of 'a good many of his sect' ('parecchi della setta sua'). The judges saw clear evidence of the guilt of those named after examining the 'writings found in their homes' ('scritture trovateli') or because some, including Donzellini, took flight forthwith. The document showing the interest of the Roman authorities in the physician, who was working for Cardinal Durante Duranti at the time, confirms Girolamo's involvement in the heterodox network that was uncovered:

> Our Lord, who wants this matter to be well known in order to discover the truth, requested me to write to you. When you receive this, order a search of the physician's writings and books, and make sure that he is thoroughly investigated. If you find any evidence that he is what he has been accused of during the investigation or in another way, have him placed under guard.[68]

These lines come from a letter sent to Duranti by Cardinal Alessandro Farnese, written five days after the discovery of Enzinas's epistle. As fate would have it, though, Duranti was in Camerino, a small town in central Italy, with his physician at the time. In this way, after being informed of what had transpired by his fellow believer Baldassarre Cazzago, Donzellini managed to escape to Venice before the Roman Holy Office could apprehend him. He was followed a few months later by Guido Giannetti, which gave 'substantial reason to suspect the archbishop' ('gran cagione che l'arcivescovo fusse tenuto sospetto'), as Pietro Carnesecchi's depositions revealed years later. Giannetti and Donzellini were then reunited at the English embassy in Venice, where the former served as an informer and intermediary between the English crown and heterodox Italians, and the latter practised as a physician.[69] In 1545, at the age of thirty-two, Donzellini could count on a growing heretical network offering support and protection. His contacts extended from Padua to Brescia and from Rome to Venice, passing through Florence and Ferrara, where his brother had worked and where he had other acquaintances. This was only the beginning.

Notes

1 On Girolamo's 'melancholy' character, see ASV, Sant'Uffizio, *Processi, Contro Girolamo Donzellini*, Bu. 39, 168r: petition by Girolamo Donzellini from prison. In the medical tradition of the time, a predominant melancholic humour was a characteristic of earth signs.

2 Giorgio Caravale, *Predicazione e Inquisizione nell'Italia del Cinquecento. Ippolito Chizzola tra eresia e controversia antiprotestante* (Bologna: Il Mulino, 2012), in particular 31–34.

3 Schutte, 'Donzellini, Girolamo.'

4 For the relationship between Donzellini and Florio, see ASV, Sant'Uffizio, *Processi, Contro Girolamo Donzellini*, Bu. 39, f. 35r: 'The man mentioned in that letter is Michelangelo Florio [at the side: Michelangelo Florio, a former conventual friar minor, now a heretical apostate]. As I was extremely young and he was in Brescia, a friar of the Order of Conventual Minors, he taught me logic. Then, when he came here to Venice, after hearing that I was here he came to see me dressed as a layman and showed himself. As he had translated Augustine's treatise on grace and free will from Latin into good vernacular language, he asked me if I could use a friend to deliver a copy to the Duchess of Ferrara. As one of my friends was Francesco Porto, who was in the service of her excellency [at the side: Duchess of Ferrara] I sent it to her using this means'; ('Questo del qual se fa mentione in quella lettera è uno Michiel Angelo fiorentino [a lato: Michiel Angelo Fiorentino già frate minore conventuale ora apostata heretico] il quale essendo io assai giovinetto et ritrovandosi lui in Brescia frate dell'ordine de menori conventuali me lesse logicha et essendo poi venuto qua in Venezia et havendo inteso ch'io era qua mi venne a trovar vestito da layco et se mi diede a conoscere, et havendo tradutto el trattato de Agostino de gratia et libero arbitrio de latino in buona lingua vulgare mi pregò ch'io volesse farne havere uno con mezzo di qualche amico alla signora duchessa di Ferrara e così avendo io qualche amicitia come Francesco Porto che stava alli serviciy de sua excellentia [a lato: duchessa di Ferrara] gel mandai per questa via'). On the figure of Michelangelo

Florio, a preacher and theologian who became a member of the Italian Church in London before having to escape to Switzerland and whose son, John Florio, was a well-known linguist at the court of James I, see Leandro Perini, entry 'Florio, Michelangelo,' in *Dizionario biografico degli Italiani*, 48 (1997); John Tedeschi, 'I contributi culturali degli esuli italiani *religionis causa* nel Cinquecento' in, idem, *Intellettuali in esilio. Dall'Inquisizione romana al fascismo*, Giorgio Caravale, Stefania Pastore (eds.), (Rome: Edizioni di Storia e Letteratura, 2012), 162–64.

5 Colleen Linda Redmond, *Girolamo Donzellino, Medical Science and Protestantism in the Veneto*, PhD thesis, Stanford University, 1984, 14.

6 ASV, Sant'Uffizio, *Processi, Contro Girolamo Donzellini*, Bu. 39, 106r.

7 Ibid., 52v.

8 Marina Caffiero, Alessia Lirosi (eds.), *Donne e Inquisizione* (Rome: Edizioni di Storia e Letteratura, 2020), 36.

9 'When I was in Venice, Christ our Lord set before my eyes this friar, a rotten Lutheran and heresiarch who forsook his order, so that he can be punished. I ran into him last Thursday at the bridge of San Tomà at the Arsenal, and also last night at the Rialto at around eleven in the evening, dressed as a layman. This proves that he does not fear God.' ('Hor al presente ritrovandomi in Vinetia, acciochè questo sfratato marcio luterano e eresiarca sia castigato, il signore christo l'ha mandato inanti gli occhi miei, impercioche giovedì sera passato, io il scontrai al ponte di San Tomà al arsenale, et heri sera ancho in Rialto, circa a 23 hore, vestito da laico, la onde dimostra che non teme Iddio.'). See the complaints lodged against Cornelio Donzellini, also known as Fra' Teodoro, contained in ASV, Sant'Uffizio, *Processi, Contro fra' Teodoro di Capodistria*, Bu. 4, specifically: complaint dated 28 September 1549 lodged by Fra' Clemente of Brescia; see also ibid., complaint lodged by Bernardo Navagerio on 25 July 1549. These complaints cannot have had much effect, however, as Cornelio carried out his pro-Protestant literary work regularly between 1550 and 1551. On Vergerio, see Anne Jacob Schutte, *Pier Paolo Vergerio: the making of an Italian Reformer* (Geneva: Droz, 1977).

10 See the complete interrogation of Lucio Paolo Rosello on 30 December 1552, from which considerable information about Cornelio Donzellini can be gathered. ASV, Sant'Uffizio, *Processi, Contro Lucio Paolo Rosello*, Bu. 10, deposition of 30 December 1552. On the figure of Rosello, see Andrea Del Col, 'Il Nuovo Testamento tradotto da Massimo Teofilo e altre opere stampate a Lione nel 1551,' *Critica storica*, 15, no. 4 (1978), 138–71; Idem, 'Lucio Paolo Rosello e la vita religiosa veneziana verso la metà del secolo XVI,' *Rivista di Storia della Chiesa in Italia,* 32 (1978), 422–59.

11 Lucia Felici, ed., *Firenze Nella Crisi Religiosa Del Cinquecento (1498–1569)* (Florence: Claudiana, 2020).

12 Massimo Firpo, *Gli affreschi di Pontormo a San Lorenzo. Eresia, politica e cultura nella Firenze di Cosimo I* (Turin: Einaudi, 1997), 375–76; Gigliola Fragnito, 'Un pratese alla corte di Cosimo I. Riflessioni e materiali per un profilo di Pierfrancesco Riccio,' *Archivio storico pratese,* 52 (1986), 42–43.

13 Gustavo Bertoli, 'Luterani e anabattisti processati a Firenze nel 1552,' in *Archivio storico italiano*, 154, no. 3 (1996), 113–15, which includes the text of a speech in support of Cornelio Donzellini by Camillo Orsini, whose daughter-in-law had been one of his pupils.

14 ASV, Sant'Uffizio, Processi, Contro Girolamo Donzellini, Bu. 39, 47r.

15 Ibid., 114r.

16 The following were all doctors in arts and medicine, and all shared heretical ideas with their family members: Giovan Battista Goineo, Nicola Antonio and Teofilo Panarelli, Agostino Gadaldino, Giovan Battista Clario, Achille and Leonardo

Benvoglienti, Niccolò Buccella, Filippo and Alessandro Capodivacca, Giovanni Grillenzoni, Giovan Battista and Antonio Francesco Pigafetta, Giovan Battista Gemma, Onorio and Sebastiano Flaminio, Nicola Gallo, Pancrazio and Matteo Gentili, and Giuseppe Moscardo.

17 Many heretics were involved in familial religious dissent, including Pellegrino and Olimpia Morato, who both fled from Mantua to Ferrara; members of the Modenese Academy, Bonifacio and Filippo Valentini; Lelio Sozzini and his nephew Fausto, leading sixteenth-century religious dissenters at an Italian and European level (Lelio also shared heretical ideas with his brothers Celso, Dario, Cornelio and Camillo); the noblewomen Isabella Frattina and Caterina Sauli, mother and daughter, who were both involved in an Inquisition trial; and the archbishop Pier Paolo Vergerio with his nephew Aurelio.

18 ASV, Sant'Uffizio, *Processi, Contro Ludovico Abioso e Teofilo Panarelli*, Bu. 32, deposition by Panarelli of 16 November 1572. On the Italian Reformer, heterodox preacher and teacher Bartolomeo Fonzio and his relationship with Panarelli see infra Chapter 4. For his biography see Fragnito, 'Fonzio, Bartolomeo.' in *Dizionario Biografico degli Italiani*, 48 (1997).

19 'When my father was in Veglia, he had a friend, Nic de Dominicucci, who likewise had certain prohibited books and, as far as I can remember, Ochino's sermons. My father had them read aloud in our house and we all saw them; sometimes my father read them himself and had my sister Virginia, who is now in Venice, read them out. I just listened as I was still only a boy of eight or nine years old'; ('Stando mio padre a Veglia haveva amicitia dì un Nic de Dominicucci il qual haveva midisimamente certi libri proibiti e per quanto mi ricordo le prediche dell'Ochino e mio padre li facea liggere in casa nostra che tutti li vedevamo e alle volte esso mio padre leggeva et li faveva ligere da mia sorella Virginia che hora sta in Venetia per il che io che ero putto ascoltavo ancora io che ero di otto o nove anni'); ASV, Sant'Uffizio, *Processi, Contro Ludovico Abioso e Teofilo Panarelli*, Bu. 32, deposition by Panarelli of 23 November 1571.

20 'The Devil tempted my father and sent my brother to Germany, together with the natural son of the above-mentioned Stefano the priest, to listen to Philip Melanchthon and Martin Luther, enemies of God. They went with a man named Matthias Flacius Illyricus, who took the place of Martin Luther and as far as I knew had been banished from Albona. I saw letters that he [my brother] wrote to my father asking for money and various other things. I also saw the improvements my brother made in literature and religion. When war came to Germany and the Emperor reached Wittenberg, my brother and the others mentioned above left the city and went to Brunswick together with Melanchthon.'; ('Il Diavolo tentò mio padre et mandò detto mio fratello insieme con un figliolo naturale di detto prete Stefano in Germania a udir Filippo Melantone e Martino Lutero inimici di Dio e andorno con uno chiamato Mattheo Illirico d'Albona che è intrato in loco di Martino Luthero il quale per quanto intendevo era bandito da Albona e ho visto lettere che scriveva a mio padre che dimandava denari e serviva diverse cose e il profitto che faceva nele littere mio fratello e nella religione loro et dopo che venne la guerra in Allemagna che l'Imperatore era in Wittenberg loro cioè mio fratello e li sopradetti se partirono da Wittenberg e andorno a Brunscich insieme con Melantone.'); ibidem.

21 Also known under the pseudonym of Alessio Piemontese, Ruscelli founded the Accademia Segreta in Naples and in 1557 published the *De' secreti del reuerendo donno Alessio Piemontese* (*On the Secrets of the Reverend Alessio Piemontese*), a hugely successful alchemy recipe book, in Venice (where he had moved to in 1548, working as a polygraph at Vincenzo Valgrisi's printing house). See Eamon, *Science and the Secrets*, ad indicem. On Virginia Panarelli and Ruscelli's

relationship see also ASV, Sant'Uffizio, *Processi, Contro Teofilo Panarelli*, testimony given by Ludovico Abioso on 4 March 1572; Federica Ambrosini, 'Libri e lettrici in terra veneta nel sec. XVI: echi erasmiani e inclinazioni eterodosse, in Achille Olivieri (ed.), *Erasmo, Venezia e la cultura padovana nel '500* (Rovigo: Associazione Culturale Minelliana, 1995), 82.

22 Ivi, *Contro Dionora Calia*, Bu. 21, testimony given by Teofilo Panarelli on 30 June 1566.

23 Ivi, *Contro Ludovico Abioso e Teofilo Panarelli*, Bu. 32, letter from Virginia Panarelli dated 25 December 1571.

24 He stated to the inquisitors that he had spent eight years in Padua, ASV, Sant'Uffizio, *Processi, Contro Girolamo Donzellini*, Bu. 39, 48r.

25 Paul F. Grendler, *The Universities of Italian Renaissance* (Baltimora: Johns Hopkins University Press, 2002), 314. On the Renaissance Italian Universities, and medical teaching see also Jerome Bylebyl, 'The School of Padua: Humanistic Medicine in the Sixteenth Century,' in *Health, Medicine and Mortality in the Sixteenth Century*, Charles Webster (ed.) (Cambridge: Cambridge University Press, 1979), 335–70; Anthony Grafton, Lisa Jardine, *From Humanism to the Humanities: education and the liberal arts in fifteenth- and sixteenth-century Europe* (Cambridge: Harvard University Press, 1986); Nancy Siraisi, *Medieval and Early Renaissance Medicine: an introduction to knowledge and Practice* (Chicago: University of Chicago Press, 1990); Robert Black, 'Italian Renaissance Education: Changing Perspectives and Continuing Controversies,' *Journal of the History of Ideas* 52, no. 2 (1991), 315–34.

26 The fact that the values of humanism were responsible for a radical upheaval of the notions that sixteenth-century scholars derived from ancient knowledge is demonstrated by Vesalius's profound knowledge of Galen. It was precisely thanks to this expertise that he was able to question the method of inquiry used by Galen, who had claimed that he dealt with the functioning of the human body by taking his cue from its animal equivalent, and was able to launch his famous anatomical revolution that has rightly been compared to Copernicus's breakthrough in the study of heavenly spheres (in a strange coincidence, the *De humani corporis fabirca* (*On the Fabric of the Human Body*) and the *De rivolutionibus orbium celestium* (*On the Revolutions of the Heavenly Spheres*) were both published in 1543). The merits of Vesalian anatomy will not be discussed here; on these matters, see the extensive existing biography, in particular Charles Donald O'Malley, *Andreas Vesalius of Brussels, 1514–1564* (Berkeley: University of California Press, 1964); Andrew Cunningham, *The Anatomical Renaissance, the Resurrection of the Anatomical Projects of the Ancients* (Aldershot: Scolar Press, 1997).

27 On the practice of dissections, see Andrea Carlino, *La fabbrica del corpo: libri e dissezioni nel Rinascimento* (Turin: Einaudi, 1994). On the anatomical theatres and anatomy studies in Padua, see Cynthia Klestinec, 'A history of Anatomy Theatres in Sixteenth-Century Padua,' *Journal of the History of Medicine and Allied Sciences*, 59, no. 3, 2004, 375–412; eadem, *Theaters of Anatomy: Students, Teachers, and Traditions of Dissection in Renaissance Venice* (Baltimore: John Hopkins University Press, 2011).

28 The physician had been asked by the students in Padua to share his anatomical expertise and he duly held dissections at his house. However, the political and religious authorities put a stop to this practice in accordance with the canon law prohibition which established that 'no one may ever cut open human bodies in private' ('nullus privatim incidere possit semel humana corpora'); Stella, *Dall'anabattismo al socinianesimo*, 136. On Buccella, see also infra Chapter 3.

29 Elda Martellozzo Forin (ed.), *Acta graduum academicorum Gymnasii Patavini: ab anno 1538 ad annum 1550* (Padua: Antenora, 1971), 97.
30 ASV, Sant'Uffizio, *Processi, Processi 1552 – Registri, Contro Gasparo Parma,* Bu. 158, 26r.
31 Dennj Solera, Howard Hotson, 'The Importance of The University Of Padova In Europe For The Early Modern Intellectual History,' in *"Libero, finalmente libero! Ma sperduto nella città." Itinerari di vita studentesca a Padova tra XIII e XVIII secolo*, Cristina La Rocca and Giulia Zornetta (eds.) (Rome: Donzelli, 2021); Paola Molino, Dennj Solera, Andrea Caracausi, *Lo spazio della* libertas. *Libertà religiosa, libertà politica, libertà del sapere* (Rome: Donzelli, 2021).
32 ASV, Sant'Uffizio, *Processi, Contro Ludovico Abioso e Teofilo Panarelli,* Bu. 32, deposition given by Panarelli on 19 November 1571.
33 Ibidem.
34 Ibidem.
35 ASV, Sant'Uffizio, *Processi, Contro Ludovico Abioso e Teofilo Panarelli,* Bu. 32, deposition by Panarelli given on 20 November 1571.
36 On German students in Padua in the context of the Counter-Reformation see Michaela Valente, 'Padova, alveare a molte api e a non poche vespe della Riforma. Gli studenti tedeschi a Padova: una sifda alla Chiesa?' in Boillet, Felici, *Dis/simulazione e tolleranza*, 105–26.
37 Ivi, *Contro Giovanni Cassinati, Francesco Gentil da Fermo e Manusso Mariano,* Bu. 27, deposition by Maran given on 21 June 1568.
38 Maran's former landlady testified that: 'Every so often [I] heard some students from Pesaro shouting at him and I said to them, "Why don't you leave him be?," referring to Manusso, and "For what reason are you shouting at him so much?." They answered me, "Dear landlady, we will tell you the truth, and we would like to lead him to good faith, as he does not want the saints to be worshipped and says that the saints are servants of God and cannot be compared to God at all. This is why we are shouting at him."'; ('Sentiva che ogni tanto quelli scholari da Pesaro gridavano con lui e io li diceva dove viene che non lo lassate stare, parlando del ditto Manusso perché causa cridate tanto insieme con lui, loro me rispondevano cara patrona vi diremo la verità el voressimo pur tirar alla bona fide lui non vol che si reverisca li santi et dice che li santi sono famegli di Iddio et che con Iddio i non possono cosa alguna che questo è il nostro cridar'); ibid., see the testimony by 'donna Angela' given on 29 July 1570.
39 Seidel Menchi, *Erasmo in Italia*, 424.
40 See the letter of 5 April 1569, which the vicar and suffragan of Heraklion, Friar Vincenzo of Lugo, sent to the Venetian judges: ASV, Sant'Uffizio, *Processi, Contro Giovanni Cassinati, Francesco Gentil da Fermo e Manusso Mariano,* Bu. 27.
41 The best known of these philosophers was undoubtedly Pomponazzi. For an overview of his thinking, see Martin Pine, *Pomponazzi Radical Philosopher of the Renaissance* (Padua: Antenore, 1986).
42 Giuseppe Speranza, *Alberico Gentili. Studi dell'avvocato Giuseppe Speranza* (Rome: Tipografia Fratelli Pallotta, 1876), 43.
43 Cunningham, *The Anatomical Renaissance*, 263.
44 'Consequently, since our days (which we endure with sorrow) the sower of cockle, the ancient enemy of the human race, has dared to scatter and multiply in the Lord's field some extremely pernicious errors, which have always been rejected by the faithful, especially on the nature of the rational soul, with the claim that it is mortal, or only one among all human beings, and since some, playing the philosopher without due care, assert that this proposition is true at least according to philosophy, it is our desire to apply suitable remedies against this infection and,

with the approval of the sacred council, we condemn and reject all those who insist that the intellectual soul is mortal, or that it is only one among all human beings, and those who suggest doubts on this topic. For the soul not only truly exists of itself and essentially as the form of the human body, as is said in the canon of our predecessor of happy memory, pope Clement V, promulgated in the general council of Vienne, but it is also immortal; and further, for the enormous number of bodies into which it is infused individually, it can and ought to be and is multiplied.'; ('Cum itaque diebus nostris (quod dolenter referimus) zizaniae seminator, antiquus humanis generis hostis, nonnullos perniciosissimos errores, a fidelibus semper explosos in agro domini super seminare et augere sit ausus, de natura praesertim animae rationalis, quod videlicet mortalis sit, aut unica in cunctis hominbus, et nonnulli temere philosophantes secundum saltem philosophiam verum id esse asseverent; contra huiusmodi pestem opportuna remedia adhibere cupientes, hoc sacro approbante Concilio damnamus et reprobamus omnes asserentes animam intellectivam mortalem esse, aut unicam in cunctis hominibus, et haec in dubium vertentes: cum illa non solum vere per se et essentialiter umani corporis forma existat, sicut in Canone felicis recordationis Clementis Papae V praedecessoris nostri in generali Viennensi Concilio edito continetur; verum et immortalis, et pro corporum, quibus infunditur, moltitudine singulariter multiplicabilis, et moltiplicata, et multiplicando sit'); see *Sacrosancta Concilia ad Regiam editionem exacta studio Philip Labbei et Gabr. Cossartii*, vol. 19 (1732). English translation in Norman P. Tanner (ed. by), *Decrees of the Ecumenical Councils*, vol. 1 (Washington: Georgetown University Press, 1990), 605.

45 Edward Miur, *The Culture Wars of the Late Renaissance: Skeptics, Libertines, and Opera* (Cambridge, Massachussetts: Harvard University Press, 2007), 37.

46 On Busale and Basalù, who were part of the group that pushed the teachings of the theologian Juan De Valdés to their most extreme doctrinal consequences (thanks in particular to Juan de Villafranca), see Addante, *Eretici e libertini*, ad indicem. On Valdesianism, see the next section and infra.

47 Ongaro, 'La scoperta della circolazione'; Leando Perini, *La vita e i tempi di Pietro Perna* (Rome: Edizioni di Storia e Letteratura, 2002), 96–98.

48 Silvana Seidel Menchi, 'Chi fu Ortensio Lando?,' *Rivista storica italiana*, 106 (1994), 501–64.

49 On Simoni, see infra Chapter 3.

50 'A young man from Lucca that I took into my house in Padua for a few months in 1553 or 1554 because he was a student – I think he was studying medicine – and did not have the means to support himself. […] He persuaded me to do him this favour much more easily as I saw that he was just as inclined to study Scripture as medicine. Indeed, as demonstration of this, he knew almost all of St Paul by heart'; ('Uno giovane luchese che io tenni alcuni mesi in casa mia in Padua ne l'anno 1553 o 1554, perché era studente – et credo di medecina – et non haveva il modo da sustentarsi da sé. […] Et mi indusse tanto più facilmente a farli questa commodità vedendo ch'era inclinato alli studii della Scrittura non meno che della medicina. Et che sia il vero, sapeva quasi tutto san Paulo a mente'); see deposition by Pietro Carnesecchi, 2 March 1567, *Processi Carnesecchi,* 1074.

51 Valerio Marchetti, 'Figure di esuli italiani del Cinquecento: Fabio Nifo,' *Critica storica*, 8 (1969), 691–705.

52 ASV, Sant'Uffizio, *Processi, Contro Giovanni Cassinati, Francesco Gentil da Fermo e Manusso Mariano,* Bu. 27. See Seidel Menchi, *Erasmo in Italia*, 220–22.

53 ASV, Sant'Uffizio, *Processi, Contro Ippolito Craya*, Bu. 15, 4r. See also Ferretto, *Il 'caso' Pomponio Algieri*, 77–79.

54 AVB, sez. 1, rep. IV, *Processo Venzo* (sic!) *1579–1580,* Bu. 11, which contains the typescript of the sentence against Agostino Vanzo of 11 June 1580, from which the quotation is taken. The sentence is now held at Trinity College Library in Dublin (Dublin, Reel 8, Sec. J, ms 1225), 344v. See also *Opera omnia Desiderii Erasmi Roterodami. I-8 Iulius Exclusus, De civilitate morum puerilium, Conflictus Thaliae et Barbariei,* Silvana Seidel Menchi, Franz Bierlaire, and René Hoven (eds.) (Leiden – Boston: Brill, 2012), 120–24. On Vanzo, see Alessandra Celati, 'Il caso di Agostino Vanzo medico condotto eretico e il suo Dialogo di papa Leon [X] e s[anto] Pietro,' *Rivista Storica Italiana*, 133, no.2 (2021), 494–530.

55 'Reading the Gospel by myself, I found that these things are not prescribed, and I also heard this argued by others. Question: Who did you hear arguing these false opinions? Answer: Being a student in Ferrara, I heard some German students discussing them at my house, and together with these students I started to read the New Testament. And they were the reason why I started to read the New Teastament'; ('Da me medemo leggendo l'Evangelio, ho trovato che queste cose non sono prescritte e ho sentito anco ragionarne da altri. Int: da chi ne habbi sentito a ragionar di queste false opinioni? R.it: Essendo in Ferrara scholaro sentii ragionarne ad alcuni scholari thodeschi che stavano li appresso di me, e insieme con quelli tedeschi cominciai a legger il testamento novo, che loro furono causa che cominciai a legger il testamento nuovo'); AVB, sez. 1, rep. IV, *Processo Venzo* (sic!) *1579–1580,* Bu. 11, deposition of 13 November 1579.

56 On Camillo Renato, see Luca Addante, entry 'Renato, Camillo,' in *Dizionario Biografico degli Italiani*, 86 (2016); Antonio Rotondò (ed.), *Camillo Renato, Opere, documenti e testimonianze* (Florence – Chicago: Sansoni – The Newberry Library, 1968).

57 On the figure of Girolamo Mercuriale (1530–1606), see Alessandro Arcangeli, Vivian Nutton (eds.), *Girolamo Mercuriale. Medicina e cultura nell'Europa del Cinquecento. Atti del Convegno (Forlì, 8–11 novembre 2006)* (Florence: Olschki, 2008); see also Girolamo Mercuriale, *De arte gymnastica*, Concetta Pennuto, Vivian Nutton (eds.) (Florence: Olschki, 2008).

58 Richard Palmer, *The Studio of Venice and its graduates in the sixteenth century* (Trieste: Edizioni Lint, 1983).

59 On this subject, see Siraisi, *Communities*, 1–36. See also infra, Chapter 5.

60 See infra, Chapter 3.

61 Richard Palmer, *Physicians and the State in Post-medieval Italy,* in Andrew Russell (ed.), *The Town and State Physician from the Middle Ages to Enlightenment* (Wolfenbüttel: Herzog August Bibliothek, 1981), 47–61.

62 ASV, Sant'Uffizio, *Processi, Contro Antonio Massimo*, Bu. 15.

63 Ivi, *Contro Stephano medico de Gardon,* Bu. 8.

64 Firpo, *Dal sacco di Roma all'Inquisizione*, 62–81.

65 *Processi Carnesecchi,* see in particular deposition CV of 6 March 1567, 1048 and ad indicem.

66 The apostolic protonotary was scandalised by this 'form of semi-hypocrisy' ('una spetie di mezza hippocrisia'). *Processi Carnesecchi*, 1049. On Borri, see Stabile, entry 'Borri, Girolamo,' in *Dizionario Biografico degli Italiani*, 13 (1971); Grendler, *The Universities,* ad indicem; Ugo Baldini, Leen Spruit (eds.), *Catholic Church and Modern Science: Documents from the Archives of the Roman Congregations of the Holy Office and the Index,* vol. 1 (Rome: Libreria Editrice Vaticana, 2009), 812–54.

67 Borri first came under investigation in 1551 for unknown reasons and was probably released. Ten years later, he published one of his most important texts, the *Del flusso e reflusso del mare* (*On the Ebb and Flow of the Sea*) (Lucca, 1561) which was targeted by the ecclesiastical censors in 1564 together with a

Ragionamento di Teofilo Filogenio della perfettione delle donne (*Reasoning by Teofilo Filogenio on the Perfection of Women*), with which it had been printed. This edition of the work was edited by the heterodox dissenter Girolamo Ghirlanda, who drew radical consequences from the Valdesian premises and who Borri included among those with whom he enjoyed learned discussions, a reference that consolidates the intertwining of Reformation, radicalism, and philosophical-scientific research. The treatise on the tides takes shape as as experiment in philosophical concordism in which the thoughts of Plato and Aristotle were aligned within a cosmological vision and an epistemological programme that envisaged the deciphering of phenomena exclusively from natural causes and regardless of any form of transcendental intervention. In this case, the action of the moon's rays on the sea and the rising tides were placed in a mechanistic relationship: the activity of God, the 'first engine' ('primo motore') who cannot 'understand or love anything other than himself' ('intendere né amare altro che se stesso'), became irrelevant for the functioning of nature. The divinity had the essential task of informing reality and accommodating 'in himself the multitude of intellects that emanate' ('in sé la moltitudine degli intelletti che emana'). Borri described this process, whose implicit consequence was the deification of man and nature, as a circle 'whose centre is everywhere and whose circumference cannot be found anywhere' ('il cui centro è per tutto e la cui circonferenza non si trova in verun luogo'), Borri, *Del flusso*, 27–29, 52. Donzellini used the same hermetic metaphor in his *Remedium Ferendarum Iniuriarum* (*Remedy for Bearing Injuries*) in 1587, as we will see in Chapter 6. At the second trial, which saw Borri in the dock between 1562 and 1565 (when he was also accused of possessing prohibited books, abstaining from Catholic rituals, and rejecting the Catholic precepts), the judges discussed these and other compromising theses with him, subjecting them to censorship. In defending his arguments, Borri invoked the theory of the double truth, which had been condemned many decades previously. Furthermore, he claimed the right to put forward innovative philosophical positions, whereby 'every man is entitled to find new things in philosophy, and therefore deserves praise and not condemnation, especially when the new things discovered are reasonable like in this case' ('ad ogni huomo è lecito ritrovar cose nuove nella filosofia, e si merita lode e non biasimo perciò massime quando le cose di nuovo ritrovate hanno del ragionevole come questo'), all the more so as 'nature wanted to conceal its things on purpose to give us a reason to exert our intelligence' ('la natura apposta ha voluto coprir le cose sue per darci ragione d'affaticar i nostri ingegni'); see Archivio Arcivescovile di Pisa, *Contro Girolamo Borri*, Busta 1, 9r–11r. This call for freedom of research asserted the legitimacy of taking the most subversive elements of Renaissance Platonism and Aristotelianism and applying them to cosmological inquiry, with disconcerting results in terms of orthodoxy. The accusations levelled against Borri also claimed that while 'reading in his cathedra' ('leggendo in cattedra') in Pisa he had stated that 'it was pitch black in paradise' ('nel paradiso era buio pesto'; ibid., 7r), meaning that there was no afterlife, and had reiterated the concept by maintaining that heaven consisted of 'mountains of cheese and macaroni' ('montagne di formaggio e maccheroni'). Borri was cleared of the accusations during the same period that saw the conclusion of the investigations involving him in relation to the Carnesecchi trial. He could thus devote himself once more to his philosophical-scientific interests, publishing works such as the *De motu gravium et levium* (*On the Motion of Heavy and Light Bodies*, Florence, 1575) and teaching pupils such as Galileo Galilei. In 1583, at the age of 71, he was locked up again in the Holy Office prisons and it was only thanks to the personal intercession of Pope Gregory XIII, who considered him 'a great man' ('un grande uomo'), that he was freed after about a year. The French libertine and physician Gabriel Naudè described Borri as an '*athée parfait* [perfect atheist], an orthodox Aristotelian and mocker of the friar-inquisitors' ('*athée parfait*, aristotelico ortodosso e sbeffeggiatore di frati inquisitori').

68 'Nostro Signore – quale vuol che questa pratica sia bene conosciuta per ritrovar il vero – ha commesso ch'io le scriva che al ricevere di questa la vogli far ricercar tra le scritture et libri di esso medico, et far che lui sia bene examinato. Et ritrovando ne l'examine o altramente alcuna coniectura che egli sia tale, quale è stato accusato, lo faza ritenere sotto bona custodia,' letter to Cardinal Duranti by Cardinal Farnese. The document is cited in Dario Marcatto, *"Questo passo dell'heresia": Pietro Antonio di Capua tra valdesiani, "spirituali" e inquisizione* (Naples: Istituto Italiano per gli Studi Filosofici, 2003), 28.

69 On Giannetti, see Guido Dall'Olio, entry 'Giannetti, Guido' in *Dizionario Biografico degli Italiani*, 54 (2000).

2 Healing the body, healing the soul: Venice, 1546–1553

Donzellini arrived in Venice in 1546. The Italian 'gateway to the Reformation' served as his home until 1553, protecting him with its dense network of *calli* (streets or alleys), bridges, and *campi* (squares). During this seven-year stay, he entered a phase of conscious heretical activism and professional fulfilment through his encounters, discussions, and experiences, with a significant overlap between medical and heterodox practice.

Venice was a driving force in the Reformed movement. Firmly opposed to the political and jurisdictional claims of Rome, the city was welcoming and relatively tolerant (for the Italian peninsula) with inhabitants from all over Europe. Furthermore, it served as an international centre for the publication and distribution of major new titles – including, naturally, medical and religious texts – and was a vital hub in the Italian intellectual and theological landscape. The city attracted the most inquiring and eclectic minds, enabling them to establish relational networks. In this way, they exchanged cultural ideas and theological reflections, learned the basics of Reformed religiosity, and formed personal views on the doctrinal debate with a large margin of freedom.

Donzellini initially described Venice as highly 'curious in matters of faith' ('curiosa nelle cose della fede'), especially with regard to 'learned and scholarly men' ('gli uomini dotti e letterati'). He consequently strove 'to make friends whenever possible' ('quanto poteva di acquistar delle amicitie'), building religious, medical, intellectual, and personal relationships with fellow sojourners, men of culture, former clerics, and local patricians. In this way, he managed to consolidate his professional reputation and create a solid religious support network, which will constitute the focus of this chapter[1] (Figure 2.1).

2.1 Venice, city of heretics

In order to explore the everyday social reality of heterodox practice in Venice, we can attempt to reconstruct the urban map of the network established by Donzellini and other heterodox physicians.[2] This can be done by examining his habitual haunts and, more generally, the places that served

DOI: 10.4324/9781003218852-3

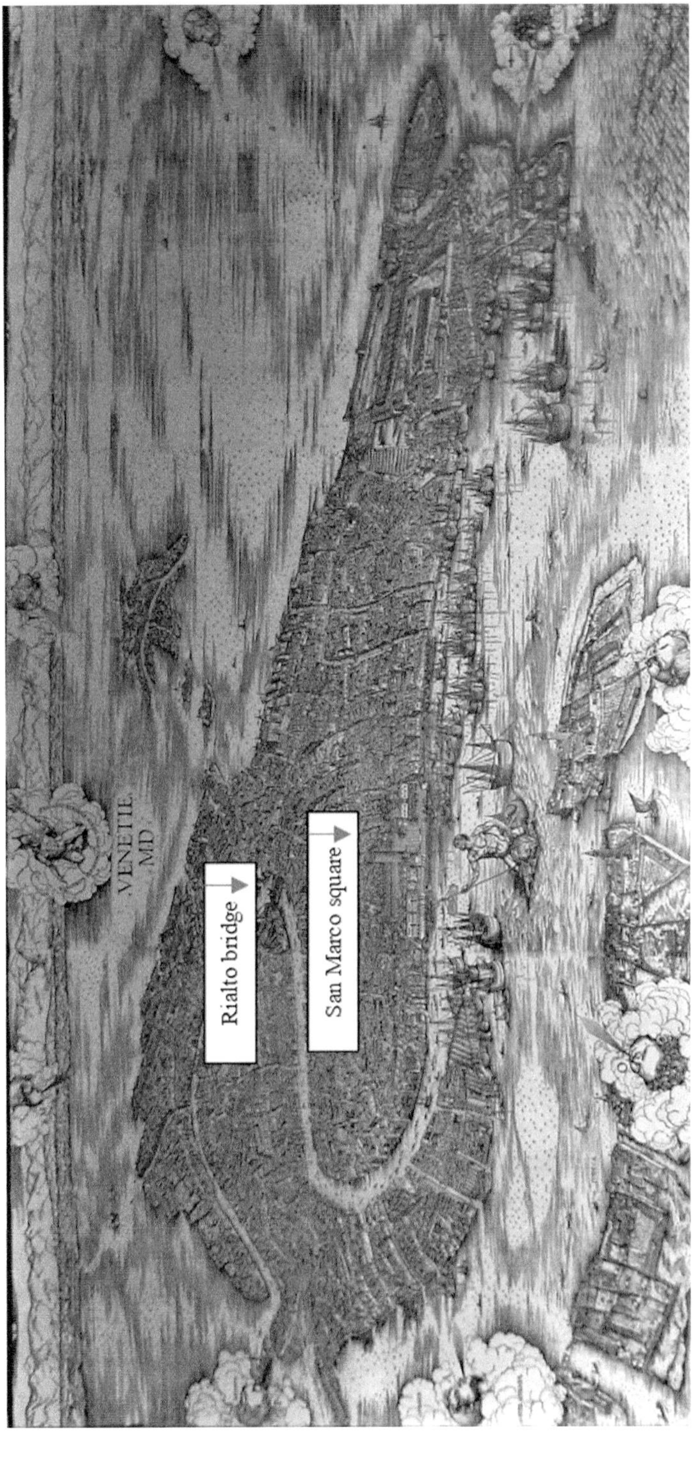

Figure 2.1 Bird's eye view of Venice produced by Jacopo de'Barberi in the fifteenth/sixteenth century (ante 1516).

as repositories of books, information, and heretical discourse. In this respect, a survey of the Venetian landscape can provide an operational overview of the heretical movement, highlighting elements of internal continuity and rupture, as well as possible relationships that are not directly documented in the sources.[3]

It is known that Girolamo's Venetian home was 'between the parishes of San Beneto and San Lio' ('tra le parrocchie di San Beneto e San Lio'), close to the Rialto market. The apothecary shop that Donzellini used as a base for his medical work – the *Spezieria del Sarasin* – was situated nearby in campo San Bartolomeo. The Rialto was located in the heart of the city, an area bustling with tradesmen and traders at the market. Girolamo thus entered the social and economic lifeblood of the city. Nearby, for example, was the Fondaco dei Tedeschi, a *palazzo* overlooking the Grand Canal that served as a headquarters for German-speaking merchants and a warehouse for their goods, as well as housing the offices of the Fugger banking family. The Fondaco played an essential role in the spread of heterodox ideas during the religious crisis in sixteenth-century Venice and was even used as a place of rendezvous and a hideout for heretical groups at the height of the Counter-Reformation.

As the city market and, most importantly, the only bridge over the Grand Canal were located in the Rialto area, it was regularly frequented by Venetian residents. The Rialto was also the nerve centre for book distribution and therefore, in many respects, the spread of heterodox ideas. While the majority of the city's bookshops and printing houses were located between the Merceria and the Frezzeria (the main thoroughfares connecting Rialto and San Marco), a plethora of small-scale vendors could be found on the Rialto bridge and in the surrounding *calli* selling inexpensive vernacular books and pamphlets with a Reformed tone. Many of these books were read aloud or sung in the street as a marketing strategy and were sold together with spices and medicine, providing a perfect blend of body and mind, and combining the learned and popular worlds.

The vibrancy of the Venetian publishing market was renowned throughout Europe and remained part of the city's appeal until the late 1540s, when the effects of censorship started to be felt.[4] The men of culture who came to Venice from all over Europe were familiar with the different bookshops. As they often knew the printers personally, they had no difficulty in locating the new titles on their wish lists. Book culture played an essential role in the heretical movement in Venice and indeed throughout the Italian peninsula. People involved or interested in the Reformation in various ways used books to build relationships, hold discussions, and initiate or strengthen their engagement with the movement. While this was true in general, for physicians in particular the book world acted as a common denominator for extremely diverse heterodox experiences. During the Reformation, the Counter-Reformation, and the subsequent period of book censorship, Italian physicians, who were often writers and, above all, readers, strove to maintain communication channels with each other and their Northern European colleagues, bridging the religious rift through the circulation of texts and ideas (as the case of Donzellini illustrates).[5]

Andrea Arrivabene's bookshop *all'insegna del Pozzo* (at the sign of the well) was one of the main dealers in Protestant texts, various anti-Catholic publications, and scientific works. Donzellini was a regular visitor in the 1540s, followed in subsequent years by other heterodox physicians such as Teofilo Panarelli. For his part, Arrivabene was also involved in the heretical movement: in 1549, he was summoned by the Holy Office and warned not to sell heterodox books; in 1551, he was denounced as a Lutheran; and in 1570, he was tried again for selling forbidden texts. On each occasion he defended himself successfully. He helped to distribute prohibited books between Venice and Viadana (a small city between Mantua and Parma) until at least 1562. His shop was a delivery point for foreign publications imported into Italy through a dense network of relations extending northwards from the Venetian Republic (most notably to Basel and Frankfurt) and established partly through the mediation of Donzellini.

Another bookshop that formed part of the city's heretical network until the end of the century was located *all'insegna di Erasmo* (at the sign of Erasmus) in the Merceria, owned by Vincenzo Valgrisi, a French-born naturalised Venetian.[6] As we will see in Chapter 6, this was the scene of one of Donzellini's final acts of reckless heretical zeal at the beginning of 1587; regarding his collection of forbidden books, it can be directly related to his execution shortly afterwards. More generally, the international scope of Valgrisi's business highlights the scale of the network that Donzellini was part of. After closing his shop in Lyon to open his Venetian *bottega* in the 1530s, Valgrisi built up a network stretching from the Venetian Republic to France. He also established connections between his bookshop in Venice and sister establishments in Padua, Bologna and in the Marche region (in particular in Macerata, Recanati, and Foligno). Both Vincenzo and his sons Giorgio (who inherited the shop) and Felice (who received the family publishing business) were also suspected of nurturing heterodox beliefs. When Giorgio was tried in the summer of 1587, a few months after the execution of Donzellini, among other things he had to account for his friendship with the physician. In addition, Valgrisi's printing house published works by Pietro Andrea Mattioli – his *Commentari* (*Commentaries*) on Dioscorides and his *Dioscoride …con i veri ritratti delle piante e degli animali* (*Dioscorides … with True Portraits of the Plants and of the Animals*, Venice, 1557) – that were highly sought-after by physicians in the peninsula and beyond. It is therefore extremely probable that the shop was also visited by many of Donzellini's colleagues on a regular basis.

This publishing enterprise also illustrates the theoretical interweaving of medicine and heterodoxy in mid-sixteenth-century Venice. Valgrisi made several reprints of *La medicina dell'anima* (*The Medicine of the Soul*) – the Italian translation of *Seelen Ärtzney* by the German Protestant theologian

Urbanus Rhegius – between 1544 and 1545 following the incredible popularity of the book during the religious crisis in the peninsula. Mainly addressing the sick and the dying, the text focused on the subject of illness as an expression of inscrutable divine will,[7] stressing that if 'medicine works well inside you, this must be attributed to the grace and help of God' ('la medicina fa in te buona operazione ciò si debbe attribuire alla gratia e aiuto di Dio'). It reminded all those with a restless conscience that while death was an inevitable and frightening scourge (a warning spelled out by the images of Hans Holbein the Younger's *Dance of Death*, reproduced at the beginning of Valgrisi's edition), 'you have no reason to be troubled by your sins, given that they have already been cancelled [...] and just as Jesus Christ cannot be damned, you cannot be either, having placed all of your trust in Him' ('tu non hai cagion di haver fastidio per i tuoi peccati, vedendo che già sono cancellati [...] e sì come Iesu Christo non può esser dannato, così non ne puoi esser tu, havendo messo tutta la tua fidanza in Iesu Christo').[8] This form of inclusive eschatology drew on the content of the best-known work of the Italian Reformation, the *Beneficio di Cristo* (*The Benefit of Christ Crucified*), which circulated widely in Venice after its publication there in 1543.[9] The ecclesiastical authorities were quick to understand that the purpose of the medical metaphor underpinning *La medicina dell'anima* was to propagate the subject of universal resurrection, guaranteed by faith in the sacrifice of Christ. As a result, the work was placed on the Venetian Index of Prohibited Books in 1554 and on the Roman Index in 1559.[10] Even in 1570, when Valgrisi was first tried by the Inquisition for possession of prohibited books, he was found to have more than four hundred copies of the forbidden work, admitting that it was still 'in great demand' ('de gran domanda').[11]

Another well-known active bookshop and printing press was owned by the Giunta family, located *all'insegna dei Tre re* (at the sign of the three kings) near the Rialto Bridge. Although there is no documentary evidence that the Giuntas were directly involved in heretical dissent in the city, they certainly did nothing to disassociate themselves from it.[12] Indeed, they established relations with book smugglers like Donzellini and the printer Pietro Perna and supported a protest against the Index of Prohibited Books together with other Venetian booksellers. Furthermore, they published Antonio Brucioli's vernacular Bible, the first translation that differed from the Vulgate. This version became one of the key texts for Italian heretical conventicles. Agostino Gadaldino, a physician with Reformed sympathies, also published and translated Galen's *Opera omnia* (*Complete Works*, Venice, 1541) for the Giuntas. The fact that Andreas Vesalius was also involved in this undertaking demonstrates that the printing house had a reputation for scientific innovation.[13]

Donzellini became involved in the production and distribution of pro-Reformation texts from the 1540s onwards, working above all with his brother Cornelio and Pietro Perna. The latter was one of the most important and active members of Donzellini's network, and the pair remained in contact throughout the physician's life. After serving in the Dominican Order for around ten years, Perna converted to Protestantism and fled his native city in 1543, settling in Basel. It was here that he opened a printing house which published an extraordinary number of works over the years, partly with Donzellini's help. These publications in the fields of philosophy, medicine, and religion were largely anti-dogmatic and non-confessional in nature. As soon as business started booming in the late 1540s, Perna relocated to Venice with the collaboration of Donzellini and another physician, Andrea de Neri, from Perugia. The latter's house near the church of Santi Giovanni e Paolo was used for book storage and served as the group's nerve centre.[14] From here, Perna distributed books 'that denied purgatory and free will' ('che negavano il purgatorio e il libero arbitrio'), works by Pier Paolo Vergerio and 'by other authors from the Capuchins printed on German soil' ('di altri autori de scapuzini stampati in le parte di Alemagna'), and texts in German that were probably distributed at the Fondaco dei Tedeschi.[15] The storehouse was situated a stone's throw from the imposing convent of the Dominican Order, the guardians of orthodoxy and the backbone of the Holy Office in Venice. Perna was caught and arrested at De Neri's house in 1549, the books were burned, and he was banished from the city. He never returned to Italy and settled in Basel, where Donzellini joined him around ten years later.

During the same period, Cornelio Donzellini joined his brother in Venice and stayed there until 1550. Cornelio worked in the city with the former priest Lucio Paolo Rosello on the Italian translation of Calvin's *Trattato sulla santa cena* (*Short Treatise on the Holy Supper*) and texts of the patristic tradition and the Gospels. Cornelio was also in contact with Perna. Indeed, a letter which is included in the records of the trial against Girolamo Donzellini – sent to him at the *Spezieria del Sarasin* in San Bartolomeo by Perna from Basel in 1550 – attests that the printer was working with Cornelio at the time to print and distribute the grammar written by the latter in Florence before his arrest. Reading between the lines of the grammar rules, an attentive reader would have perceived the author's openness towards the main tenets of the Reformation and his desire to proselytise in a clandestine yet determined manner. However, at first sight the censor would have found 'nothing bothersome' ('nessuna cosa fastidiosa') in it. The letter shows the high level of trust and collaboration between Perna and the Donzellini brothers. It also includes some information about life in Basel. The printer reports that an unidentified friend of Girolamo from Verona had recently visited his group, staying with the exiled humanist Celio Secondo Curione, who in turn sent his greetings. There are details about Perna's personal life too, namely the extent of his restlessness, which is described as worse than the previous year when he had been in prison, as well as information on the distribution and price of texts.[16] Donzellini was told to keep anything that interested him and take the remaining books to their storehouse, which was clearly still operative despite the Inquisition raid the year before. While Perna intended to work on the publication of Cornelio Donzellini's translation of the *Testamento novo* over the following months, Cornelio's grammars were to be sold at twenty *marchetti* each. When Perna referred to this, he also expressed regret that he could not send a copy of the grammar to Cornelio in Florence (due to lack of intermediaries) before distributing the other volumes.

Donzellini and De Neri also acted as Pietro Perna's personal physicians; the bookseller suffered from syphilis and required frequent treatment. On the basis of this relationship and Donzellini's expertise in treating the "French disease," it can be assumed that he was familiar with the *Ospedale degli Incurabili* (Hospital for Incurables), an institution established in Venice in 1522 on the Fondamenta delle Zattere on the southern outskirts of the city. The hospital treated patients with serious conditions who were not self-sufficient or could not pay their medical expenses, those with chronic, repellent, or dangerous diseases, and orphaned children.[17] In 1528, the founder, Girolamo Miani, also established the *Ospedale dei Derelitti* (Hospital for the Destitute) together with a group of laymen inspired by devout Christian ideals.[18] Adjoining the church of Santi Giovanni e Paolo, this became the first hospital in the city with an important medical role. Between 1547 and 1549 Guillaume Postel, the visionary French humanist, Kabbalist, astronomer and mystic who was later put on trial by the Inquisition, was the Derelitti's chaplain.[19]

With no clear boundary between pastoral care and bodily care, material charity in such institutions was contingent on spiritual charity. In the sixteenth century, the poor, orphans, syphilitics, and 'penitent women' ('penitenti') were gathered there to be redeemed through the 'community discipline of the closed institution' ('disciplina comunitaria dell'istituzione chiusa').[20] Despite the intentions of their governors, however, hospitals were not immune to the spread of heretical ideas. Indeed, they offered fertile ground for the reception, discussion, and propagation of non-conformist religious ideas precisely because of the combination of the pious atmosphere with the suffering and forced isolation of the sick.

One case in point is that of Zanetto Cipolla, a twenty-eight-year-old barber surgeon at the *Ospedale degli Incurabili* who preached heterodox ideas to patients gathered around the fire at night in the 1560s. Cipolla did not enjoy the social status of a learned physician: he lacked Donzellini's university education and philosophical calling and had always lived at the hospital, where he had been raised as a foundling. Despite (or perhaps as a result of) spending so many years in such an uncompromisingly Catholic environment, Cipolla converted to the Reformation and started introducing radical doctrines into the hospital. In addition to preaching, he showed his proselytes 'a sheet with paintings of ten heads of men with lines in their mouths showing the commandments' ('una carta dove erano dipinte 10 teste di uomini con alcune linee in bocca che mostravano i comandamenti') that he had acquired 'in the

Merceria.' When addressing his audience of patients, paupers, and hospital nurses, he denied the divinity of Christ and the value of the Gospels as a revealed text, teaching that it was necessary to believe 'only in God' ('solamente in Dio') and in 'the ten commandments of ancient law' ('li 10 comandamenti della legge antica').[21] He also argued that priests should feed the poor instead of waking them for Mass early in the morning, and that clerics deceived paupers about the truth of Catholic doctrine, claiming that they had established the Church and 'said anything they liked to earn money' ('facevano quei versi che li pareva alloro, per guadagnar').[22] He did not attend religious services and as his room was close to the altar, he locked himself inside to avoid hearing anything. The charisma deriving from Cipolla's medical role meant that he could spread his views in a similar way to learned physicians.[23] Furthermore, his daily contact with the sick allowed him to carry out a persuasive propaganda campaign on a regular basis. Coupled with his blatant intolerance of the religious life at the hospital and his stubborn refusal to admit his wrongs, this heterodox campaigning led to a long trial that ended in a public recantation before all those that he had 'scandalised.'[24]

There is no direct evidence that Donzellini ever worked at the *Ospedale degli Incurabili* in a medical capacity, but he certainly played an active role at other hospitals in the city. Shortly before his death, a few prohibited books bearing his name were found in a secret hiding place in one such institution.[25] Many years before, in an unspecified Venetian hospital, he had also provided treatment and discussed religious matters with Marchetta Zotta Schiavona, an erudite Dalmatian lady who also knew Donzellini's like-minded friends Gasparo and Pantasilea Parma (Marchetta, the Parmas, and the other members of this heretical circle will be examined in greater detail in the following sections).

Fresh from his experience as physician to two illustrious Roman cardinals, Donzellini made the most of his contacts when he arrived in Venice. He found work there as personal physician to Edmund Harvel, the English ambassador, a position he retained when Pietro Vanni took over the role. In the late 1540s, the wars of religion were raging on German soil, the Council of Trent was yet to conclude, and even a *spirituale* like Reginald Pole could entertain the idea of becoming pope. Against this backdrop, the English crown held out great hope for Italian heterodox dissenters.[26] Many of the latter (such as Bernardino Ochino and Alessandro Citolini) moved to England, where Edward VI duly appointed the former Augustinian monk, Reformed theologian, and religious exile Peter Martyr Vermigli as a religious adviser. In Venice, the English embassy served as a base for political and religious activists such as Guido Giannetti from Fano, who Donzellini had already associated with in Rome. Harvel's secretary, Baldassarre Altieri, was the Venetian agent of the Schmalkaldic League and the Resident in Venice of the Landgrave of Hesse and the Elector of Saxony. He corresponded with Luther and Bullinger on doctrinal and political issues, hoping that the Venetian Republic would openly support the Reformation and the

Protestant princes. Altieri was in close contact with Giovanni Andrea Ugoni, a Brescian friend of Donzellini and godfather to Altieri's son. Donzellini met Altieri and Harvel through Ugoni and possibly Vincenzo Maggi, who was also from Brescia and worked as a diplomat.[27] At the English embassy, Altieri provided him with a copy of Philip Melanchthon's *Loci communes theologici* (*Common Places in Theology*, Wittenberg, 1535) after the physician had read Melanchthon's 'logic and natural philosophy' ('la logica e la filosofia naturale'). It came naturally to Girolamo to move from a humanistic cultural perspective to the Reformed doctrine, crossing the permeable boundary between medicine-philosophy and theology. At the embassy Donzellini also received, read, and discussed many other books including the *Pasquino in estasi* (*Pasquino in Ecstasy* – first latin edition Geneva, 1544) by Celio Secondo Curione, the *Tragedia del libero arbitrio* (*Tragedy of Free Will*, Basel, 1546) by former Benedictine Francesco Negri, the *Homeliae in Evangelium Lucae* (*Homilies on the Gospel of Luke*, Basel, 1544) by Johannes Brenz, a work seen as a standard of Nicodemite thinking, the *Catechismo* (*Catechism*, Frankfurt, 1545) by Urbanus Rhegius, and the *De admirabili Dei consilio* (*On the Admirable Judgement of God*, Basel, 1545) by Johann Rivius.

Like all physicians in Italian urban environments, Donzellini required a reliable *spezieria* for assistance in preparing medicinal products and in his daily work. At a time when traditional medicine was starting to recognise the contribution of practical knowledge, apothecary shops became places of experimentation and scientific innovation.[28] They were also hubs of Italian city life in an extensive network; in their pronounced social dimension, they were used to exchange scientific information and to stay informed about local events and the latest developments in politics or religion (a function that pharmacies would continue to have until the eighteenth century).[29] Together with barber shops, they played a fundamental role in the spread of Reformed ideas, providing a vital link in the heretical chain by storing and distributing prohibited books, offering shelter to dissidents, and acting as centres for the circulation of heterodox ideas. Donzellini's apothecary shop of choice in the 1540s was the *Spezieria del Sarasin* in San Bartolomeo, owned by Marco and Ippolito Fenari. The Fenari brothers stood out for their innovative professional approach and interest in medical matters, which they naturally shared with Donzellini. Marco travelled around the Mediterranean collecting medicinal simples, seeds, bulbs, and plants to prepare pharmacological remedies. He shared his findings in correspondence – yet to be published – with the humanist, naturalist, and collector, Ulisse Aldrovandi between 1569 and 1573. In 1562, Ippolito was the first Prior of the newly established *Collegio degli Speziali* (Guild of Apothecaries) and was one of the founders of the botanical garden in Venice, opened in 1566. Donzellini was on excellent terms with both brothers, and Ippolito defended him at his first trial, describing him as a learned and 'temperate' ('morigerato') person.[30] While this shop does not seem to have played a major role in heterodox practice, Donzellini, together with the Maggis and the Parmas, was also a regular customer at *the Spezieria all'Insegna della Torre*, whose owner was considered 'the most profligate in these worldly matters' ('il maggior tristo de queste cose del mondo').

The dense network of *spezierie* in Venice provided the heretical movement with meeting places for debating doctrinal questions, reading forbidden texts, and even hiding.[31] In 1567, Antonio Moscardo, the third heterodox brother together with Paolo and Giuseppe (who were in the same heretical group as the physician Panarelli), was protected in a *spezieria* owned by a fellow believer named Carlo. Although Antonio managed to escape through Carlo's vegetable garden at night, evading the Inquisition's henchmen, he was subsequently caught and put on trial. During the same period, Ludovico Abioso, another member of the same circle, was called to the *Spezieria alla Borsa* and warned about the case being prepared against him. From the 1560s onwards, the same apothecary shop was also frequented by Vincenzo Negroni, a physician who was ordered to recant, Alessandro Guerini from Crema, a former friar and empirical physician accused of practising judicial astrology and making 'extremely rare poisons' ('veneni rarissimi'), and the heretics Ludovico Abioso and Teofilo Panarelli, who forged their heterodox friendship both here and in Arrivabene's shop.[32] Panarelli mainly used the *Spezieria di Castello*, where he met the goldsmith Giulio di Stan in the late 1560s, leading to joint readings of the *Beneficio di Cristo*. This text was also available in other *spezierie*: Panarelli stated that he had found it at the *Spezieria dell'Elmo*, where he had also taken his friend, colleague, and fellow heterodox dissenter Francesco Pegolotto. They read the 'sweet little book' ('dolce libriccino') together and discussed predestination, free will, and justification by faith.

Panarelli also used the *Spezieria delle Due Colombine* and the *Spezieria della Gatta*, in San Marcuola, both of which were owned by the Gemma family. The *Spezieria delle Due Colombine* was managed by Silvestro and his sons, Giambattista and Marcantonio (at least until the latter became a dyer), while the *Spezieria della Gatta* was owned by Silvestro's brother, another Marcantonio, who left the family business to open his own shop after his nephews grew up and adopted an 'arrogant' ('superbo') approach.[33] Both *botteghe* were located in the north-eastern *sestiere* of Cannaregio on the right bank of the Grand Canal near the Jewish ghetto. The local inhabitants were mostly poor people, migrants, servants, and maids.[34] The area was also home to several embassies and foreign visitors from all over Europe, who exchanged their books and ideas with the Venetians. As the local police had no jurisdiction in areas surrounding embassies in the city, contraband could flourish. Moreover, the number of shops in this part of Venice increased dramatically over the course of the century (a phenomenon that exploded in the seventeenth century), contributing to the increased footfall in the *calli* of Cannaregio. These social and geographical features might well have contributed to the success of the Reformed movement in the area. One local resident in the 1570s was Caterina Sartora (previously known as Caterina Colbertalda, a former servant to Donzellini and his friend Lucrezia Pansa, who we will return to shortly). In the trial against her, the witnesses dissuaded the judges from interrogating her neighbours as they were all members 'of the same sect [as her]' ('della stessa setta').[35] The Gemmas' *spezierie* therefore served as heretical hubs in an area that was already difficult for the Holy Office to monitor.

There is some documentation of the heretical socialising that occurred in such places. Silvestro and Marcantonio Gemma organised chess matches between members of the heterodox network at the *Gatta*,[36] while there was a hidden copy of a text by 'Savonarola about the *Miserere*' ('Savonarola sopra il *Miserere*') at the *Due Colombine*. In addition, people 'spoke ill' ('parlava male') of friars, the intercession of the saints, indulgences, Mass, and Catholic sacraments.[37] Marcantonio Gemma's sisters-in-law were scandalised whenever they visited their sister, Marita, the apothecary's wife. On a typical day in the Gemma household, one might have heard imprecations against the clergy or witnessed irreligious behaviour (such as eating meat on eves of feast days) and the mocking of Catholic rituals and sacraments. In addition to Silvestro, open religious dissent was also displayed by the rest of the family at the *Due Colombine*: his 'daughters who are brainless' ('putte che non hanno cervello') and his sons Marcantonio and Giambattista – the latter was decribed as being engrossed in heretical reading even while 'he was eating' ('manzava').[38]

Besides bookshops, apothecary shops, and private houses, churches also offered opportunities for spreading heterodox ideas. Acting as social meeting points as well as – and perhaps even more than – Catholic places of worship, Venetian churches and sermons regularly brought the faithful into contact with theological discourse, often introducing them to nonconformist opinions or providing a stage for anti-Catholic behaviour. Donzellini's friend Gasparo Parma, for example, used to 'meet up in church' ('ritrovarsi in Chiesa') but left as soon as Mass started.[39] The physician Vincenzo Negroni turned his back on the preacher in the church of San Polo as a mark of protest whenever the priest expressed theological doctrines that he disagreed with.[40] Instead, during his first deposition Gianbattista Gemma stated that he had regularly gone to listen to the sermons in the church of San Geremia in Cannaregio, seizing the opportunity to 'discuss something in a Christian way' ('ragiona*re* di qualche cosa cristianamente') with Sebastiano Malipiero and Gian Battista Trevisano; the three friends even went as far as questioning the preacher about the doctrine of predestination.

A rough map can be plotted showing the Venetian churches with the most extensive and effective links between the Catholic and Reformed worlds. The church of the Santi Apostoli, also located in the Cannaregio district, was a centre of heterodoxy, most notably between 1539 and 1542 but also subsequently. It was here that Bernardino Ochino stayed during Lent in 1539 and 1542 as the guest of the parish priest, Marco Santo, who introduced him to the evangelical circles in the city.[41] Those who regularly attended the church and listened to Ochino's preaching included Pietro Aretino and Pietro Bembo, who brought along the painter Titian for the sermons, and two figures associated with Donzellini, the bookseller Gabriele Giolito and the humanist Celio Secondo Curione. This group was 'contaminated by the preaching of Fra Bernardino' ('contaminati per il predicar di frate Bernardino'), seeking fresh spiritual nourishment in his words, while Santo's pastoral work was said to have transformed the church into an environment as pure as the primitive Church.[42] When Donzellini was in Venice in 1547, non-conformist readings of Scripture were still being preached in the Santi Apostoli. The physician Stefano De Giusti, an Anabaptist convert who was forced to recant in 1550, stated

> I started having bad religious views after hearing two or three sermons by Master Marian of Crema in the church of the Santi Apostoli three years ago. Since then, I have gone from bad to worse, persisting with these wicked opinions.[43]

The The area near the Santi Apostoli was also home to Grazioso Percacino, a friend of the heretical physician Panarelli who was connected to dissident religious groups by the production of compromising texts (and who will reappear in a later chapter). Finally, the physician Agustino da Modena discussed St Paul with a converted Jew in the same church in 1563, 'pulling out a book from his breast' ('cav*andosi* un libro dal seno') that he considered 'highly valuable' ('molto prezioso') and did not want to 'show to anybody as it will be taken from him' ('mostrar a persona del mondo che gli sarà tolto').[44] Agustino later invited the converso to dinner at his home after enquiring whether he 'knew Hebrew' ('sapeva ebreo') and could help him to read the precious book, entitled 'More Nebuch,' which 'speaks against the faith and against images' ('parla contro la fede e contro le immagini'). The work in question was the *Guida dei perplessi* (*Guide for the Perplexed*, in Hebrew *More Nevukhim*), written in the twelfth century by Mosè Maimònide, the Andalusian philosopher, rabbi, physician, and jurist. This text attempted to rationalise Judaism through the philosophy of Aristotle by addressing the 'perplexed,' who were unable to explain the contradictions between philosophical teachings and the literal meaning of the Torah. It is not clear how Agustino acquired the volume, but his curiosity about the Jewish tradition, also shared by other members of the heretical movement, suggests a desire to return to the original text of the Bible and to understand it with philological precision. More specifically, the interest in the *Guida dei perplessi* shows a rationalistic resolve that was a forerunner to the intellectual approach of seventeenth-century thinkers like Baruch Spinoza, who was an attentive reader of Maimonide. The fact that a text like this could be found at the Santi Apostoli, becoming a means for forging new heterodox friendships, speaks volumes about the social relations in Venetian churches.

Donzellini told his judges that during the period in question he 'took communion in his parish church, which was in San Beneto and San Lio' ('pigliava la comunione nella *sua* parrocchia che stava a San Beneto e San Lio') between San Marco and Castello, while he confessed to a 'father from Tolentino' ('padre di Tolentino') at the Basilica dei Frari on the (opposite) left bank of the Grand Canal in San Polo.[45] Although it can be assumed that a heterodox dissenter like Donzellini did not assiduously reveal sins to his confessor, he was probably not lying about confessing at the Frari as it was vital for defendants to demonstrate their observance of confession during an inquisitorial trial. Having grown accustomed to Nicodemite practices during his Roman sojourn, Donzellini probably saw confession at the Frari as the best way to appear orthodox. Other Venetian inhabitants troubled by religious disquiet also confessed at the same church. Girolamo Parto, a notary sentenced to death by the Inquisition in the 1570s (jointly responsible for the heterodox letters sent to the preacher of San Polo, for which the physician Vincenzo Negron was condemned – see Chapter 4), confessed at the Frari, whereas the rest of his family went to the nearby parish church of San Pantalon. Caterina and Francesco Sartori, a married couple tried by the Holy Office in 1574, travelled from their home in Cannareggio to the Frari to confess. Dionora Calia, a housekeeper in contact with Teofilo Panarelli, lived in San Samuele (on the right bank near San Marco); when she was tried for heresy in 1566 and 1578, she told her suspicious judges that her confessor came from outside Venice and that she observed the precepts of the faith when he visited the Frari once a year.[46] Finally, Claudio Textor, a French alchemist that had immigrated to Venice, also chose to confess in the Frari; he was sentenced to death in 1587 a few days after Donzellini. The sources do not enable us to explain these repeated mentions of the church with any certainty, but its size and the constant flow of people meant that witnesses could always confirm that someone had confessed. It is also feasible that priests at the church had some form of connection to the heterodox world. An apothecary named Francesco told the judges in 1560 that he had learned heretical views from the preacher at the Frari, who frequented his *spezieria* in San Raphael (probably the area close to the church of the Angelo Raffaele in Dorsoduro, a ten-minute journey from the Frari). In addition, there was a *spezieria* inside the Frari building that was both owned and frequented by men involved in the movement. For instance, one regular visitor to this *spezieria* was the heterodox priest Don Fedele, who was connected to Teofilo Panarelli's group. At this pharmacy, the empiric Antonino Volpe and the physician Decio Bellebuono prepared medicines obtained through distillation and other alchemical procedures. This suggests that the Basilica dei Frari formed the backdrop for practices that were both religiously heterodox and medically unorthodox. Volpe and Bellebuono were the key figures in an Inquisition case that featured professional rivalry, alchemical chimeras, and religious heterodoxy (which will be examined in Chapter 4).

As the heretical groups in Venice were closely monitored by the repressive authorities, they were regularly forced to seek safe new meeting places. Teofilo Panarelli's circle went to great lengths to read heterodox books between 1565 and 1570, hiding in the vegetable garden on the island of San Giorgio Maggiore, on the Giudecca, or at the Fondaco dei Tedeschi. The houses of Venetian patricians involved in the movement such as Marcantonio Da Canal and Alvise Bembo also provided safe environments.[47] These aristocrats were active members of the group led by Panarelli in the 1560s. Most notably, Da Canal entrusted the education of his children to the aforementioned Don Fedele, who lived with the family for a year; when the priest went on trial in 1568, he accused his former employer of being a clever dissimulator.[48] It is significant that the same two patricians, Da Canal and Bembo, had associated with the Donzellini brothers a decade beforehand, above all Cornelio, who worked as a tutor at their respective homes in San Lorenzo and Rio Marin. Even at the height of the Counter-Reformation, they continued to host heterodox meetings and dissidents.

2.2 Women and the network

One useful way to contextualise Donzellini's medical and heretical activity in Venice is to examine how female members contributed to his network. Women had traditionally been forced into monasticism or marriage, conditioned by 'roles they had not assumed and expectations they had not realized,' but the general upheaval in the sixteenth century caused by the religious crisis prompted some to embark on their own independent religious experiences.[49] They did this by joining heterodox groups and following unorthodox figures, partially breaking free from their enforced intellectual and social subordination. This section will illustrate this female involvement in heretical networks, with some women playing a bridging role between different groups. Physicians like Donzellini became close to their female patients due to frequent contact and the fact that their relationship was based on trust and reliance. In this respect, women enabled physicians to extend their social circles and proselytise more extensively.

Women first took on a more important social role in Venice in the sixteenth century, which partially compensated for their political and financial inferiority.[50] The emergence of a nascent sense of gender identity can be perceived in the growing female demands for freedom of appearance, showcasing their beauty with jewellery and revealing clothes, and perfecting it with hair dye and other forms of make-up.[51] Although this dynamic consolidated the exclusion of women from top-level roles, it ushered in the slow process of emancipation, which was also facilitated by changes in the material structure of city life.[52] When the demand for labour in the city increased between 1540 and 1630 (thanks to the development of the manufacturing industry), the new employment opportunities attracted a high number of female migrants from the rural hinterland with a consequent rise in urban density.[53] These new arrivals modified the social fabric of the *sestieri* and bolstered neighbourhood communities, the heart of female life in the city, which in turn favoured the creation of new networks and social relations.[54]

In this context, female involvement in heterodox networks was far more than a secondary element of arbitrary importance.[55] Two of the women that joined Donzellini in heretical practice as a result of his professional activity were Marchetta Schiavona and Pantasilea Parma, the wife of his heterodox friend Gasparo Parma. A native of Modena, Gasparo was considered 'a man of subtle intelligence who wanted to understand matters of Scripture' ('homo sotil che voleva intendere delle cose della Scrittura').[56] After marrying Pantasilea, who was already a widow, in Venice, they welcomed various fellow heterodox dissenters into their house, first in San Pantalon and then in San Canzian. It was said that this group spoke 'freely' ('liberamente') and 'read all kinds of books' ('leggevano libri di ogni sorte'). Donzellini had first met the couple when he treated Pantasilea Parma, who 'suffered greatly from sickness' ('pativa infermitade assai'). He also attended to Schiavona's health in the same house. Schiavona had come to Venice to seek legal recourse after being tricked by her relatives, deprived of her inheritance, and left down and out in Zara (present-day Zadar, Croatia). Donzellini had already treated Schiavona in hospital and her intellectual sharpness – a quality also recognised by Gasparo Parma and the Inquisition judges – might have led him to introduce her to the group. Gasparo and Pantasilea Parma were deeply touched by the misfortunes of the elderly lady and decided to take her in and provide help. They did so in order to perform an act of generosity (as Gasparo told the judges) and, in all likelihood, for the sake of confessional solidarity between Italian heretics.

The Parmas' landlord, Agostino dal Lion Bianco (or Lion Albo) stated that a secret conventicle met at the house in San Canzian: 'Anytime I passed by, I heard their discussions, but as soon as they saw me, they fell quiet' ('segondo che passava, i sentiva rasonar, ma come mi vedevano se quietavano').[57] The whole neighbourhood 'suspected them of being heretics' ('li haveva per sospetti heretici') and the parish priest of San Canzian even warned Lion Albo not to 'keep such people in his house' ('tenissi simil gente in casa'), prompting the landlord to evict the couple.[58] The Parmas moved to Padua in the mid-1550s, where Pantasilea died in 1556, and at the end of the decade Gasparo was in the service of Caterina Sauli, a noblewoman with connections to dissident religious groups.[59] He was investigated by the Holy Office in 1568 and forced to recant following the proceedings that involved his employer. For her part, Sauli had previously also offered work to Alessandro Citolini, another of Parma and Donzellini's friends and cohorts. Citolini was employed to tutor her daughter, Isabella, who in turn was also investigated by the Inquisition in 1568.[60] All of this network, including its female members, formed a close-knit support group.

Together with Pantasilea Parma and Marchetta Schiavona, Girolamo Donzellini was involved in one of the most effective acts of heretical propaganda documented by the Holy Office: the conversion and escape of two nuns of aristocratic origin – Suor Paola, born Paola Marcello, and Suor Febronia, born Cecilia Morosini – from the convent of Santa Lucia. The episode came to light during the third trial against Donzellini in the mid-1570s when the judges examined his heretical past in Venice around twenty-five years before. The main accuser on this occasion was another woman, Marietta Cagnon, who had been part of the group that met at the Parma house in the 1550s. Twenty-five years later, she was urged by her confessor to admit her sins and report her accomplices to the judges. Contrite and afraid that salvation was now impossible, Cagnon issued a gushing deposition that revealed compromising details about all the members of her old heterodox circle, who had since dispersed. She even claimed that she had been 'rebaptised' ('ribattezzata') by Donzellini at the Parma house. The physician denied any connection with Anabaptist groups and the judges did not pursue this line of inquiry, showing at least in this instance that they believed his statement. The accusation is relevant; however, as it demonstrates that different strands of the movement could blend together in mid-sixteenth-century Venice, combined in the memories of an old lady. What is certain is that in the 1550s Donzellini was in close contact with Cagnon, who knew many details about the flight of the nuns. When the judges accepted her deposition as valid, the trial entered a new phase in which Donzellini's position was seriously compromised.[61]

Marietta Cagnon's testimony reveals that 'the treacherous physician' ('quel traditor del medego') brought prohibited books into the convent, partly by exploiting his professional role and partly with the help of the female members of the Parma household. She then explained that he had encouraged the two nuns to develop ill-advised opinions about ecclesiastical authority, convincing them that 'the Lord God had not asked for either nuns or friars' ('messer Domineddio non aveva comanda' né munage né frati').[62] Having been engaged by the Moresini family as Cecilia's personal physician, he paid regular visits to the convent together with two other men not identified by the judges (one was the barber surgeon who worked for Donzellini, while nothing is known about the other). Taking advantage of his medical role, he advised Cecilia to 'change air' ('mudare aire') and leave the convent, extending the invitation to her inseparable friend.[63] Cagnon stated that the physician had 'damned' ('fatto dannar') the two nuns 'with these books' ('con questi libri'), reiterating the point through the fact that, once outside the convent, Paola Marcello 'went around daubed in make-up with her breasts visible and dyed her hair blonde' ('andava sbelleta coi petti fuori et che la se biondizzava').[64] Perhaps in an attempt to downplay her (and her companions) guilt, Marcello admitted that she preferred to talk to Pantasilea 'more readily about matters of love than of faith' ('più presto de cose de amor che de fede'):[65] her theological awareness and confessional affiliation must have lacked solidity. Donzellini clearly perceived the broad potential scope for action and did his utmost to convert the two nuns to new ways of thinking.

As Marcello told the inquisitors in 1575, her family had sent her to the convent against her will when she was a child (considering the outcome of the episode, it seems probable that Morosini had suffered the same fate).[66] In this context, according to the testimony given by the former Suor Paola, the tipping point was the inflexibility of their new confessor, Fra Lorenzo Pegolotto, which threw them 'into great confusion' ('in confusion grande').[67] At the time of their flight, many cloistered nuns in Venice lived as "sinners," secretly developing romantic and sexual relationships with aristocratic men. While, outside convent walls, the authority of the clergy was being questioned throughout the city and heretical books and opinions circulated widely.[68] Against this backdrop, Donzellini drew on his professional role and his connections with various women to spread Reformed doctrines from within, triggering a desire for freedom in the nuns. Additional factors that should not be underestimated are the characteristic intimacy of the physician-patient relationship and the charisma that a humanist like Donzellini must have exerted on poorly educated women relegated to the margins of city life. It was easy for the physician to ensure that the two nuns did not 'like the ceremonies and religion as much as they used to' ('ghe piacesse così le cerimonie e la religione come erano solite de far').[69] With heretical ideas penetrating the convent walls, the two nuns (Morosini was in her thirties, Marcello in her forties)[70] found suitable ideological support for their designs on freedom.

When they fled one night in April 1551, Cecilia and Paola cleared out their cells, much to the great disappointment of the inquisitors, who, even after more than two decades, still hoped that an interrogation might reveal the titles of any forbidden books left behind. Morosini died shortly after her escape, while Paola Marcello returned to live with her family. Although forgiven, she was forced to serve her brother-in-law for the rest of her life.[71] Living in Cannareggio, she continued to be accostumed with those involved in religious dissent – which was almost unavoidable in Venice.[72]

In 1550, at the time when he regularly visited the convent of Santa Lucia, Donzellini started living with Caterina Strozzi (known as Strozza), who was the owner of his house and 'of the things' ('della robba') inside it except for the books. He paid her sixty-one ducats a year for rent and household services. Strozza was interrogated by the judges in her capacity as Donzellini's housemate and probable mistress.[73] Her deposition provides important information about the day-to-day nature of heretical relations in Venice in the 1540s and 1550s. Caterina took her name from her former partner of six years, Francesco Strozzi, another of Donzellini's cohorts. A native of Tuscany, Francesco was arrested in Venice in 1546 soon after the physician arrived in the city (although it is possible that they had already met in Rome, where Strozzi lived before moving to Venice).[74] Prior to his capture, Francesco Strozzi lived at Pietro Carnesecchi's house and completed an Italian translation of the *Pasquino in estasi* (*Pasquino in Ecstasy*), a fiercely polemical anti-Roman work by Celio Secondo Curione, another member of Donzellini's network.

Although Caterina Strozza attempted to gloss over her former relationships during the first trial against Donzellini in 1553, held in absentia, certain details emerged during questioning. For example, she was forced to admit that she had been the partner of someone who 'was blamed for having written a book about something or other' ('si incolpava che l'aveva fatto un libro di non so che cosa'). Not only did she not suggest any bond of intimacy with the physician, but she also complained that he owed her money. Nevertheless, she tempered the virulence of the accusations by specifying that Donzellini had never spoken about anything other than 'the sick and medicine' ('de malati e de medicina') in her presence. Furthermore, while it was true that he had encouraged her to eat meat during Lent, to her knowledge he had not violated the precepts of the Church in any other way. She replied promptly to the judges' questions about his social habits, which must have been familiar to the Holy Office in any case. She confirmed that Donzellini had been part of the English ambassador's social circle and that Gaspare Parma and Pietro Perna had visited their house. The fact that Perna had been there only a few months before demonstrates the continuity and solidity of Donzellini's extended network as the printer had already emigrated to Basel. She reiterated, though, that Donzellini's social habits were essentially related to his profession. This statement did not soften the judges' approach at all. On the contrary, they used it to collect valuable information to explore the relationship between physicians and heresy in Venice. This phenomenon must have been familiar to them considering the numerous attempts to pass legislation against the entire professional body in Venice, and indeed medicine itself, during the Counter-Reformation (which will be focused on in more detail in Chapter 4).

Caterina Strozzi's deposition can be cross-checked with the information provided by her namesake, Caterina Colbertalda, who had been Donzellini's 'housekeeper' ('massara') before he cohabited with Strozzi. Colbertalda was a young working-class woman of around twenty who had migrated to Venice from the rural hinterland.[75] For girls of her age and social standing, working as a maidservant was an opportunity to acquire a dowry and a husband; she duly married Pietro De Megis, a heretical empirical physician and alchemist from Rome, in the early 1550s. The couple stayed together until 1554, when Pietro was banished from Venice as a radical heretic.[76] According to the witnesses, De Megis 'did not believe in God' ('non crede*va* in Dio'), did not receive Holy Communion, did not confess, ate meat 'during Lent, on Fridays, Saturdays, and vigils' ('la quaresima, li veneri, li sabbati, et le veglie'), denied purgatory, 'which is imposed as a tax on souls by the pope' ('che è messo per gabella alle anime dal papa'), rejected the value of the sacrament of the Eucharist, 'scorned the Virgin Mary' ('*dis*prezzava la Vergine') and the intercession of the saints, refuted free will, and 'always spoke badly of the pope and all the most illustrious prelates, saying that they are thieves and ministers of the devil and that the pope is the Antichrist' ('diceva sempre male del pontefice e di tutti li illustrissimi prelati dicendo che sono ladroni et ministri del diavolo e che il papa è Anticristo').[77] The same accusations were then levelled against his wife, who was accused of Anabaptist-style marriages to two other men, one in Verona and one in Vicenza.

The judges did not explore the matter of polyandry and Colbertalda was careful not to reveal details of her personal situation during the interrogation in the Donzellini trial. It is certain, however, that she was connected to the heretical network. It is not known whether she met Donzellini through De Megis, or whether Donzellini ever met De Megis through her, but this is a significant relationship: a possible friendship with De Megis would potentially date the physician's interest in magic and Hermeticism to his first stay in Venice (whereas it is only documented from the late 1550s onwards). Moreover, one of De Megis's closest associates – Giovan Battista De Freschi Olivi, a converted Jew – was another physician that might have known Donzellini.[78] After studying in Padua and becoming a renowned physician, De Freschi Olivi practised in Cannaregio, where the Jewish ghetto was located. He was a neighbour of De Megis and Paola Marcello, after Donzellini had encouraged her to leave the convent in 1550. The details of Giovan Battista's life emerge from the records of the trial against his mother, Elena (in which he did everything in his power to defend her against the accusations of Judaism, partly by drawing on his medical experience). Paola Marcello also appeared as a witness, testifying that Elena 'scowled and grumbled' ('faceva brutti visi') and threatened to 'take by the throat' ('prendere per la gola') the priest of San Marziale when he spoke about the mystery of the incarnation of Christ during Mass.[79] The emergence of a network potentially connecting a radical alchemist from Rome, a physician that was a converted Jew, a former nun, a housemaid, and a heterodox physician illustrates the dense Venetian web with its intricate blend of medical practice and religious dissent.

Colbertalda worked for Donzellini until 1550. After this, her husband 'no longer [wanted her] to stay with them as a housekeeper' ('più che stia con loro per massara') and obliged her to stop working. This might perhaps have been out of jealousy, as Caterina also testified that Pietro forbade her from leaving the house and engaged a woman to follow all her movements from a boat.[80] She was thus forced to abandon not only her position working for Donzellini but also what must have been her main job. Indeed, for just over three years Colbertalda had served as personal maid to Lucrezia Maggi, Donzellini's friend and cohort and the wife of Vincenzo Maggi, the aforementioned diplomat. Young housemaids became integral parts of the families they worked for during the Renaissance period, acquiring certain privileges and even assuming the identity of the household.[81] As Colbertalda seems to have been close to the Maggis, her deposition is especially useful for reconstructing the day-to-day activities of the group and was certainly valuable to the judges. Furthermore, after her radical husband was arrested (he died soon afterwards), she broadened her heterodox circle and ended up in the dock herself in 1574. Even though she attempted to play down any personal involvement in the network during the 1553 trial, it is clear that her religious feelings were strongly influenced by her experiences in the Donzellini and Maggi households.

Lucrezia Maggi, a physician's daughter whose maiden name was Pansa, came from the Friuli region. After marrying Vincenzo – already an apostate, an ambassador in France and a diplomat in Turkey – in San Vito in 1548, she moved to Venice and lodged with the Parmas (probably while her husband was on his travels) in San Pantalon. She also moved with them to a new house in San Canzian in the heart of the city, not far from the Rialto, where Donzellini also lived and worked. The latter became her physician in 1546, so it is possible that she introduced him to her husband Vincenzo in Venice (although Girolamo might have already encountered him, at least by reputation, in the early 1530s in Brescia).[82] As a diplomat, Vincenzo had the opportunity to make numerous contacts and distribute or procure new books. The presence of a diplomat, a physician, and several printers in this heretical network enabled the group to access a variety of social environments (from courts to embassies, literary circles, private houses, and female monasteries) and conduct an extensive and pervasive proselytism campaign. Caterina Colbertalda stated that Vincenzo distributed pamphlets by Vergerio and received (and sent) many letters from England. This correspondence was with 'a friar named Michelangelo who was in prison [...] and then went off to England, where he preaches in the Italian language' ('uno frate chiamato Michielangelo che è stato in prigione [...] et poi se ne andò in Inghilterra, donde el predica in lingua italiana'). The man in question was Donzellini's former tutor, Michelangelo Florio.[83]

Colbertalda also stated that Vincenzo and Lucrezia Maggi, Gasparo and Pantasilea Parma, Alessandro Citolini (who we will return to shortly), Girolamo Donzellini, and Caterina Strozzi were all 'new Christians' ('christiani novi') who practised their religion together and 'exchanged their secrets with each other' ('fac*eva*no li suoi segreti l'uno con l'altro').[84] The characteristic features of Donzellini's network in the 1540s and 1550s were underground complicity and clandestine activism, intellectual debate, and practical support. In this context, private events like marriages constituted opportunities to consolidate personal ties based on religious solidarity. The whole group attended Lucrezia and Vincenzo Maggi's wedding and Donzellini even acted as the best man. The celebrations probably involved jokes at the expense of the clergy and anti-Catholic satire, elements which played a role on other similar occasions. One such event was the wedding of the daughter of another heterodox physician, Niccolò Machella, a member of the Accademia Modenese, a hotbed of humanists won over by evangelical ideas that included at least six physicians. The best-known heterodox figures in Modena gathered to celebrate at Machella's house (which was already a safe haven for heterodox reading). During this feast, criticism and mockery were heaped upon Don Serafino da Fermo, who had condemned the *Sommario de la sacra Scrittura* (*Summary of the Holy Scripture*) shortly before.[85]

Regardless of their lower level of theological awareness and intellectual refinement, women acted both as important links in the network and valuable sources of information when summoned by the Inquisition.

2.3 Books, doctrines, and practices: The growth of heresy in 1540s Venice

Caterina Colbertalda's testimony reveals that the Maggis owned numerous prohibited books. We can reconstruct the reading list of group members from this deposition and the statements made by Caterina Strozzi, Gasparo Parma (who was questioned about these events in 1574), and Girolamo Donzellini. The titles included a *Testamento novo* – probably the copies of Cornelio Donzellini's translation that Perna had sent to Donzellini in 1550 – and classic works of the Italian Reformation such as the aforementioned *Pasquino in estasi.*

Caterina Colbertalda also testified that the Maggis used to read a 'great book' (libro grande).[86] Although she did not specify its title, it might have been Giorgio Siculo's work of the same name, the *Libro grande*, which was already in circulation in the 1550s. If this were the case, it would demonstrate a connection between Donzellini's Venetian circle and radical groups in Ferrara. Such a link is likely to have involved Donzellini, who was in contact with the heterodox Greek scholar Francesco Porto and Duchess Renée in the latter city. His brother Cornelio was also there at precisely this time (before he moved on to Florence). Giorgio Siculo's doctrine, described as an 'effective synthesis of mysticism and rationalism, predestinarianism and Pelagianism,'[87] attracted those who sought a fresh theological perspective and disliked the confessional barriers dividing Christian Europe. It seemed to offer a comprehensive and reassuring spiritual solution to the long-term religious crisis afflicting the Italian peninsula. Physicians played a notable role in Siculo's secret sect: Pietro Bresciani, Marcantonio Florio, Francesco Severi, and Pietro Giudici were all members.[88] The popularity of Siculo's ideas in the medical profession derived from his emphasis on the power of human nature in relation to the origin and destiny of the soul.[89] Siculo claimed that God had only created the soul of Adam; all the other souls had been born from 'parents by propagation' ('parenti per propagazione'). Human seed was thus the only agent involved in the generation of both body and soul. With regard to the afterlife, Siculo offered a solution that shares similarities with psychopannychism: after death, souls wandered the 'caliginous air' ('per aerem caliginosum')[90] until judgement day, when only those of the elect would be resurrected. Ideas of this type were probably particularly well suited to the humanistic sensibilities of physicians. As well as coinciding with their scientific inquisitiveness, such concepts were familiar to them from their studies at Italian universities. A further element that might have favoured the spread of Siculo's doctrine among physicians was the central role played by books and reading. While the former were used in the different stages of the initiatory process, the latter was attributed with a 'mystical and salvific' ('mistico e salvifico') connotation.[91] Siculo's doctrine incorporated an evolved form of the most radical elements of the Italian Reformation: denial of the Trinity, the sacraments, baptism, and the ecclesiastical institution. Although there is no evidence that Donzellini took his theological speculation to such extremes, it is plausible that he read Siculo's *Libro grande* out of curiosity as a man of culture and an established heterodox dissenter without deepening his involvement in the group. When Donzellini had to serve a long custodial sentence in Venice in the 1570s, he forged close ties with the Ferrarese humanist Nascimbene Nascimbeni, one of the most active members of Siculo's group. It is likely that this friendship flourished partly from discussing and sharing doctrines of a radical and secret nature.

Many Valdesian books also circulated in Donzellini's Venetian group such as the *Beneficio di Cristo*, and the *Cento e dieci divine considerazioni* (*One Hundred and Ten Divine Considerations*). These works provide further proof of the group's versatile doctrinal leanings and spiritualistic orientation. Valdesian theology could be read and embraced on various levels, but the most attentive readers did not fail to grasp its potential to subvert orthodoxy. Théodore de Bèze, Calvin's second-in-command, harshly criticised the *Cento e dieci divine considerazioni*, claiming that the text embodied the perfidious Anabaptist spirit; it is certainly true that the book circulated in Venetian Anabaptist circles. Pietro Manelfi (an Anabaptist minister who later became an Inquisition informer) sent the text to Pier Paolo Vergerio, who in turn passed it on to Celio Secondo Curione. The latter then edited the first edition, published in Basel in 1550, the same year in which there are records of his acquaintanceship with Donzellini.[92] For his part, Curione had already praised the Spanish theologian, the 'knight of Caesar's who became a knight of Christ' ('cavaliere di Cesare divenuto cavaliere di Cristo') in the *Pasquino in estasi*, a work read and admired by the physician. Although there is no concrete evidence that Girolamo read other Valdesian works, given his leading role in producing and smuggling books it is perfectly feasible that he came across other works published or written in 'Spiritual' ('spirituali') circles.

As we have seen, Donzellini had previously frequented Valdesian groups in Rome in the early 1540s. In Venice too, the common denominator in his group's heterodox experiences was the search for a personal approach to religion and the eschatological problem, in which exploration of the Reformed doctrine did not take shape as an alternative to Valdesian ideas. In his 1560 trial, for example, he described a discussion on free will he had witnessed at the monastery of the Carità in Venice: an exchange of views on 'spiritual regeneration' ('rigenerazione spirituale') between Girolamo Zanchi and the philosopher Marcoantonio Passeri. The debate centred on whether such rebirth originated 'in us and thus from free will' ('in noi e cioè dal libero arbitrio') or whether, instead, God was 'the first to actuate free will in us' ('il primo a mover libero arbitrio in noi'). As was often the case in these environments, the exchange followed a similar format to a university debate. After scriptural passages were cited to support the two theses, the dispute was settled by quoting St John's 'judgement [...] at the beginning of his Gospel' ('sententia [...] nel principio del suo evangelio'), drawing on the common belief in the spiritual regeneration of all those with faith in Christ's sacrifice, who 'were born of God' ('ex Deo nati sunt'). In the perspective shared by Donzellini and his group, the harshness of the Reformed doctrine, which paved the way to predestination by denying free will, was mitigated by the image of an infinitely merciful God, a source of grace for those who believed in the salvific value of the 'benefit of Christ.'[93]

Donzellini's probable frequent visits to Pietro Carnesecchi's house and his contact with Francesco Strozzi, who had translated Curione's *Pasquillus extaticus* with help from Carnesecchi, are further indicators of his ongoing involvement in Valdesian circles in Venice.[94] During his years in the city, Girolamo also forged friendships with Ludovico Manna and Bartolomeo Spadafora, both involved at the time in Valdesian circles. In addition, he was mentioned in the list drafted by the Roman Inquisition containing 'those named by Giulio Basalù' ('nominati per dominum Iulium Basalù'), thereby becoming associated with others connected to the Neapolitan Valdesian group like Isabella Bresegna and Germano Minadois.[95] This list was compiled from the Venetian dossier for the trial against the radical heretic Giulio Basalù in 1555. Girolamo's name is crossed out, probably because the judges had given up hope of finding him after he had been in hiding for two years. The names on the list were divided into nine groups on the basis of the accusations against them. The physician appeared in the third of these alongside those that not only affirmed justification by faith alone and drew the resulting conclusions ('de iustificatione et consequentiis') but also held heterodox opinions about the sacraments. As Luca Addante has demonstrated, Basalù and several others (members of the Neapolitan Valdesian group who had adopted the radical teachings of Juan de Villafranca) moved 'from consequence to consequence' ('di consequentia in consequentia'). In this way, starting from the article of justification by faith, they went on to deny the virginity of Mary and the divinity of Christ, eventually claiming that the soul was mortal.[96]

According to Valdés, success in the 'Christian business' ('negotio christiano') was the result of personal 'inspiration' ('inspirationi') through 'experience' ('experientia') and revelation.[97] The religious trajectory was therefore subject to change over time and liable to reach higher planes of theological awareness. Although Girolamo never developed the extremist tendencies of Basalù, the Valdesian framework that influenced his devout feelings might have led him further down the path of religious subjectivism. In 1559, as a member of the Basel group connected to Pietro Perna's printing house, Girolamo contributed to the promotion of religious tolerance with the short treatise *De succesione doctrinae ab origine mundi* (*On the Succession of Doctrine since the Origin of the World*), which focused on issues of Christian humanism and *prisca theologia* (ancient theology). In this, he again cited figures associated with Valdesianism like Marcantonio Flaminio and Reginald Pole as examples of those who had contributed to the rebirth of primordial knowledge and embodied the ideal of religion and philosophy that he advocated. Then, in his *Remedium ferendarum iniuriarum sive de compescenda ira* (*Remedy for Bearing Injuries, or On Containing Anger*), published in Venice in 1586, a year before his execution, Donzellini expressed a vision of the divine with pantheistic overtones, verging on modalism. These Latitudinarian and radical developments, which will be examined below, should be interpreted in the context of the intellectual milieu in which his religious thinking evolved. His heterodox take on Christianity derived more from the humanism of Erasmus than the belligerence of Luther. Indeed, both the references to Valdesianism and his endorsement of more openly Reformed articles of faith should be placed within this humanistic framework.[98] The spiritual profile of a heterodox physician and humanist like Donzellini cannot be reduced to any single movement in the Italian Reformation; it remained nuanced and eclectic throughout his life.

To gain some measure of such a complex religious stance, it will be useful to profile a few of his close friends and associates during this period. The experiences of these humanists and physicians in 1540s Venice highlight the link between philosophy, medicine, heresy, and daily religious practices. We will start with the humanist Alessandro Citolini. He lived in Calle dal Forno and was easily recognisable with 'only one eye' ('un solo occhio'). Citolini was a regular visitor at Gasparo Parma's house and a personal friend of Donzellini. Born in Serravalle in the Treviso area, he was tutored in the 1530s by one of the most interesting figures in sixteenth-century Italian culture, the erudite visionary Giulio Camillo Delminio. The latter's *Idea del Theatro* (*Idea of The Theatre*, Venice, 1550) aimed to include all human knowledge, offering the opportunity to consult the cultural heritage produced over the preceding two thousand years. It is difficult to say exactly how Camillo's Theatre was supposed to take shape in concrete terms – was it a building, a model, or a purely abstract plan?[99] Drawing on Neoplatonic, Kabbalist, astrological, and alchemical influences, his project fell within the realm of the art of memory, a discipline, which aimed to enhance the human ability to acquire knowledge and dominate the existent.[100] Camillo drew on the Hermetic tradition by viewing the intellect as divine as it emanated directly from God. In this vision, man (as a microcosm) was able to perceive the entire universe (as a macrocosm), understanding and remembering it through his *mens* or memory.[101]

In 1561, the Valgrisi printing house published a text by Citolini – the *Tipocosmia* (*Typocosmy*) – modelled on Camillo's doctrine. This encyclopaedic classification of knowledge aimed to overcome the instability of human memory through correlations between the micro- and macrocosmos. The texts by Citolini, Camillo, and indeed Donzellini when he started publishing philosophical works in 1559, are all characterised by Hermetic and Platonic overtones: 'a spiritualistic and esoteric "religion" [...] not so far removed from certain classic contemporary records of Italian "heresy"'.[102] Unsurprisingly, the content of the *Tipocosmia*, which also featured ironic, biting attacks on the Catholic Church, was the main reason why Citolini was convicted in absentia by the Venetian Inquisition in 1565. By then, however, he was already safe in England, where the *Tipocosmia* had earned him a warm welcome. European humanists saw the work as 'a valuable tool' for maximising the potential of human reason.[103] Donzellini was later involved in the republication and distribution of his friend's texts in the 1570s and 1580s.

Giulio Camillo influenced several physicians connected to the Venetian Reformed movement that knew Donzellini. One of these, Agostino Abioso, was even granted exclusive access to Camillo's Theatre.[104] A member of an illustrious family originally from Ravenna, Abioso was never tried by the Holy Office but mixed in heterodox circles. He was added to a list of active 'Lutherans' in Venice in 1551 by Pietro Manelfi, who had stayed at Abioso's house in 1547 while on the run (Abioso was sandwiched between Girolamo Donzellini and Andrea Arrivabene on the list).[105] Furthermore, Abioso was in contact with Pietro Carnesecchi, and his son, Ludovico, as we shall see, was one of the most active members of the heterodox group led by the physician Teofilo Panarelli.[106]

Camillo also became acquainted with Ortensio Lando following their first meeting in Bologna in the 1530s. A versatile writer and self-taught physician, Lando, alias *Turchetto*, alias Giorgio Filalete, was in turn a friend and colleague of Donzellini, as well as a fellow heterodox dissenter; in the 1550s, he was employed in the Sauli household like Parma and Citolini.[107] After abandoning the Augustinian Order in around 1534, Lando set off down a complex cultural and religious path. Along the way he developed doctrines steeped in radical and spiritual elements (as is evident in his *Dubbi religiosi* [*Religious Doubts*]), fostered an interest in astrology and medicine, and drafted a theological text entitled *Una breve pratica di medicina per sanare le passioni dell'animo* (*A Brief Practice of Medicine to Cure the Passions of the Soul*). As already mentioned, copies of Michele Servetus's *Christianismi restitutio* (*Restoration of Christianity*) were distributed in northern Italy through Giorgio Filalete, Pietro Perna, and the radical jurist Matteo

Gribaldi. Finally, Ortensio Lando was one of the most active readers and supporters of the thinking of Heinrich Cornelius Agrippa, the ultimate magician. He 'borrow[ed] certain themes from the *De incertitudine et vanitate scientiarum et artium* [*Declamation Attacking the Uncertainty and Vanity of the Sciences and Arts*, Antwerp, 1530] that appeared socially and politically subversive' and all his own writings were indeed inspired by this text.[108] He also guided his friend Gaudenzio Merula – a physician, astrologer, and historian – in the same direction: through the mediation of members of the esoteric circle established by Agrippa in northern Italy, Merula received an intellectual education despite his humble origins.[109]

Donzellini's Venetian network thus blended Hermetic and Neoplatonic ideas, as well as religious and "philosophical" spiritualism. These concepts continued to circulate in Donzellini's group of contacts in the 1560s and indeed in the following decades. In 1562 the aforementioned heretic from Brescia Giovani Andrea Ugoni wrote a treatise, published by another of Donzellini's friends, Publio Francesco Spinola, about the 'assignment of names' (*Trattato della impositione de' nomi*). In this work, he debated the origin of words in relation to the alleged inherent meaning of the things to which they referred, grounding his argument in the Kabbalist and Pythagorean traditions. When Ugoni was put on trial by the Inquisition in 1565, the investigation soon led the judges onto the trail of Spinola, who was executed in 1567.

The Venetian network of Donzellini was also animated by many heterodox physicians. Girolamo daily shared with them medical practice, the reading, discussion and distribution of prohibited books and an intense form of religious propaganda. One of such physicians was Francesco Stella. Inter alia, he gave Girolamo a copy of Francesco Negri's *Tragedia del libero arbitrio*. Just as Stella embodies the intellectual and religious attitude of heretical physicians in Venice, his library reflects the ways in which books and ideas circulated in the heterodox movement they supported. A key player in the spread of the doctrine preached by Pier Paolo Vergerio, like Cornelio Donzellini and Vincenzo Maggi before him, Stella was described by his judges as the 'head of all heretics that are in this country' ('capo di tutti li heretici che sono in questo paese').[110] Together with Francesco Pirrochini, he 'spread these wicked and diabolical thoughts among poor countryfolk and unlettered people, to whom they preach [...] that a dog is worthier of worship than an image of Our Lady' ('dilata*to* queste cattivissime e diaboliche operazioni in poveri contadini e persone idiote, a quali predicano [...] che un cane è più degno di esser riverito che non è immagine di Nostra Donna')[111], winning the majority of the population over to the Reformation. Being part of the heretical fabric of Venice, Stella also helped to distribute Vergerio's works in the city with the assistance of the bookseller Andrea Arrivabene. His heterodox contact network included medical colleagues, booksellers, publishers, commoners, and peasants alike, extending from his house in a village near Treviso – described as a 'synagogue where the Christian religion is debated' ('sinagoga dove si ragiona della religion cristiana')[112] – to Venice, where he lodged at

Giovanni Giacomo Sforza's house in San Samuele.[113] As with many other physicians, Stella comes across as an intellectual with a voracious cultural appetite and a troubled relationship with religion. As a result, he was willing to risk his freedom to peruse the latest major publications and spread Reformed views as widely as possible. His library featured around sixty prohibited books, including volumes by the best known Italian Reformed thinkers, theological texts printed in Zurich and Basel, and works by Lorenzo Valla and Erasmus.[114] After attracting the attention of the Inquisition in 1549, Stella did not appear at his trial and was the focus of a decade-long judicial process (during most of which he remained at large, managing to continue his heterodox activities). Eventually, in 1558, Cardinal Ghislieri asked for his extradition to Rome, which duly happened in April 1560. Before he was transferred to the papal capital, Stella was imprisoned in Venice and he drafted his will, which shows that his Protestant faith was still unshaken. He commended his soul to 'his guardian, the Lord God, the supreme shepherd' ('suo curator Signore Dio supremo pastore') without expressing the desire for his memory to be celebrated in the years to come or referring to the Catholic Church in any way. He also pledged to leave some of his wealth 'to prisoners' ('alli prisoneri'), one of the many expressions of solidarity between detainees in the inquisitorial records.[115]

Another interesting figure in Donzellini's Venetian network who was equally adept at combining medicine and Reformed ideas was Agostino Gadaldino. The son of Antonio, a bookseller from Modena, who had taken part in the heterodox meetings held at the Academy of Modena in the late 1530s and early 1540s, Agostino developed a friendship with Donzellini in the 1540s and 1550s. He embraced heterodox ideas during this period while they were 'practising together as physicians every day' ('praticando insieme tutti i giorni come medico') and attended gatherings at the *Spezieria del Sarasin* and Gasparo Parma's house, before recanting in 1555. *Doubt* played a key role in Gadaldino's heterodox experience; he explained to the inquisitors that 'I never knew that doubting faith is heresy, because I saw a statement that it is not heretical to doubt faith' ('io non ho mai saputo che il dubitar della fede sia heresia perché io ho visto questa proposizione che dubitar di fede non haereticum esse'),[116] adopting a skilful strategy during his spontaneous appearance (*spontanea comparizione*) in 1555.[117] Appearing before the judges to avoid a probable inquisitorial summons and benefit from the leniency promised by Julius III's edict, he hid behind the smokescreen of a man of culture whose only sin had been a degree of scepticism on religious matters (not accompanied by any real profession of heretical faith) and unwarranted curiosity about theological discourse, which was common at the time. From Donzellini's testimony, however, we know that Gadaldino was more deeply involved in the world of heterodoxy than these rote confessions would suggest. Indeed, he is frequently mentioned as one of the fellow believers with whom Girolamo shared heretical books and beliefs in the early 1550s.

While Gadaldino's statements clearly followed a defensive logic, it is also true that he was a man of culture, an avid reader who questioned scholastic knowledge through critical and philological methodology. As a boy, he had been educated in book culture by his father, who was involved in distributing and printing heretical publications. Then, between 1541 and 1542, the Giunta brothers commissioned him to coordinate the work for a critical Latin edition of Galen's *Opera omnia* (*Complete Works*) in Venice.[118] In his introductory letter to the volume, Agostino explained that the team assembled by the printers collected and collated Greek manuscripts from libraries all over Italy. The texts were then translated by experts in languages and medicine such as Andreas Vesalius. As the editor-in-chief of this huge undertaking, Gadaldino was responsible for ascertaining the philological accuracy of the texts, which involved painstakingly comparing the Greek and Latin versions, and checking for mistakes during the printing process. The exertion required for this laborious task took its toll on the physician, who fell ill and was debilitated for months; he specified in the introduction that any flaws in the text were the result of lack of time rather than absence of effort.[119] As a humanist, bibliophile, and philologist, as well as a physician, it was a natural transition for Gadaldino to move from criticising medieval medical culture in philological and humanistic terms to questioning the Catholic religious paradigm. The connection between his scientific-philological and theological-scriptural experiences was largely methodological in nature.

Gadaldino's brand of Reformed heresy was quite distinctive. For example, he accepted the doctrinal authority of the councils and the sacrament of confession, and only criticised the rite of Mass when it was officiated by a sinful priest.[120] Just as compliance with Protestant orthodoxy did not seem to be one of his priorities, forced recantation was probably not a millstone around his neck. Although he read heterodox books and discussed 'matters of faith [...] in the street, at sermons, and in *spezierie*, speaking to different people' ('delle cose della fede [...] in strada, alle prediche et nelle spezierie parlando con diversi'), he took care not to 'scandalise the uneducated' ('scandalizzare i semplici').[121] Attracted to the heterodox movement by his intellectual curiosity, he examined sacred texts freely and read forbidden books with the restless, elitist attitude of an academic. This also prompted him to take a back seat and immerse himself in his private religious realm – which might have embraced spiritual influences too. In this way, there was no risk to his intellectual, scientific, and medical work, and he could continue to contribute to the heterodox movement, albeit marginally and sporadically. One such contribution was his endorsement of the irregular doctoral candidacy of Manusso Maran – the aforementioned young Cretan medical student with Calvinist leanings – out of professional and confessional solidarity.

The topos of attraction to the Reformation triggered by cultural leanings was part of a well-orchestrated defensive strategy. Indeed, the physicians making such statements were on trial and their safety, freedom, and reputation were in serious danger. It is striking, however, how frequently the motif appears in depositions made by heterodox physicians, including Donzellini. While intellectual curiosity was the mainstay used by medical practitioners to justify their religious deviance, it is safe to assume that their heretical tendencies were rooted in concrete foundations built on familiarity with knowledge and humanist methodology; a propensity for dialectical reasoning; an inclination for criticising scholastic truths; philological and philosophical grounds; and a fascination with books and major cultural innovations, including developments in the theological field.

Manusso Maran offered a twofold justification for possessing and reading prohibited books. While he stressed that he was 'goaded by the devil into wanting to see these opinions of his' ('instigato dal demonio per voler veder dette sue opinioni'), he also admitted that it happened 'out of curiosity' ('per curiosità'). His inquisitiveness was so uncontrollable that he even took home a text on religious matters from a public urinal so that he could study it at leisure.[122] Gianbattista Goineo, another heterodox physician from Pirano in the Venetian Republic, also used intellectual curiosity as a justification and basis for his interest in Reformed ideas.[123] After playing an active role in heretical and intellectual networks in the 1540s, travelling around Europe, graduating from Padua University, and spreading heretical beliefs among his patients, Goineo was arrested by the Holy Office in 1550. His attempts to defend himself, drawing precisely on the idea that it was legitimate for a man of culture to study religious matters, were somewhat clumsy. The judges were not satisfied and pursued the proceedings, forcing him to choose religious exile in Ljubljana without ever returning to Italy.[124]

As we will see, Donzellini used the same topos to justify his involvement in the Reformed movement when he appeared before the judges many years later.[125] He too was eventually forced to leave Italy. The suspicions of the Inquisition were first raised in 1553 and he was summoned by the Holy Office together with Vincenzo and Lucrezia Maggi. At this point, he decided to flee from Venice and subsequently opted to leave the Italian peninsula, benefiting from all the resources that his network could provide. He first went to Padua to catch up on the latest developments in the academic world from the philosopher Vincenzo Maggi and perhaps to stock up on books. Then, he travelled to Ferrara, where he probably obtained some money from Duchess Renée and enjoyed every 'comfort like before' ('comodità come prima'). Finally, he stopped off at his father's house in Orzi Nuovi to rest before his long journey and say goodbye to his family.[126] For the following six years, he was a fugitive on German soil.

Notes

1 'As this city of ours is extremely curious in matters of faith and is not satisfied or appeased by the faith of its forebears, it goes in search of new sects, especially the learned and scholarly men. It is no great surprise that many of my friends

and people I have met have been condemned there for their beliefs.' ('Hora essendo questa nostra città tanto curiosa nelle cose della fede, che non si contentando né si quietando nella fede dei suoi maggiori, va cercando nuove sette e massime gli huomini dotti e letterati, non è gran meraviglia che in tanti amici e persone de quali ho avuto conoscenza molti ve ne siano stati per la loro dottrina condannati'); ASV, Sant'Uffizio, *Processi, Contro Girolamo Donzellini*, Bu. 39, 48v.

2 A map of the main places mentioned in this one and the following chapters can be found in the book's "Appendix: visualisations", see infra, figure A.1.

3 On the distribution, organisation, and function of spaces in Venice see Ennio Concina, *Venezia nell'età moderna. Struttura e funzioni* (Venice: Marsilio, 1989).

4 On book censorship, see Mario Infelise, *I libri proibiti da Gutenberg all'Encyclopédie* (Rome-Bari: Laterza, 2013).

5 Siraisi, *Communities*; Alessandra Quaranta, 'Exile Experiences 'Religionis causa' and the Transmission of Medical Knowledge between Italy and German-Speaking Territories in the Second Half of the Sixteenth Century,' in Vincenzo Lavenia, Cornel Zwielein (eds.), *Fruits of Migration. Heterodox Italian Migrants and Central European Culture 1550–1620* (Leiden-Boston: Brill, 2018); see also Marcus, *Forbidden Knowledge*, which suggests that ideas also circulated through the work of physicians appointed to censor prohibited texts, who thus reflected on the benefit and scientific value of new publications.

6 In 1559, the Holy Office forced Valgrisi to remove the sign of Erasmus, and his *bottega* was renamed 'at the sign of the Tau,' the letter that featured on his publications.

7 This view was established in the Middle Ages, with disease seen as an instrument to test the patient and the faith of a Christian; only God could decide 'to make it leave through medicine [...] and other things made effective by him' ('di farla partire per il mezzo delle medicine [...] e altre cose da Lui fatte efficaci'). See the volume published by Vincenzo Valgrisi that contains: *Simolachri, historie, e figure de la morte. La medicina de l'anima [di Urbanus Rhegius]. Il modo, e la via di consolar gl'infermi* (*Depictions, Stories, and Figures of Death. The Medicine of the Soul [by Urbanus Rhegius]. The Method and the Way of Consoling the Sick*), see in particular the section: *Il chiamare i medici e usar le medicine nelle malattie non essere peccato* (*Calling physicians and using medicine for diseases is not a sin*).

8 Ibid., in the chapter *De la consolazione Evangelica, e come ogni nostra salute, perdono, e remission de peccati sia in Cristo* (*On the consolation of the Gospel and how all our health, absolution, and remission of sins is in Christ*).

9 *La medicina dell'anima* was followed by an *Oratione a Dio da dirsi appresso l'ammalato mentre si visita* (*Prayer to God, to be recited while the sick person is examined*), which reminded the physician or the invalid's relative of their duty to provide comfort through the subject of the "benefit" of Christ, 'who paid dearly on the wooden Cross, not only for this sick man but also for all the rest of us' ('il quale ha pagato il fio su il legno de la Croce, non pur per questo infermo, ma etiandio per tutti noi altri'). On the *Beneficio di Cristo* see Massimo Firpo, *Tra alumbrados e "spirituali". Studi su Juan de Valdés e il Valdesianesimo nella crisi religiosa del '500 italiano* (Florence: Olsckhi, 1990); idem, 'Il *Beneficio di Christo* e il concilio di Trento (1542–1546),' in *Rivista di storia e letteratura religiosa*, 31 (1995), 45–72; Giorgio Caravale, 'Il *Beneficio di Cristo* e l'Inquisizione romana: un caso di censure tardive,' in *Cinquant'anni di storiografia italiana sulla Riforma e i movimenti ereticali in Italia (1950–2000)*, Susanna Peyronel ed. (Turin: Claudiana, 2002), 151–73.

10 See Silvano Cavazza, 'Libri in volgare e propaganda eterodossa: Venezia 1543–1547,' in Adriano Prosperi, Albano Biondi (eds.), *Libri, idee e sentimenti religiosi nel Cinquecento italiano* (Panini: Modena, 1987), 22.
11 Massimo Firpo, *Vittore Soranzo vescovo ed eretico: riforma della Chiesa e inquisizione nell'Italia del Cinquecento* (Rome-Bari: Laterza, 2006), 296. On Vincenzo Valgrisi, see Ilaria Andreoli, entry 'Valgrisi, Vincenzo,' in *Dizionario Biografico degli Italiani*, 98 (2020). The Valgrisi storehouse was located near the church of Santi Giovanni e Paolo, which was also the area where Donzellini's book-related activities were concentrated. 1277 forbidden books were found there in 1564 during the searches in relation to the promulgation of the Tridentine Index.
12 On the Giunta family and their activity in the context of the Venetian heterodox movement see Firpo, *Artisti, gioiellieri, eretici*, 102–06.
13 On Gadaldino, see this chapter, infra.
14 Perini, *La vita e i tempi*, 72.
15 Ibid., 73.
16 Letter from Pietro Perna to Donzellini, dated 13 November 1550, ASV, Sant'Uffizio, *Processi, Contro Girolamo Donzellini*, Bu. 39, 1r. On Curione, see Lucio Biasiori, *L'eresia di un umanista. Celio Secondo Curione nell'Europa del Cinquecento* (Rome: Carocci, 2015).
17 Brian Pullan, 'La nuova filantropia nella Venezia cinquecentesca,' in Bernard Aikema, Dulcia Meijers (eds.), *Nel regno dei poveri. Arte e storia dei grandi ospedali veneziani in età moderna, 1474–1797* (Venice: Arsenale editrice, 1989), 22.
18 Richard Palmer, 'L'assistenza medica nella Venezia cinquecentesca,' in Aikema, Meijers, *Nel regno dei poveri*, 35.
19 On Postel see Marion Kuntz, *Guillaume Postel: Prophet of the Restitution of All Things, His Life and Thought* (La Haye: Martinus Nijhoff, 1981); Yvonne Petry, *Gender, Kabbalah and the Reformation: The Mystical Theology of Guillaume Postel (1510–1581)* (Leiden: Brill, 2014).
20 Pullan, *La nuova filantropia*, 24. On pauperism in the early modern world see Marina Garbellotti, *Per carità: poveri e politiche assistenziali nell'Italia moderna* (Rome: Carocci, 2013).
21 ASV, Sant'Uffizio, *Processi, Contro Zanetto barberotto dell'Ospedale dell'incurabili*, deposition by Giorgio Veneto on 14 February 1568.
22 Ibid.
23 On Cipolla's medical work at the hospital, see Palmer, *L'assistenza medica*, 40, 42. On his heretical activity, see Alessandra Celati, '*Contra medicos*: Physicians Facing the Inquisition in Sixteenth-Century Venice,' *Early Science and Medicine*, 23, no. 1–2 (2018), 96–97.
24 In addition to the case of Zanetto Cipolla at the *Ospedale degli Incurabili*, evidence of heretical infiltration can also be found at the *Ospedale di San Giovanni e Paolo*, for example in the experiences of its apothecary, Francesco Castellano, on which see ASV, Sant'Uffizio, *Processi, Contro Francesco Castellano speziale*, Bu. 32, and its steward, Antonio Columban; ivi, *Contro Antonio Columban*, Bu. 22. Both believed in radical doctrines that denied the trinity (Columban) or rejected the difference between the "law" of Christians, Turks, and Jews (Castellano). They also read and exchanged books such as *Pasquino in estasi* (*Pasquino in Ecstasy*). On Castellano, see Celati, *Contra medicos*, 97–98.
25 Quaranta, *Medici italiani*, 90.
26 On the relationships between England and Italian religious dissenters, see Diego Pirillo, *The Refugee-Diplomat: Venice, England, and the Reformation* (Ithaca,

London: Cornell University Press, 2018). See in particular chapter 2 (29–55) on the English embassy in Venice.

27 Maggi had worked in France and Turkey, see: ASV, Sant'Uffizio, *Processi, Fascicolo no. 3*, Bu. 11, 11 July 1553, testimony of Caterina Colbertalda.

28 Filippo De Vivo, 'La farmacia come luogo di cultura: le spezierie di medicina in Italia,' in Maria Conforti, Andrea Carlino, Antonio Clericuzio (eds.), *Interpretare e curare. Medicina e salute nel Rinascimento* (Rome: Carocci, 2013), 129–44.

29 Filippo De Vivo, *Information and Communication in Venice* (Oxford University Press: Oxford, 2007); idem, 'Pharmacies as Centres of Communication in Early Modern Venice,' in Sandra Cavallo, David Gentilcore (eds.), *Spaces, Objects and Identities in Early Modern Italian Medicine* (Hoboken: Blackwell Publishing, 2007), 505–21. The phenomenon was not limited to Venice. For example, heterodox groups met at *spezierie* owned by Viano de Viani in Viadana and Giuseppe Ranialdi in Bologna. In Modena, a city that was particularly active in the spread of heterodox doctrines, the *bottega* of Pietro Curioni, a 'plague doctor' ('medico di piaghe'), served as a meeting place, while the heretical meetings of the *Accademia Modenese* were held at the *spezieria* owned by the family of the founder, the physician Giovanni Grillenzoni; Archivio di Stato di Modena, *Inquisizione*, Bu. 5, 22; Matteo Al Kalak, *L'eresia dei fratelli, Una comunità eterodossa nella Modena del Cinquecento* (Rome: Edizioni di Storia e Letteratura, 2011), ad indicem and in particular 21, footnote no. 70. Finally, the Anabaptist Pietro Manelfi testified that he had discussed matters relating to faith at *spezierie* in Ferrara and Venezia.

30 ASV, Sant'Uffizio, *Processi, Contro Girolamo Donzellini*, Bu. 39, 13v.

31 It would be quite an undertaking to comprehensively reconstruct (and pinpoint) the phenomenon as it appears in Inquisition documents. Instead, here follows a brief sample of cases: in addition to what is outlined in the text, we know that in 1549 the *speziale* Camillo Orsin from Milan denied the presence of Christ in the Eucharist in his *Spezieria all'Orsa* (ivi, *Contro Camillo Orsin Milanese*, Bu. 7); in 1551, Emiliano Bonifacio, a *speziale* in *San Foca* persuaded a small audience that Purgatory did not exist and that the doctrine of free will was unsustainable by reading from the Bible (ivi, *Contro Emiliano Bonifacio*, Bu 9); in the mid-1550s, the apothecary at the *Spezieria alla Chioccia* was forced to recant (ivi., *Contro Marco Jacomo Darina*, Bu. 15); in around 1560, heretical conversations were often conducted at the *Spezieria al Cagnoletto* (for which the owner's father was tried), at the *Spezieria del Pardo*, at the *Spezieria all'Insegna di San Rocco*, popular among workers (for which Domenico Gottardo was tried; ibid., *Contro Domenico Gottardo*), at the *Spezieria alla Duchessa*, where the preacher from the Frari converted the owner, Francesco, who was later tried (ibid., *Contro Francesco Speziale*); and at the *Spezieria all'Aureola* and *Spezieria allo Spinon*, where Teofilo Panarelli denied the value of the invocation of saints (ivi, *Contro Teofilo Panarelli e Ludovico Abioso*, Bu. 23, 12 June 1567, deposition by Andrea Calatario). In 1574, Bernardin Legge, the apothecary at the *Spezieria alle Tre Colonne*, was denounced for his 'diabolical art' ('arte diabolica'); ivi, *Contro Bernardin Legge*, Bu. 38.

32 Ivi, *Contro Teofilo Panarelli e Ludovico Abioso*, Bu. 23, deposition by Ludovico Abioso, 24 May 1568.

33 Ivi, *Contro Giambattista Gemma*, Bu. 37, testimony by Marcantonio Gemma sr, 11 October 75.

34 Philippe Braunstein, 'Cannaregio, zona di transito?,' in Donatella Calabi, Paola Lanaro (eds.), *La città italiana e i luoghi degli stranieri (XIV-XVIII secolo)* (Rome – Bari: Laterza, 1998), 52–62. Heresy could propagate following the

social urban fabric; see also Martin, *Venice's hidden enemies*, 91, which locates radical artisans in San Moisè, close to San Marco.

35 ASV, Sant'Uffizio, *Processi, Denuncia contra Caterina 1574* [in *Contro Giambattista Gemma*], Bu. 37, complaint by Ottaviano Navarta.

36 These included Gian Battista Michiel, who will feature again in Chapter 5.

37 ASV, Sant'Uffizio, *Processi, Contro Teofilo Panarelli*, Bu. 32, deposition of 20 November 1571.

38 Ivi, *Contro Giambattista Gemma*, Bu. 37, 1v

39 Ivi, *Contro Gasparo Parma*, Bu. 25, 26r.

40 Ivi, *Contro Vincenzo Negroni medico*, Bu. 22, testimony by Antonio Mercadante, 22 March 1567.

41 On the Church of the Santi Apostoli and Ochino's experience, see Michele Camaioni, *Il Vangelo e l'anticristo. Bernardino Ochino tra francescanesimo ed eresia (1487–1547)* (Bologna: Il Mulino, 2018), 347–66, especially 354–55. Thanks to Dr Camaioni for providing me with this information about the church before the publication of his book, thereby allowing me to further my research.

42 Ibid., 355–57. The definition 'contaminated' comes from Dionigi Zanettini, known as *Il Grechetto*, who described the group thus in a letter to Rodolfo Pio dated Venice, 14 January [1546], cited in Karl G. Bushbell, *Reformation und Inquisition in Italien um die Mitte des XVI. Jahrhunderts* (Paderborn: Druck und Verlag von Ferdinand Schöningh, 1910), quoted in Camaioni, *Il Vangelo*, 355.

43 'I started having bad religious views after hearing two or three sermons by Master Marian of Crema in the church of the Santi Apostoli three years ago. Since then, I have gone from bad to worse, persisting with these wicked opinions' ('Il principio di questa mal opinione che vedo che fusse due over tre prediche che fecer quel maestro Marian da Crema in San Apostolo da tre anni in circa e da quella volta in qua se pur sono andato de male in peggio continuando in questa mala opinion'); ASV, Sant'Uffizio, *Processi, Contro Stephano medico de Gardon*, Bu. 8, deposition of 13 December 1550. The subject of preaching heterodox content either directly or indirectly is too broad to be addressed here. See to this end Giorgio Caravale, *Preaching and Inquisition in Renaissance Italy: Words on Trial* (Leiden-Boston: Brill, 2016). It is worth mentioning, however, the Church of San Cassiano, where Giulio da Milano preached the Lent sermons in 1541, which led to his arrest, and the Observant Franciscan church of San Francesco della Vigna, home to the theologian and cabalist Francesco Zorzi. The latter was the author of the *De harmonia mundi* (*On the Harmony of the World*, Venice, 1525) and the treatise *In Sacram Scripturam problemata* (*Problems in the Holy Scriptures*, 1536), in which he expressed doctrines comparable to Latitudinarianism and discussed the chances of salvation for those who had not received Christ. Although these doctrines were not Reformed, they were considered heterodox, and Zorzi's works were subsequently censored.

44 ASV, Sant'Uffizio, *Processi, Contro Agostino di Modena Medico*, Bu. 17, testimony by Gian Battista dal Cairo, 16 October 1563.

45 Ivi, *Contro Girolamo Donzellini*, Bu. 39, 31v.

46 Dionora alternated between this church and San Francesco della Vigna. ASV, Sant'Uffizio, *Processi, Contro Dionora Calia*, Bu. 21, deposition of 16 July 1566.

47 On the diffusion of heterodox ideas among aristocrats, see Federica Ambrosini, *Storie di patrizi e di eresia nella Venezia del '500* (Milan: Franco Angeli, 1999).

48 ASV, Sant'Uffizio, *Processi, Contra Pre Fidelem*, Bu. 23, 54v. Don Fedele was born in the Marche region. He was put on trial and died in prison in 1568. About him see Ambrosini, *Storie di patrizi*, ad indicem.

49 Patricia H. Labalme, 'Women's roles in early modern Venice. An Exceptional Case,' in eadem (ed.), *Beyond Their Sex: Learned Women of the European Past* (New York: New York University Press, 1980), 129.
50 On this subject see Stanley Chojnacki, *Women and Men in Renaissance Venice. Twelve Essays on Patrician Society* (Baltimore: John Hopkins University Press, 2000); idem, 'La posizione della donna a Venezia nel Cinquecento,' in *Tiziano e Venezia. Convegno internazionale di studi (Venezia 1976)* (Vicenza, Neri Pozza, 1980).
51 On Venetian women's sixteenth-century fashion see Alvise Zorzi, *La vita quotidiana a Venezia nel secolo di Tiziano* (Milan: Rizzoli, 1990), 38–39.
52 Labalme, *Women's roles*, 134–35.
53 On the manufacturing industry in Venice, see Frederic Lane, *Storia di Venezia* (Turin: Einaudi, 2015, first edition 1973) 355–68.
54 Monica Chojnacka, *Working Women of Early Modern Venice* (Baltimore: John Hopkins University Press, 2001), 19. See below the case of Caterina Colbertalda and infra, Chapter 5.
55 Moreover, the Inquisition records document various trials for heresy against women in sixteenth-century Venice, although no inventory or systematic study has ever been attempted. Some of these are cited in Chojnacka, *Working women*, others in Ambrosini, *Mediterranean Urban Culture*. See also the trial against Caterina Sauli and Isabella Frattina. Outside Venice, the best-known cases are those involving heretical noblewomen such as Giulia Gonzaga, Vittoria Colonna, and Caterina Cybo (all involved in Spiritual circles), and above all Renée of France. The latter's court was also the scene of the extraordinary religious and intellectual experience of Olympia Morata. On Renée, see Belligni. On Olympia, see Lisa Saracco, entry 'Morato Olimpia Fulvia' in *Dizionario Biografico degli Italiani*, 76 (2012); Lucia Felici, 'Olympia Fulvia Morata: 'Glory of Womankind both for Piety and for Wisdom',' in Lavenia, Zwielein, *Fruits of Migration*, 147–77.
56 ASV, Sant'Uffizio, *Processi, Contro Gasparo Parma*, Bu. 158, 26r.
57 Ivi, *Contro Girolamo Donzellini*, Bu. 39, 134v.
58 Ibid., 134r.
59 Federica Ambrosini, *L'eresia di Isabella. Vita di Isabella da Passano, signora della Frattina (1543–1601)* (Milan: Frnaco Angeli, 2005), ad indicem and in particular 76–78.
60 Ibid., ad indicem.
61 See infra, Chapter 5.
62 ASV, Sant'Uffizio, *Processi, Contro Girolamo Donzellini*, Bu. 39, f. 124*r*.
63 Ibid., 123v.
64 Ibid., 124r.
65 Ibid., 136v.
66 'It'll be twenty-four years this April since I left the convent. When I entered, I was really little and in reality I did not want to go; I played with dolls and my heart was never in it' ('Credo che sto avril sia compiuto 24 che sono ussita "dal convento" et quanto andi dentro era puta puta de fatto che non ghe voleva andar, che ziogava alle piavole, ma mai el mio cor è stato cotesto'); ibid., 137*v*.
67 Ibid., f. 138v.
68 On the condition of female convents in Venice, see Zorzi, *La vita quotidiana a Venezia*, pp. 266–69.
69 ASV, Sant'Uffizio, *Processi, Contro Girolamo Donzellini*, Bu. 39, 127r.
70 Ibid., 129v.
71 Ambrosini, *Storie di patrizi*, 191.

72 ASV, Sant'Uffizio, *Processi, Contro Elena De Freschi Olivi*, testimony by Paola Marcello, 27 March 1555, Bu. 12.

73 'You can obtain information from Gasparo Parma and his wife, and also from Mr Girolamo Donzellini and Mrs Caterina Strozza, who is with the aforementioned physician' ('Potete informarve da detto Gasparo Parma e da sua moglier e ancho da messer Hieronimo Donzellino medico et da madama Caterina strozza che sta con el ditto medico'); ivi, *Fascicolo no. 3*, Bu. 11, testimony by Caterina Colbertalda, 18r.

74 Martin, *Venice*'s *Hidden Enemies*, 47.

75 Colbertaldo, in the Treviso area.

76 ASV, Sant'Uffizio, *Processi, Contro Pietro De Megis*, Bu. 12; ivi, *Fascicolo no. 3*, Bu. 11, testimony by Caterina Colbertalda, 14r.

77 ASV, Sant'Uffizio, *Processi, Contro Pietro De Megis*, Bu. 12, complaint against Pietro De Megis.

78 On the relationship between medicine, hermeticism, religion and the jewish world see Germano Maifreda, *Italya. Storie di ebrei, storia italiana* (Rome-Bari: Laterza, 2021), 45–48.

79 ASV, Sant'Uffizio, *Processi, Contro Elena De Freschi Olivi*, testimony by Paola Marcello, 27 March 1555, Bu. 12.

80 ASV, Sant'Uffizio, *Processi, Denuncia contra Caterina 1574* [in *Contro Giambattista Gemma*], Bu. 37, 11 October 1575, deposition by Caterina [Colbertalda] Sartora. The identification of Caterina Colbertalda with the woman who is called 'la Sartora' twenty-five years later is made possible by the reference that Sartora makes to her first marriage to Pietro De Megis.

81 Nicholas Terpstra, *Ragazze perdute. Sesso e morte nella Firenze del Rinascimento* (Rome: Caroccci, 2010), 130.

82 Vincenzo Maggi's sister, Laura, was the wife of Donzellini's old friend Giovanni Andrea Ugoni, tried by the Inquisition in 1565. She might also have facilitated the friendship between Vincenzo and Girolamo.

83 ASV, Sant'Uffizio, *Processi*, Bu 11, testimony by Caterina Colbertalda, 18r.

84 Ibid., 17v.

85 The book is the Italian vernacular version of a Protestant Dutch work by the Lutheran theologian Heinrich Bommelius. It was printed for the first time in Modena by the members of the Academy without any information about the year and the publisher. Many copies of the book were burnt in 1538. See Cesare Vasoli, 'Il processo per eresia di Oddo Quarto da Monopoli,' in Civitas Mundi. *Studi sulla cultura del Cinquecento* (Florence: Olschki, 1996), 157; Peyronel Rambaldi, *Dai Paesi Bassi all'Italia*.

86 ASV, Sant'Uffizio, *Processi, Fascicolo no. 3*, Bu. 11, testimony by Caterina Colbertalda 17v, 18r; 'He has some books at home like the *Benefit of Christ Crucified*, the *Charon* and the New Testament, and also has another great book, and it is said that they are prohibited' ('lui ha delli libri in casa, come el Beneficio di Cristo, il Caronte et Testamento novo, et ha un altro libro grande che si dice che sono prohibiti').

87 'Sintesi efficace tra misticismo e razionalismo, predestinazionismo e pelagianesimo,' Belligni, *Renata di Francia*, 312.

88 After Bresciani converted to the Reformation in the early 1540s, he was tried for heresy in Milan in 1547 and sentenced to life imprisonment. However, he somehow managed to escape this punishment as he was later involved in religious dissent once again, first in Cremona and then in Chiavenna, where he frequented the radical circles associated with Camillo Renato. On returning to Italy, he appeared before the Holy Office and abjured, but subsequently became a member of Giorgio Siculo's heretical group. He avoided the trials against

Siculo's followers in the late 1560s by fleeing, probably travelling abroad again, after which there are no more traces of him; on Bresciani, see John Tedeschi, 'Bresciani, Pietro,' in *Dizionario Biografico degli Italiani*, 14 (1972); Federico Chabod, *Lo Stato e la vita religiosa a Milano nell'epoca di Carlo V* (Turin: Einaudi, 1971), ad indicem, in particular 337–41. Florio was also a member of Giorgio Siculo's sect and had contact above all with Francesco Severi, a physician from Argenta with whom he discussed the *Libro grande* even after the death of their leader. He was involved in the major trial against Siculo's followers in 1567–1568 and was sentenced to perpetual imprisonment on 29 August 1568. His sentence was subsequently reduced and in 1574 he was allowed to 'take off his *abitello* [a penitential garment] and practice medicine publicly' ('deposto l'abitello possi medicare pubblicamente'); Adriano Prosperi, *L'eresia del Libro Grande. Storia di Giorgio Siculo e della sua seta* (Milan: Feltrinelli, 2000), 271–81, 448 footnote 88. On Severi, see ibid., ad indicem and Archivio della Curia Patriarcale Venezia, Archivio Segreto, *Inquisizione, Contro Francesco Severi*, Bu. 2, (on 83r there is a description of the book-based relationship between Florio and Severi), see also infra, Chapter 5. Giudici was Duchess Renée's confidant. After joining Siculo's sect, he was sentenced to death in 1567. Before the trial, he supported Siculo's supposed successor, a monk named Stefano, along with Pietro Bresciani. He also safeguarded the writings used by the monk to reveal the secret of his divinity, before repenting and realising the deception thanks to guidance from Nascimbene Nascimbeni; see Carlo Ginzburg, *Due note sul profetismo cinquecentesco,* (Naples: Edizioni scientifiche italiane, 1966), ad indicem; Prosperi, *L'eresia del Libro Grande*, ad indicem, in particular 280.

89 Ibid., 264–65.

90 Ibidem.

91 Ibid., 271.

92 See the aforementioned letter sent to Donzellini by Pietro Perna on 13 November 1550, which first refers to a man from Verona for whom the physician made arrangements to stay with 'messer Cel.' in Basel and then sends greetings from 'messer Celio' and his family. ASV, Sant'Uffizio, *Processi, Contro Girolamo Donzellini*, Bu. 39, 1r. The letter was used as evidence against Donzellini in the 1560 trial.

93 Ibid., 50r.

94 Massimo Firpo, *Dal sacco di Roma all'Inquisizione. Studi su Juan de Valdés e la Riforma italiana* (Alessandria: Edizioni dell'orso, 1998), p. 113.

95 ASV, Sant'Uffizio, *Processi, Contro Giulio Basalù*, Bu. 13, list of 'nominati per d. Iulium Basalù.'

96 Addante, *Eretici e libertini*, 25–30.

97 Juan de Valdés, *Le cento e dieci divine considerazioni di Giovanni Valdesso,* Eduard Boehmer (ed.), (Halle: Ploetz, 1860 – first edition 1550), 266.

98 When Donzellini recanted before the judges after his third trial for heresy, he repented for denying the authority of the pope, the intercession of saints, and ritual fasting. He also rejected the belief that Mass was no 'more than a memory of the sacrifice made by Our Saviour on the cross' ('altro che memoria del sacrificio fatto dal salvator nostro in croce') and the idea that 'Christians are not bound by the traditions of the Church which are not found in the Holy Scriptures' ('le traditioni della chiesa che non si trovano nella scrittura santa non obbligar li christiani'), ASV, Sant'Uffizio, *Processi, Contro Girolamo Donzellini*, Bu. 39, 182r-183v.

99 It must have been something like a chessboard, with the seven planets arranged vertically and images related to these celestial bodies arranged horizontally, taken from the philosophical, mythological, and religious traditions. Thanks to

the movement and combination of its components, it was supposed to be able to generate new meanings and new knowledge. On Delminio's theatre see Lina Bolzoni (ed.), *L'idea del Theatro con "l'idea dell'eloquenza" il "de transmutatione" e altri testi inediti* (Milan: Adelphi, Milano, 2015).

100 For a history of the art of memory, starting from classical sources and moving through the medieval and Renaissance traditions to Descartes, Leibnitz, and the beginning of the eighteenth century, see Francis Yates, *L'arte della memoria* (Turin: Einaudi, 2007 – first edition 1966), in particular 121–60.

101 Ibid., 139.

102 'Una "religio" spiritualistica ed esoterica [...] non molto lontana da alcuni classici documenti contemporanei della "eresia" italiana'; on the connections between the figure and the thought of Giulio Camillo and the world of Italian heterodoxy see Cesare Vasoli, 'Tra retorica, arte della memoria ed eresia: ipotesi su Giulio Camillo Delminio e i suoi discepoli,' *Bollettino della Società di Studi Valdesi*, 138 (1975), 81–95.

103 Massimo Firpo, entry 'Citolini, Alessandro' in *Dizionario Biografico degli Italiani*, 26 (1982).

104 Thanks to Prof. Adorni Braccesi for providing me with information about this figure to supplement Giorgio Stabile, entry 'Camillo, Giulio detto Delminio'; ibid., 17 (1974).

105 Ginzburg, *I costituti*, 48, 70, 71.

106 Historiography has them as brothers. However, Ludovico stated in 1568 that he was 36 years old, meaning that he was born in the early 1530s, while Agostino was born at the end of the fifteenth century. It is therefore more probable that they were father and son.

107 Ambrosini, *L'eresia di Isabella,* ad indicem.

108 Simonetta Adorni Braccesi, 'L'"Agrippa arrigo" e Ortensio Lando: fra eresia, Cabbala e utopismo. Ipotesi di lettura,' «*Historia philosophica. An International journal*," II (2005), 1–17, in particular 109. Agrippa's book was translated into Italian in 1547 by Lodovico Domenichi.

109 Simonetta Adorni Braccesi, *Gaudenzio Merula tra Erasmo e Calvino: ricerche in corso*, in Susanna Peyronel Rambaldi (ed.), *Giovanni Calvino e la Riforma in Italia: Influenze e conflitti* (Turin: Claudiana, 2011), 245–74.

110 ASV, Sant'Uffizio, *Processi, Contro Francesco Stella,* Bu. 7, the complaint is not dated but was probably made in 1549, the year in which the trial against Stella started. However, he was not arrested until ten years later. On Francesco Stella and his heretical activity, see Andrea Del Col, 'Un territorio sotto l'Inquisizione. Conegliano e la diocesi di Ceneda nel Cinquecento,' in Gian Domenico Romanelli, Giorgio Fossaluzza (ed.), *Un Cinquecento inquieto. Da Cima da Conegliano al rogo di Riccardo Perucolo. Conegliano, Palazzo Sarcinelli, 1° marzo - 8 giugno 2014* (Venice: Marsilio, 2014), 48–63, in particular, 53–54. Seidel Menchi describes him as a lawyer (Seidel Menchi, *Erasmo in Italia*, 323), but the sources clearly state that he was a physician.

111 ASV, Sant'Uffizio, *Processi, Contro Francesco Stella,* Bu. 7, complaint against Francesco Stella.

112 Ibidem.

113 Andrea Del Col, entry 'Stella, Francesco,' in Dizionario Biografico degli Italiani, 94 (2019).

114 ASV, Sant'Uffizio, *Processi, Contro Francesco Stella*, Bu. 7, inventory of books seized at the trial of 1549.

115 ASV, Notarile, *Testamenti*, Bu. 194, will of Francesco Stella, 28 April 1560.

116 ASV, Sant'Uffizio, *Processi, Contro Agostino Gadaldino*, Bu. 13.

117 In 1550, to mark the Jubilee, Julius III issued two edicts that established

clemency and private abjuration for anyone who appeared spontaneously before the judges: the prospect of avoiding the humiliating punishment of public recantation and the physical and moral suffering of an inquisitorial trial led many heterodox dissenters to denounce themselves. However, the fact that, in the event of suspected heresy, "spontaneous" appearance was imposed in sacramental confession with the threat of a trial and a death sentence from the Holy Office gave the procedure a coercive character, see Elena Brambilla, entry 'Spontanea comparizione (procedura sommaria),' in Adriano Prosperi, Vincenzo Lavenia, John Tedeschi (eds.), *Dizionario Storico dell'Inquisizione*, vol. 3 (Pisa: Scuola Normale Superiore: 2010), pp. 834–36.

118 On the Giunta edition, see Stefania Fortuna, 'The Latin Editions of Galen's Opera Omnia (1490–1625) and Their Prefaces,' *Early Science and Medicine*, 17 (2012), 391–412; see also O'Malley, *Andreas Vesalius*, which on pp. 102–04 features an English translation of some of Gadaldino's introductory letter to Galen's works dedicated to medical students.

119 'Nevertheless, I do not hesitate to assert that I did everything with the greatest care and diligence, never evading labor or vigilance, and because of my assiduous concern and too-great solicitude I fell into a long and grave illness and for many days and months it was necessary that this task be carried on by another. As a result of my diligence, you have all except the introductory matter, spurious works, and a large part of the fifth section of the work, of which the corrections and emendations were overseen by that learned who substituted in my place. If you should find anything in these works that may seem to have slipped by with too little consideration and that does not fully satisfy your very sharp judgment, I beseech you to ascribe it to lack of time rather than to any lack of diligence on my part, and – such is your kindness- that you will pardon me who, with whatever knowledge and capability I possess, and I freely confess that it is slight, was responsible for all this'; ibid., 104.

120 ASV, Sant'Uffizio, *Processi, Contro Agostino Gadaldino,* Bu. 13, deposition by Gadaldino of 3 August 1557.

121 Ibid., spontaneous appearance, 29 July 1557.

122 Ivi, *Contro Giovanni Cassinati, Francesco Gentil da Fermo e Manusso Mariano*, Bu. 27, plea by Manusso Maran, undated (but 1571). Manusso's library was substantial. It consisted of volumes of pasquinades (like the 'songs against the state and ecclesiastical order' ['canzoni contro el stato et ordine ecclesiastico']), philosophy and astronomy books, texts by classical authors such as Cicero and Aristophanes, works by Reformed writers like Melanchthon, Brucioli and Castellio, as well as writings by Agricola, Machiavelli, and Erasmus. Manusso had the latter's critical edition of the New Testament, commentaries on the Acts of the Apostles, and the *Adagia* (*Adages*); ibid., 'inventario delli scritti et libri eretici ritrovati in mano di Manusso Maran.'

123 Silvano Cavazza, entry 'Goineo, Giovan Battista,' in *Dizionario Biografico degli Italiani*, 57 (2001).

124 On Goineo see ASV, Sant'Uffizio, *Processi, Contra Ioannem Baptistam Goyneum*, Bu. 4; ivi, *Pirano, comunità*, Bu. 8, passim.

125 See infra, Chapter 5.

126 We know that this was his last stopover because he received a letter from Traian da Crema dated 4 December 1553 while he was in Orzi Nuovi. The missive was about the purchase of a horse, for which he acted as an intermediary; ASV, Sant'Uffizio, *Processi, Fascicolo no. 3*, Bu. 11, "sottoscritture." In 1554, he was already in Tübingen.

3 The diaspora

In a letter to his father included in his Inquisition trial, Girolamo Donzellini explained that

> driven by the enemies of God, […] as I wanted to continue in my usual condition, I would have had to refute Christ and say that His divine doctrine was heretical, and in the end I would have had to become a renegade Christian ('condotto dalli nemici de Dio, […] volendo io perseverar nel mio stato come prima, bisognava che ve negasse Christo et che decesse che quella dottrina che egli ha posto di cielo fosse heretica, et finalmente che io deventasse un christiano renegato').[1]

His only remaining option was to leave Italy and he fled at the beginning of 1554. This chapter focuses on his experience as a religious refugee, in the wider context of Italian physicians' religious exiles.

3.1 Italian physicians and religious migration

The sixteenth century was characterised by a high level of mobility, which had significant repercussions on cultural and intellectual history.[2] Voyages of exploration and conquest took Europeans to new worlds. New commercial outposts were established by consolidating trade routes and a network was thus created linking cities like Antwerp, Lisbon, and Seville to Africa and Asia. In the same period, the ongoing diaspora of Iberian Jews reshaped the ways in which Europeans cohabited with the 'other,' often to a dramatic extent.

The confessional rift in Europe was a significant mobility trigger too. Migrants were driven both by religious repression, with large numbers moving from the Catholic south to the Protestant north, and the confessional uniformity triggered by the principle of *Cuius regio, eius religio* (1555), which forced families and individuals to move from one region of Central Europe to another. All this mobility facilitated the long-term spread of different forms of knowledge over a wide area. Ideas and books travelled across Europe together with merchants and migrants on their

DOI: 10.4324/9781003218852-4

horses, carts, and carriages. Discussions and exchanges ensued at fairs and whenever the opportunity arose: travellers at inns and hostelries, chance encounters at Alpine passes, and correspondence between migrants and their contacts back home. This was the environment that Donzellini and many of his colleagues and fellow believers became part of in the mid-sixteenth century.[3]

Protestant lands could only be reached after tiring journeys over Alpine passes, a constant source of fear for travellers. The mountain environment was fraught with dangers and difficulties ranging from the weather to encounters with wild animals like bears and wolves, as well as the sense of disquiet triggered by the vast open spaces and unnatural silences of Alpine peaks.[4] Besides these natural perils, wayfarers had to take care not to fall victim to robbers or bandits, ensure that they had sufficient material resources (money, clothes, provisions, and drinks), and learn about their intended routes by securing help from local people or organising themselves in advance. Despite the difficulties inherent in leaving a personal comfort zone, religious exile was an experience shared by many at the time. In recognition of this fact, the heterodox physician Guglielmo Grataroli wrote one of the first known travel guides, the *De regimine iter agentium* (*Regimen of Health for Travellers*). This handbook reflected the author's strong practical spirit and the sense of solidarity among exiles, a group to which he belonged as a native of Bergamo living in Basel.[5] He offered readers practical advice (such as the technique for preserving wine by soaking pieces of bread in it and letting them harden into 'biscuits,' before melting them in water), medical guidance (how to treat sores caused by walking for hours), and magical-spiritual suggestions (spells for warding off demons and evil spirits). He also offered geographical tips: as communication was so vital for travellers, he translated place names that might be needed on a journey from Italy to German-speaking countries from Latin into the local languages.[6]

Migrants were transformed by their journey and the process of acclimatising to a new environment. They not only had to learn a language and adopt new customs and ways of thinking but, from the sixteenth century onwards, were also forced to conform to religious rules, which changed from place to place and had specific behavioural consequences (such as diet).[7] As Rita Mazzei noted, foreigners who were alone, uprooted, and disoriented were more likely to practise dissimulation, adapting to traditions and habits imposed by Churches and states with an agility seldom seen in their homeland. More generally, the experience of life abroad made travellers more adaptable and flexible, with new ideas and beliefs developing rapidly along with religious and ideological affiliations.[8] This pattern is visible in Donzellini's experience too. When he decided to leave the Italian peninsula, he was moved by the strong motivation of preserving his Reformed faith. However, his exile modified his religious attitude and was a decisive turning point in his spiritual and intellectual path.

Girolamo Donzellini shared the same experience with numerous peers and younger colleagues. For many of these émigré physicians, exile marked a point of no return in their professional, scientific, and religious careers. As they all had to engage with new cultural and religious contexts, they redefined the boundaries of their spiritual and scientific leanings. While settling on German soil strengthened Protestant views in some cases, direct contact with the ideas, protagonists, and institutions of the Reformation prompted the majority, including Donzellini, to devise new spiritual solutions or abandon theological discourse altogether. Many did not settle permanently in the Grisons, other parts of Switzerland, or Germany and continued their travels, often moving to the eastern fringes of Europe. These distant, mysterious lands offered a healthy dose of religious freedom and a high level of professional satisfaction and prestige.

It was also common for Italian exiles on Protestant soil to publish works in the fields of medicine, general science, philosophy, or religion. They produced critical-philological editions of ancient texts or distributed Italian works that could not be published in the peninsula (see, for example, Guglielmo Grataroli's contribution to the edition of Pomponazzi's *De incantationibus* [*On Incantations*] printed in Basel).[9] Donzellini followed a similar path, using his friend Pietro Perna's printing press in Basel to publish an edition of orations by the rhetorician Themistius, which we will return to in the last section of this chapter. The extent of the involvement of Italian exiles in the publishing world might suggest that they all endorsed a single cultural programme to disseminate the key themes of the Italian Renaissance – with their radical nuances – in northern Europe. As we will see below, however, the community was actually characterised by strong tensions and controversies that also affected physicians, often putting them against each other and the religious authorities.

The tone and subject matter of the theological works by physicians show their active engagement in the battle against Rome, or their search for new doctrinal solutions. Sometimes their works even demonstrate a detached attitude towards all confessional Churches that champions freedom of belief. In the field of science, exile physicians achieved prominence for their familiarity with the philosophical tradition and their humanistic approach, learned at Italian universities. In some cases, their texts blended medical discourse and religion, offering pastoral care and legitimising their spiritual intervention by referring, for example, to St Luke's experience as a physician, tending to the health of souls by writing his Gospel, and by drawing on the passage in Ecclesiasticus (38:1) that established physicians as God's helpers.[10] The decision to leave Italy strengthened the intellectual liveliness of physicians: applying the instruments of their education and profession to the theological field came as second nature.

3.2 Exile physicians and their networks

The fact that physicians were particularly prone to mobility is a broad, complex phenomenon that cannot be explored in detail here.[11] However, it is worth outlining some common traits and biographical profiles of Italian physicians in exile by analysing their religious militancy and medical work, and by exploring the network of relations they established between Italy and Central-Eastern Europe bound by ties of language, kinship, friendship, religious solidarity, mutual assistance, professional support, and indeed rivalry.[12] This overview will show that exile was extremely common and help to contextualise Donzellini's experience.[13]

The first interesting case is the aforementioned Guglielmo Grataroli, notable for his pragmatic attitude to treating the body and studying nature.[14] He was born in Bergamo in 1516 and graduated in Venice in 1539 after studying at Padua University. He fell afoul of the Holy Office on two occasions and emigrated to Basel in 1550. The city embraced and promoted the most radical and liberal religious ideas, and Grataroli found himself in the minority. He adopted a position that defended Calvin, his doctrine, and the death sentence handed down to the anti-Trinitarian Michael Servetus, triggering a long-running dispute with Sebastian Castellio, the humanist and theologian from Savoy who was a prominent voice of anti-Calvinist dissent.[15] It is possible that Donzellini met Grataroli, either in the Republic of Venice or through the network in Basel. In any case, although they both belonged to the same group of Italian physicians in exile, they did not share the same religious outlook. What united them was their interest in Hermetic philosophy, partly channelled through their publishing collaborations with Pietro Perna. Indeed, Grataroli's most important work, the *Verae alchemiae artisque metallicae, citra aenigmata, doctrina, certusque modus*, (*On the Enigmas, Doctrine, and Certain Way of True Alchemy and the Metallic Art*, Basel 1561), published by Perna, established a connection between medieval alchemy and late Renaissance Hermetic and Paracelsian traditions. Grataroli also explored esoteric and occult disciplines such as physiognomy and the art of memory in his *Opuscola* (Basel, 1554), a collection of texts with a strong Hermetic influence published by Nikolaus Episcopius.[16]

Religious and scientific elements were closely interwoven in Grataroli's work. His books revealed the practical implications of this blend, which derived from his self-perceived status as one of the predestined elects. In the preface to the *Verae alchimiae*, he explained that only those loved by God could explore and understand the secrets of nature and perform alchemical transformations with 'great results.' He also connected his scientific and publishing work to his desire to act for the glory of God, for which he had endured many risks and sacrificed a comfortable life in his homeland. He felt that he was now being rewarded for this, as the Lord had chosen to 'speak' to him rather than to others.[17]

In the historiography on Italian exiles, on the basis of his correspondence and scientific output Grataroli was described as an intransigent Calvinist who was willing to denounce his fellow exiles as heretics to the religious and academic authorities. However, the originality of his work and his contribution to scientific renewal suggest that this is an overly simplistic image.

Indeed, it does not take sufficient account of the education he received in Italy or the potential impact of his experience as an exile. During his university years he was influenced by Paduan humanistic culture with its impetus on open-minded, independent philological research. He developed a particular interest in the thinking of Pomponazzi, whose radical naturalism was a major inspiration for his scientific thought.[18] On Reformed soil, he subsequently strengthened his Calvinist faith and his sense of belonging to those 'loved by God' ('a Deo amati') as a result of his relationship with Calvin (to whom he became a medical consultant) and other reformers like Bullinger and De Bèze, awareness of his sacrifice, and the success of his personal undertaking. At the same time, though, it is apparent that this penchant for free, experimental research into the mysteries of nature stemmed from ideas first nurtured in Italy. Furthermore, given the prevalence of Hermeticism in Basel and in Pietro Perna's circle, it is difficult to believe that Grataroli, as an Italian among Italians on foreign soil, shared such ideas by chance. In these specific circumstances, though, the Hermetic framework was not combined with a tolerant religious approach, as it happened in the case of the Basel group of humanists who were part of Perna's network (about which I will speak in detail below). Instead, it reinforced the understanding that he was on the right side of history and religion.

Giorgio Biandrata, a native of Piedmont, was also deeply involved in the doctrinal disputes. As a specialist in gynaecology, a shrewd politician, and a theological expert, he was a fundamental point of reference in the medical and religious network in Central and Eastern Europe for at least two decades. Born in 1516, he graduated from the University of Montpellier in 1533 and worked in the Polish and Transylvanian courts from the early 1540s to 1552 as a personal physician and adviser to Bona Sforza, Isabella Jagiellon, and King John Sigismund Zápolya. He probably converted to the Reformation in the first half of the 1550s while staying in Lombardy and the Venetian Republic. After he moved to Geneva in 1556, his contact with the Calvinist world prompted him to choose a different path from Grataroli: he abandoned Reformed orthodoxy and took on an active role in developing new theological thought. He became a key figure in the debate triggered by the execution of Servetus, standing in opposition to Calvin's intransigence along with many other Italians.[19] When this dispute heightened, Biandrata fled Switzerland shortly before radical Italians were forced to sign a profession of Trinitarian faith (1558) and returned to Eastern Europe, moving from Pińczów to Kraków and then to Alba Iulia.

The journey from Italy to Poland was especially tough, taking in almost a thousand kilometres of frequently freezing and desolate terrain. However, the large number of Italian exiles who migrated there in the sixteenth century shows that there were valid reasons for undertaking it.[20] Kraków was a major European capital with close ties to Italy in terms of art, architecture, and a range of Renaissance cultural influences (particularly strong links existed with Padua University and the d'Este court). There were also solid diplomatic and trade relations nurtured, respectively, through strategic marriages and the gradual establishment of a sizeable community of Italian merchants.[21] Furthermore, Reformed ideas circulated widely in Eastern Europe. With their diverse blend of communities including Jews, Muslims, Catholics, and Orthodox Christians, these lands boasted a consolidated tradition of peaceful interreligious cohabitation. The combination of this confessional pluralism and a weakened monarchy, undermined by the local nobility, created fertile ground for the success of the Reformation in Poland, Lithuania, and Transylvania.[22]

After making contact with prominent members of the Reformed community, Biandrata exploited the support of the monarch and the local nobility to implement a shrewd political and diplomatic strategy, exerting notable influence on the Polish Reformed Church and carving out a leading role in the process of establishing the Transylvanian anti-Trinitarian Church. As often happened in the medical profession, the religious propaganda he was involved in as an exile was bolstered by the persuasive tools and opportunities for proselytism available to him as a physician (for example, he transmitted radical views to Francesco Lismanini, Bona Sforza's Franciscan confessor, using medicine as a pretext – 'praetextu medicinam').[23] At the same time, he nurtured a close relationship with his royal patients in accordance with the Hippocratic canon, thereby corroborating his excellent reputation at court. After coming to the throne in 1559, King Sigismund Zápolya abandoned Catholicism three years later and, with Biandrata's influence, embraced anti-Trinitarian ideas over the following years. He then agreed to organise public debates on the Trinitarian dogma, culminating in the Edict of Torda in 1567. This stated that 'faith is a gift of God' and prohibited persecution on religious grounds, establishing a regime of coexistence between Catholics, Lutherans, Calvinists, and Unitarians.

In this context, Biandrata also drafted theological works to lay solid scriptural foundations for the new Unitarian Church. His starting premise was that the Holy Scriptures had to be interpreted using rigorous philological criteria and that any dogma not clearly substantiated therein could not constitute an article of faith.[24] In this respect, he collaborated with Ferenc David, co-founder of the Transylvanian Unitarian Church, to publish the *De vera et falsa unius Dei, Filii et Spiritus Sancti cognition* (*On the True and False Knowledge of the One God, Son, and Holy Spirit*, Alba Iulia, 1567), described as 'one of the most important works produced by the Italian and European heretical movement in the sixteenth century.'[25] Biandrata also published the *Antithesis pseudochristi* (*Antithesis of the Pseudo-Christ*, Alba Iulia 1568) and the two-volume work *De regno Christi* and *De regno Antichristi* (*On the Kingdom of Christ* and *On the Kingdom of the Antichrist*, Alba Iulia, 1569). He was clearly familiar with Servetus's *Christianismi restitutio*, one of the founding texts of the anti-Trinitarian tradition, as he borrowed entire passages from it in the latter publication. These anti-Trinitarian manifestos offered a Christological position staunchly opposed to both the Catholic and Protestant stances, emphasising the historical continuity of the anti-Nicene doctrine. Furthermore, Biandrata forged a fruitful friendship with Fausto Sozzini after the latter arrived in Poland, making an active contribution to the Socinian doctrine through their religious discussions. The first Minor Reformed Churches were established from 1565 onwards with Socinian leanings, embodying a successful compromise between Central and Eastern European reform and the Italian tradition.[26]

Biandrata also produced many medical texts, which, unfortunately, have not survived. The titles and basic content of these works can only be accessed through (sometimes unreliable) nineteenth-century commentators like Vincenzo Malacarne. It is known that they were based on the latest major developments in anatomy and the direct observation method of symptomatology, taking gynaecological knowledge in directions previously unexplored by the Aristotelian canon.[27] More generally, in terms of physiological research, Biandrata's focus on the biological dynamics associated with the generation of life reflects a religious yearning to solve the mystery of the relationship between God, man, and creation. He shared this interest with Gabriele Falloppia, an anatomist from Modena who was acquainted with the heterodox world, while the radical Simone Simoni (who we shall return to shortly) also drafted a treatise on the conformation of the foetus (*De partibus animalium* [*On the Parts of Animals*], Leipzig 1575).

Although Biandrata was in his element in noble and princely palaces, he continued to help his persecuted fellow countrymen. He not only recommended colleagues like Niccolò Buccella and Marcello Squarcialupi at court but also sent financial aid to Italian communities, thereby earning a reputation as a man who 'pleases all and embraces everyone, especially the people of this country' ('fa piacer a tutti e abbrazza ogniuno massime del paese de qui').[28] Two thousand ducats were sent to Venice in 1574 by Biandrata and Prospero Provana, a businessman who lived in Kraków. The money was received, counted, and put into circulation through Iacopo Gattis and Decio Bellebuono (a physician to whom we shall return in Chapter 4).[29]

The dispute between Biandrata and Calvin in Geneva needs to be contextualised. Throughout the century, the Calvinist capital held a compelling attraction for Italians as a model of piety, discipline, and harmony. The legendary reputation of the city also spread thanks to the description by Pier Paolo Vergerio in his *Epistola nella quale sono descritte molte cose della città e della Chiesa di Geneva* (*Epistle with Descriptions of Many Things in the City and the Church of Geneva*, Geneva, 1550).[30] Even before this, Bernardino Ochino helped to attract many exiles by describing Geneva as a place without sin or poverty, in which

> every day [...] the Holy Scriptures are read out and explained constantly, and public discussions are held about them where everyone is allowed to say whatever the Holy Spirit suggests in the way that was done in the primitive Church ('ogni dì [...] si legano et expongano di continuo le Scripture sacre et sopra esse si fanno publici ragionamenti, dove a ognuno è licito dire quello che 'l spirito santo li sugerisce al modo che si faceva nella primitiva Chiesa').[31]

In Geneva, Italian exiles shaped a community fully equipped with its own places of worship and religious ministers.

As with all myths, however, the legend of Geneva also harboured a dark side. The city soon became overpopulated, leading to serious consequences in terms of hygiene, health, and provisions with numerous famines and epidemics, including plagues (leading to the establishment of the chair in medicine, first occupied by the exile Simone Simoni in 1567).[32] For Italians, there was the added difficulty of complying with the rigid morality and discipline imposed by the Calvinist Church. They were often punished for their libertine sexual habits or for playing cards, going hunting, or throwing snowballs during religious services.[33] However, playful frivolity was the least of the problems they created for Calvin. While Basel became the driving force of opposition to Calvin over the years, there was also an active group of Italians who were reluctant to embrace the Reformed dogma in Geneva until at least the late 1550s. During the dispute between Biandrata and Calvin in 1558, the physician shared his radical views with other Italian exiles, including two colleagues, Nicola Gallo and Filippo Rustici. Neither caved in to Calvin's pressure on Italians to profess the Trinitarian faith, and while the former was tried with the better-known Giovanni Valentino Gentile from Calabria (who was later executed in Bern in 1566), the latter returned to the fold of the Calvinist Church only when he was threatened with a second exile.[34]

Nicola Gallo is an interesting case not only for his religious radicalism but also because of his background in Sardinia, a culturally backward environment steeped in anticlericalism. Little is known about him, but it is likely that his theological leanings stemmed from personally undertaken research that benefitted from contact with other Italian exiles in Geneva. Born in Iglesias in 1530, he probably first encountered heterodox ideas as a medical student in France. He then emigrated to Geneva and, like many of his colleagues, continued his religious research with an anti-dogmatic spirit, becoming involved in the theological clash. When he was arrested and tried, he was interrogated six times but did not confess his heterodox beliefs. He was subsequently released on condition that he would reappear before the Council of Geneva if summoned. The only other subsequent information available about his life is that his brother joined him in Geneva in 1589.[35]

Rustici, on the other hand, was one of the first to arrive in Geneva in 1555 with his wife and baby. He was married to Caterina, the daughter of a merchant from Lucca, Francesco Cattani, who had emigrated to the same city.[36] Biandrata acted as godfather when a second child was born, showing the close ties between physicians in exile whether for reasons of cultural and professional affinity or shared religious views. Rustici was chief physician (*medico maggiore*) at the hospital in Geneva and practised there during the plague in 1570. As with many heterodox physicians, his experience was defined by an inseparable blend of medicine, religious inspiration, and humanistic culture. He was heavily involved in the 'culture of the book' ('cultura del libro') so dear to sixteenth-century humanists and physicians, epitomised by Donzellini. Indeed, he was a hugely cultured man with a knowledge of ancient languages, including Hebrew, and translated the Psalms into French and both Testaments into the vernacular. According to Rustici, printed books were like 'dead doctors who teach everything that man wants to learn' ('dei dottori morti i quali insegnano tutto quello che l'uom imparar vuole'); they made it possible to 'see and re-examine what someone else has forgotten due to weakness of memory' ('vedere e rivedere quel che per debolezza di memoria altrui si scorda').[37] While this was true in general, printed versions of holy texts were even more valuable as they could be translated into the vernacular languages, thereby becoming instantly accessible to a much larger readership. Driven by this ideological framework, Rustici channelled all his financial resources and intellectual energy into his edition of *La Bibia, che si chiama il vecchio Testamento, nuovamente tradutto in lingua volgare secondo la verità del testo hebreo* (*The Bible, which is called the Old Testament, newly translated into the vernacular language in accordance with the truth of the Hebrew text*, Geneva, 1562). His source text was the Bible translated into Latin by Sante Pagnini, a disciple of Savonarola, whose prologue contained 'an exaltation of the divine word and bitter criticism of all schools of philosophy, fomenters of conflict.'[38] It is surely no coincidence that Servetus had used the same version of the Bible as a point of reference in his theological work.[39]

The *Bibia* was published anonymously four years after the dispute with Calvin, and it is likely that the two events were connected. The underlying aim of the publication was to defend a form of Christianity exclusively based on reading Scripture and the idea that individual believers should be able to determine the principles of their faith. The text showed Rustici's conscious, active commitment to the religious emancipation of his compatriots back in Italy; the introduction featured an 'appeal to the princes and republics of Italy' ('appello ai principi e repubbliche d'Italia'), urging Italian authorities to break free from the Roman 'yoke' ('giogo'). His ties with the motherland were clearly not broken. Indeed, it is possible that they were strengthened by his dispute with Calvin and his awareness that the Swiss Reformation had already taken shape in new authoritarian forms. He thus attempted to involve the Italian political powers in defending the 'poor faithful' ('poveri fedeli'), the 'uneducated and unlettered people' ('degli idioti e delle persone senza lettere') who were deprived of the opportunity to read the Scriptures in the vernacular by the will of Satan, namely the Roman Catholic Church. It was 'blasphemy' ('bestemmia') to claim that only ecclesiastics were capable of understanding the Bible, thereby 'restrict[ing] the efficacy of the spirit of God, who enlightens whomever He wants' ('restringere l'efficacia dello spirito di Dio, il quale illumina chiunque vuole').[40] Rustici recognised the divine origin of the legitimacy of political power, with princes assigned the role of 'lieutenants of Christ' ('luogotenenti di Cristo'). In this capacity, they were entrusted with protecting and supporting the population in both material and spiritual terms. By providing 'spiritual food' ('cibo spirituale') – access to the Holy Scriptures – they enabled people to learn God's will (which was fundamental for the moral and civil stability of society) and understand that the Church had corrupted the holy texts to conceal its prevarication of the Word and will of God. Rustici then made a historical excursus on the ecclesiastical councils and the role played there by the political authorities. His aim was to discredit the coeval Council of Trent, which had not admitted representatives of the Protestant Churches and had been interrupted and moved with the specific purpose of preventing any real doctrinal discussion. Attentive to the burning issues in the religious debate and contemporary politics, he hoped that an Italian assembly chaired by the emperor would be convened, to which 'all the Churches would be allowed to send their ministers to speak freely' ('tutte le Chiese potessero mandar i loro ministri a parlare liberamente').[41] Although he claimed to have adopted a Calvinist stance in the religious controversy, his list of past councils that had protected this fundamental right included a series of cases in which the floor had been given to heresies that denied the Trinity. Albeit through dissimulation, he nurtured the ideas of religious tolerance generated by the debate on the execution of Servetus, and in his 'appeal to the princes' he opposed any form of coercion of conscience.[42] In view of this, it is perhaps not surprising that it was not straightforward for Rustici to obtain an *imprimatur* (printing licence) either for his *Bibia* or his edition of the Psalms. Regarding the latter, the Genevan authorities only granted authorisation to publish the first part. As for the Bible, it did not leave Francesco Durone's printing press until the autumn of 1562 after much 'dithering' ('tentennamenti'), although Rustici had finished it and received a printing permit at the beginning of 1561.[43]

Despite currying favour with the municipal authorities by helping the community and its poorest members through his medical services, he was subjected to disciplinary measures by the Consistory and was even placed in a state of arrest as a result of his uninhibited private conduct. When he was convicted of adultery in 1571, he was sentenced to remain 'for three hours with a noose around his neck' ('per tre ore con il laccio al collo') and imprisoned for twelve days on a diet of bread and water. His legal problems continued six months later when he insulted and slapped a colleague, Charboneau.[44] Such behaviour illustrates Rustici's aversion to Calvinist moral rigidity and his tendency – common practice in the Italian peninsula – to combine heterodox beliefs with libertine sexual practices.[45]

The aforementioned Simone Simoni offers an extreme example of the development of radical ideas that stemmed from Italian academic culture and came to fruition in exile.[46] A native of Lucca twenty years younger than Donzellini, Simoni was a physician and philosopher of European renown with a haughty, polemical character. He graduated in medicine and philosophy at the University of Padua in 1562 and left the peninsula permanently three years later when he emigrated to Geneva. Here he married Angela, another of Cattani's daughters, thus becoming Filippo Rustici's brother-in-law; in exile, the Lucchese community joined forces in kinship ties that were also significant in religious terms.[47]

When Simoni arrived in Geneva, there was no more margin for theological discussion. In 1565, Calvin and Castellio had been dead for, respectively, one and two years, the Italian exiles had lost their theological dispute with the former, and Valentino Gentile, the only protagonist of the conflict that was still alive and active in Western Europe, would be executed the following year. After settling in the Calvinist capital, Simoni first achieved prominence for his immense culture and expertise but soon also attracted attention for a lifestyle that was incompatible with the rules established by the Consistory. While abstaining from worship and attending sermons infrequently, he assembled a group of youngsters around him who shared his opposition to the authority of the pastors. He was eventually forced to leave the city after he clashed with the minister of the Italian Church, Niccolò Balbani (who he defined as an 'ox and a beast'), and Théodore de Bèze, who had even protected him by establishing the first chair in medicine at the university especially for him. He then achieved success and prestige in Paris but was forced to move on again following an edict banning Protestants from holding university chairs. His travels then took him to Basel, Heidelberg, Leipzig, Prague (where he re-embraced Catholicism to obtain the position of personal physician to Rudolf II), Kraków, and Brno. This international mobility was accompanied by doctrinal instability: he converted from Catholicism to Calvinism and then to Lutheranism before returning to his original confession. Throughout these shifts he continued to sympathise with radical positions. As a result, his religious path was interpreted by his peers as that of an 'atheist' ('ateo') whose only god was Aristotle.

In early modern age society, the term 'atheism' was mostly used with derogatory intent to refer to different opinions questioning the existence of God with varying degrees of radicality.[48] What seems indisputable in Simoni's case is that orthodoxy gradually lost its meaning for him, along with any form of religious feeling. Unlike other Italians who settled in Eastern Europe to freely profess their personal faith, which was often individualistic and incompatible with any confession, Simoni effectively returned to Catholicism. That said, he continued to forgo Catholic rituals.

Having seen for himself the bitter dogmatic polemics that afflicted the Protestant Churches, he ultimately renounced any specific affiliation and chose to subscribe to the confession that could guarantee the best social position. The Jesuits, who were attempting to lead Italian exiles in Poland back to Catholicism, were somewhat baffled by Simoni's sarcasm when addressing his Reformed compatriots (claiming, for example, that they would all end up 'roasted' ['arrostiti'] by the Inquisition), or the self-celebratory displays in which he underlined his own intellectual restlessness. This outcome suggests that he did not join the Reformation movement because of any fervent religious ardour but out of necessity and the search for the freedom to philosophise (*libertas philosophandi*). First acquired in Padua, these factors were the underlying driving force throughout his religious and intellectual career. As Simoni stated, his passion for Aristotle's thought derived from the latter's ability to explain reality 'from the foundations of nature' ('ex fundamentis naturae'). This type of philosophical approach also influenced his religious beliefs, which strayed into unbelief as the years passed. As his philosophical, metaphysical, and moral output shows, at the end of his life he probably identified with a 'religion of nature' in which the divinity was no longer identified with the first cause, as established in the scholastic tradition from Thomas Aquinas onwards, or the peripatetic characteristics of immobile perfection and the final cause. It was instead reduced to the 'warmth' ('calore')[49] that animated living beings, while nature itself was glorified as the energy fuelling the whole of reality, the power that guided individual experience.[50] The need to conduct theological research with tools of rational inquiry and to find doctrinal solutions not weighed down by pointless dogmatism led Simoni to transcend the religious problem and focus on understanding creation rather than the creator.

With many of his compatriots settling in Poland, Simoni associated with several Italian physicians who worked at the court. King Stephen Báthory, who had studied in Padua, chose Italian émigrés as his court physicians because he valued their humanistic culture and professional expertise extremely highly. Notable among them was the Paduan Niccolò Buccella, with whom Simoni worked jointly as court physician in Kraków. Since the 1560s, Buccella had rejected Catholicism and converted to Anabaptism, which he practised during his first stay in Moravia (where he put his medical and religious vocation to good use by working in poverty-stricken communities for no remuneration). He was first tried by the Inquisition in 1562 when he came back to Italy. Unlike his fellow believers, he agreed to recant and subsequently adopted a cautious Nicodemite stance, concentrating exclusively on the medical profession and anatomical research. As a graduate of Padua University, he distinguished himself above all for his proficiency and experience in the field of anatomy. In the early 1570s he organised anatomical dissection sessions at his house in Padua which were extremely popular among students (many of whom were German).[51] During the same period, however, he was investigated for the second time by the Holy Office. He soon contacted Giorgio Biandrata with an eye to escaping to Poland and this correspondence was used against him in court when it was intercepted. Buccella only evaded the judges by leaving the peninsula; Biandrata made arrangements so that he 'came gladly' ('venisse allegramente') to Poland and helped him find employment at the royal court.[52] He acquired wealth and prestige in Poland thanks to privileges granted by the king and through other financial and business interests. He also helped his brother and sister to settle with their respective families in Poland and Lithuania. Although he never returned to Catholicism, he also rejected any new confessional affiliation and was described as 'a sect unto himself' ('fa una setta da sé).[53] Like Biandrata before him, he developed a close friendship with Fausto Sozzini, offering him valuable support through his resources.

Shortly after his arrival in Kraków, Buccella was joined by Fabio Nifo, the Aristotelian grandson of the philosopher Agostino Nifo. After studying at the School of Medicine in Padua, Nifo was awarded the chair in practical medicine in 1575, only to be imprisoned by the Inquisition a year later. When his students helped him to escape, he took refuge first in Vienna and then in Poland, where he worked alongside Buccella (who he might have known from his days in Padua). However, the two colleagues quarrelled over medical matters in 1578, and Nifo was forced to move to England. Buccella became embroiled in an even more heated clash with Simone Simoni, with whom he shared responsibility for treating King Stephen Báthory at the end of his life. The king's death triggered a bitter dispute that dragged on for years. When Buccella emerged victorious, Simoni was dismissed from the court and moved to Brno, where he worked for the next two years. After this, he returned to Kraków, where he died in 1602. The sudden death of King Stephen resulted in a reciprocal blame game in which each focused on the other's heterodoxy to discredit his standing as a physician. Marcello Squarcialupi, a physician from Leghorn also in exile in Poland, adopted the same tactic when he joined the quarrel in 1588 by publishing a fierce pamphlet that accused Simoni of atheism, the *Simonis Simonii … Summa religio*.[54] Squarcialupi was less successful than his colleagues in Kraków and never achieved a great professional reputation or financial comfort. Indeed, he continued to relocate throughout his life (moving to Poschiavo, Piuro, Basel, Třebic, Kraków, and Alba Iulia) in search of a settled serenity that he never found.[55] From this point of view, his experience highlights the inherent problems, tensions, and emotional and material effects of the choice of exile, with failure, second thoughts, harrowing family separations, frustration, and even a shipwreck.

Although Squarcialupi had to cope with difficult circumstances, his works and contact network are both noteworthy. Throughout his many hardships he was helped by the German humanist and imperial physician Johannes Crato von Krafftheim and the Swiss scholar and physician Theodor Zwinger. He also collaborated on innovative publishing projects with

Andreas Dudith, the Erasmus of Central and Eastern Europe. After moving to Transylvania in the late 1570s, he gradually lost interest in theological matters and increasingly focused on the realm of science, where he developed an original approach to a variety of interests. Through Dudith, for example, he joined the astronomical debate about the Great Comet of 1577 and contributed to *De cometis dissertationes* (*Dissertations on Comets*, Basel, 1580), which also attracted the interest of Tycho Brahe. He used the text to reassure readers that the comet was not an ominous premonition, stressing that this phenomenon had to be studied in purely naturalistic terms like any other and that comets were stars rather than streams of vapour (as they were perceived in the Aristotelian tradition). He also published another astronomy book, the *De coeli ardore* (*On the Fire of the Sky*, Cibin, 1581), the first work that provided detailed scientific analysis of the aurora borealis.[56] In addition to his astronomical pursuits, Squarcialupi is notable for his interest in the Hermetic tradition, which can be seen in certain events in his life and in his written output. In Basel, he worked for Pietro Perna and Nikolaus Episcopus, two of the most influential printers in the mid-century Hermetic revival. Furthermore, in his *Difesa contro la peste* (*Defence against the Plague*, 1565), Squarcialupi referred to the idea of the man-microcosm – 'another little world' ('un altro picciol mondo') – when speaking of an animated Nature that was living and active, imprinting 'all of the strengths of the soul' ('tutte le forze dell'anima') into human beings. This was a key concept in the tradition of alchemy and Paracelsus.[57]

The shifting views and stances of Simoni and Squarcialupi stand in contrast to Grataroli's solid confessional affiliation and Biandrata's coherence. From the 1570s onwards, Simoni and Squarcialupi found the religious disputes suffocating. Although the former took a far more radical path that subverted Christianity, it is striking that both Tuscan exiles were born in the 1530s and emigrated in the mid-1560s. Compared to physicians from the previous generation such as Donzellini, Biandrata, and Grataroli, both Simoni and Squarcialupi shared a detached and disillusioned attitude towards doctrinal controversies tending towards, respectively, unbelief and religious individualism. While the Counter-Reformation in Italy had accelerated their decision to migrate (they left at around thirty years old, ten years younger than Biandrata or Grataroli when they went into exile), the progressive consolidation of the confessional Churches and the exacerbation of religious polemics did not motivate them to join the conflict (in order to promote anti-Trinitarianism, for instance). Instead, they simply abandoned the field altogether.

This was not the case for Donzellini; like his colleagues born in the 1510s, he never left the religious arena. Unlike Grataroli with Calvinism and Biandrata with Unitarism, however, Donzellini reworked his relationship with religion during his period of exile to focus on tolerance and irenicism. He did not forsake religious militancy per se but relinquished any confessional affiliation. As the next section will show, the religious ideas he encountered in Basel were a key factor in this process; once again, differently from Grataroli, he assimilated them not only into his scientific work but also and above all into his spiritual outlook.

3.3 Donzellini as a religious exile: From Venice to Basel

On Thursday 17 August 1553 at 11 pm, Donzellini arrived home out of breath, packed a makeshift 'bundle' ('fazeto'), left his Venetian abode hurriedly, boarded a ferry, and 'left alone without anyone else' ('si part*iva* solo senza nessuno').[58] Two days later, his housekeeper Caterina Strozzi was summoned by the Court of the Holy Office. The judges asked her for everything she knew about the physician and his friends Vincenzo and Lucrezia Maggi, with whom he had already left the city. As we have already seen, this was the moment when she revealed some important details about Donzellini's network, ideas, and religious practices. Her summons had been issued on the basis of information provided a few days previously by Giordano Ziletti, a bookseller whom Donzellini had known since childhood. Ziletti might have tipped off the Holy Office to divert their suspicions about him and his publishing work; he had already been imprisoned and forced to recant in around 1550 for trading in prohibited books.[59] When the judges searched Donzellini's house, they found numerous forbidden texts. After failing to respond to the summonses that followed in late summer and autumn, Donzellini and the Maggis were banished from the city on 16 December 1553.

As was often the case in the heretical movement, Donzellini was given advanced warning of the trial being prepared against him and managed to escape in good time. He thus evaded persecution thanks to the solidarity network built up over the years and initially took refuge with the English ambassador, Pietro Vanni. Safe in the embassy, he spoke 'to various people' ('con diversi') about the right strategy to adopt in the delicate task of preparing for the trial. However, the verdict was unanimous: he was advised to flee.

Little is known about the details of Donzellini's life in his seven years outside the Republic of Venice. However, the records of his trials in 1560 and 1574, and some letters written during his exile can be used to draw a broad outline of his movements between 1553 and 1560, the year in which he returned to Venice and appeared before the Court of the Inquisition voluntarily. Following the sentence, which was described as 'crueller than death' ('più acerba che la morte')[60] for banishing him from the Republic, he prepared for his long journey by visiting various northern Italian cities in the last few months of 1553. He was already on Protestant soil in 1554 and remained there for six years.

Donzellini's foreign itinerary took in German cities including Nuremberg, Regensburg, and Augsburg, where he held prestigious positions at the imperial court and associated with Giulio Alessandrini and Pietro Andrea

Mattioli, Italian physicians that he had probably already met in Padua. His work also allowed him to extend his support network through individuals that could intervene on his behalf and pave the way for his return to Italy. He duly obtained character references from Cardinal Otto Truchsess von Waldburg, Prince-Bishop of Augsburg, Michael von Kuenburg, Archbishop of Salzburg, and Paolo Tiepolo, the Venetian ambassador. He also met the artist and antiquarian Jacopo Strada in 1558, perhaps in Nuremberg, with whom he shared anti-dogmatic religious sensibilities. After an education in Erasmian humanistic religion, Strada left Italy and his effigy was later burned by the Mantuan Inquisition in 1581. During his life as an exile, he gained the protection of Hans Jacob Fugger and then of the emperor and covered an active role in book distribution throughout Europe. Thanks to his considerable material resources, Strada provided concrete help to his compatriots in exile (such as Mino Celsi and Giovanni Bernardino Bonifacio, Marquis of Oria). Donzellini also took advantage of this patronage.[61] In 1558, Strada arranged for an apologia that the physician had written in his defence to be delivered to Antun Vrančić, Bishop of Eger, who was duly impressed. The document also enabled Donzellini to gain an audience with the emperor, who finally granted the coveted safe-conduct that allowed him to return to his homeland.

Before obtaining prestigious professional positions at court and earning the respect and protection of influential archbishops and the emperor, Donzellini had stayed with Pier Paolo Vergerio, the former Bishop of Capodistria, in Tübingen. Although this is not included in the account of his exile given to his judges in 1560, it is mentioned in a letter that Vergerio sent to Bullinger in 1554. In the missive he described the physician as a prudent man, who fled his homeland for the sake of the Gospel ('propter evangelium') and was well informed about events in Italy.[62] Every defendant accused of heresy had to decide which details should be revealed or hidden in court in order to appear collaborative without giving away too much. As a result, Donzellini also omitted another significant aspect of his exile from Italy: his collaboration with Pietro Perna on an edition of the works of Giovan Battista Da Monte and an original text between 1557 and 1559. There is no evidence that Donzellini actually lived in Basel in the years in question, but it is likely that he stayed there at various times during the period in which he focused on publishing. His friendship with Perna, who helped Italian émigrés by offering work at his printing house, and his acquaintanceship with Celio Secondo Curione suggest that Donzellini was indeed one of the exiles and men of culture who gathered in Basel. Therefore, while he was banished from Venice, Girolamo did not only make contact with influential figures that could intervene on his behalf at the Holy See and the Venetian Senate but also consolidated relations with other Italian religious exiles and German colleagues with whom he remained in contact over the following years (above all Joaquim Camerarius the Younger and Theodor Zwinger). The experience of exile had a dramatic impact on his status as a heterodox physician both in theological and philosophical terms and with regard to his relationship network. When he fled in 1553, he had nothing more than his degree in medicine, a decent professional track record, and a deep-rooted interest in Protestant doctrines. By the end of his experience abroad, however, he had become an internationally renowned physician. His contacts extended from Brescia to Nuremberg, also including Ferrara, Veneto, and Basel, while his religious identity increasingly blurred the doctrinal boundaries to embrace non-denominational spiritualism.

In 1560, Donzellini told his judges that he had been a 'confessionist' ('confessionista'), in reference to the *Confessio Augustana* (*Augsburg Confession*) written by Philip Melanchthon in 1530. At the same time, though, he demonstrated a tendency to interpret the cornerstones of the Reformation personally, by specifying that he had not 'believed *everything* that confessionists say' ('creduto *tutto* quello che dicono i confessionisti').[63] He then abandoned this doctrine during his sojourn in Germany when he was persuaded of the importance of preserving the unity of the Church by a certain Dr Lucrezio and, above all, a book given to him by the latter.[64]

The work in question was the *Concilium Coloniense*, which collected the canons of the provincial Council of Cologne in 1536 and was published together with the *Enchiridion christianae institutionis* (*Manual of the Christian Institution*) by Johann Gropper. The questions addressed at this assembly mostly dealt with the discipline of the clergy, severely criticising their sins while maintaining a soft approach towards Protestants. The fourteen articles on clerical misconduct were extremely similar in tone to Donzellini's anti-ecclesiastical polemic, outlined in his apologia, which expressed disapproval of trading and accumulating benefits, as well as the ignorance, avarice, lasciviousness, and negligence of many men of the Church.[65] At a doctrinal level, the *Concilium Coloniense* tended towards Reformed ideas by asserting the primacy of faith over works. The text affirmed that only those with a pure conscience who embraced the body of Christ with true faith could understand the genuine significance of the Eucharist. It is no surprise that the instigator of the Council, Hermann von Wied, Archbishop of Cologne, abandoned Catholicism completely in 1542 to openly embrace the Lutheran doctrine. The *Enchiridion* discussed justification from positions akin to the Protestant perspective although it stayed in line with the Catholic tradition in ecclesiological terms (and Gropper became a cardinal shortly afterwards). Gropper had clear Erasmian leanings and had participated in the Colloquies of Worms, Hagenau, and Regensburg in the early 1540s in an attempt to repair the rift in Christianity. Blending an irenic theology and ideas for renewal, his text was warmly received by members of the Italian clergy who were open to the idea of reform such as Gian Matteo Giberti, Giovanni Morone, and Vittore Soranzo. Later, however, in the changed Counter-Reformation climate of 1598, the *Concilium Coloniense* was placed on the Index of Prohibited Books by Clement VIII.

It cannot be excluded that Donzellini referred to this work during his trial to define his stance in a way that would be both credible and acceptable to the judges. Nevertheless, it coincided with his religious outlook in several places: there were similarities with the religious and biographical profile of the authors; their openness towards the pillars of Protestant doctrine and opposition to the rift in Christianity; the harsh criticism of ecclesiastical abuse; and the irenic spirit running throughout the work. Donzellini was totally opposed to the confessional controversy. The judges expressed surprise at the 'confessionist' physician's desire to make friends with Catholics, wondering 'how can there not have been religious discord?' Donzellini replied that he did not see why he had to 'break off friendships with those who were also his friends before.'[66] More generally, the desire for religious peace was frequently expressed in his literary and philosophical output.

It was therefore probably after Donzellini encountered Dr Lucrezio and read the *Concilium Coloniense* that he joined forces with the group of radical humanists who gathered at Perna's printing house in Basel. Since Erasmus and Froben's publishing collaboration, which played a significant role in launching the debate on the need to reform the Church, the city was a powerful magnet for humanists and scholars from all over Europe.[67] Located on the bank of the Rhine River and at the junction of several international trade routes between Switzerland, France and Germany, Basel was a great centre for the production and irradiation of advanced knowledge and culture. It was a sixteenth-century 'world city,' culturally restless and economically dynamic;[68] a free city, seen as a 'symbol of finesse, critical spirit, and tolerance,' with a lively programme of cultural activities and academic debate, a booming trade sector, and a thriving publishing industry.[69] In the sixteenth century, its printing industry was the most progressive in Europe and it produced humanistic, political, religious and scientific works, which were frequently subversive of the tradition (books by Postel, Machiavelli, Castellion, Sozzini, Vesalius, Paracelsus, Patrizi just to mention a few). The typographer Johannes Oporinus, who in 1544 published a Latin edition of the Koran, had often trouble with the censorship authorities and Perna was defined as the «most dangerous» printer.[70] The lively and liberal atmosphere of the city attracted numerous religious exiles, who found the opportunity to sustain themselves by being employed as authors, translators, editors, and reviewers in the city printing industry, from where they also drew the resources to start a new social and intellectual life. In the second half of the century, the city provided asylum to those who most stubbornly opposed the intransigence of the new orthodoxies, and it progressively became the capital of the European debate on religious tolerance. In 1544, Sebastian Castellio had moved there and in the following years he gathered a group of exiles who blended humanist rationalism with spiritual, Latitudinarian religiosity. A 'coalition of opinion' ('fronte di opinione') was formed by the Anabaptist leader David Joris, Erasmus's friend Bonifacio Amerbach, the academic Martin Borrhaus, the humanist from Piedmont Celio Secondo Curione, and, at certain times, the preacher Bernardino Ochino and the theologian Lelio Sozzini, as well as Pietro Perna; they were actively engaged in drafting polemical booklets and pamphlets against any form of confessionalism and intolerance.[71] In this way, ideas from the humanistic tradition implemented by the Italian Reformation were kept alive in Basel: the value of doubt, critical thinking, and dialogue; the certainty of God's infinite mercy; faith in the universal nature of the benefit of Christ; and belief in individual opportunities to contribute to salvation in an ethical rather than theological conception of Christian faith. With its atmosphere 'of prophetic inspiration' ('di ispirazione profetica'), the city also offered Donzellini the opportunity to further his knowledge of alchemy and the Hermetic doctrines circulating there.[72] It was during this period that he teamed up with Perna, championing religious tolerance through his own original contribution.

3.4 Donzellini's *On the Continuity of Doctrine since the Origin of the World*

The most significant result of this collaboration was the 1559 Latin edition of the orations of Themistius, the fourth-century Greek rhetorician and commentator on Aristotle (*Themisti Euphradae ... Orationes octo*).[73] The work is augmented by an extensive preface dedicated to Ulderico Fugger that focuses on the philosophical concept of the *docta religio* (learned religion). The physician used this expression to refer directly to the doctrine of *prisca theologia*, which became well known in the fifteenth and sixteenth century during the philosophical Renaissance instigated in Florence by Marsilio Ficino and Pico della Mirandola, but had ancient roots in Christian patristics and works by exponents of late Neoplatonism.[74] The doctrine claimed that there was a learned religion or pious philosophy with homogeneous religious content that had originated at the dawn of time; it was present in all cultural manifestations over the centuries, first embodied by the 'ancient theologians' ('prisci theologi'), Chaldeans like Zoroaster, Jews like Moses, Egyptians like Hermes Trismegistus, and Greeks like Homer, Hesiod and above all Plato. Ficino used this doctrine in Renaissance Florence as the basis for renewing Christianity on a philosophical basis. Aware that theology would wither away into sterile superstition if detached from philosophical thought, and that philosophy without religious content would lead to evil and pride, he equated the two disciplines and identified a perpetual revelation culminating in Christianity. Pico della Mirandola went a step further by using this *pax philosophica* (philosophical peace) to reassert the primacy of philosophy over religion as a guide to the afterlife.

The most recently published precedent to Donzellini's preface was the *De perenni philosophia* (*On Perennial Philosophy*, Lyon, 1540) by Agostino Steuco. This work speculated about the unity of Being and knowledge thereof, mirrored by the close connection between primordial wisdom and the Catholic Christian tradition. After serving as a Canon Regular of the Lateran, Steuco was appointed Bishop of Kisamos (Crete) and Prefect of the Vatican Library; according to Leandro Perini, he was Donzellini's main source of inspiration.[75] The physician knew him personally and referred to his philosophical work directly in the preface. The continuity between the thinking of the Catholic Steuco and the heterodox Donzellini should not come as a surprise. Indeed, Steuco's text, published on the eve of the Council of Trent, was essentially an attempt to heal the wounds in Christianity, adopting an irenic perspective wholly compatible with the physician's views. Furthermore, not too much should be read into Steuco's polemic against Lutherans, who he blamed for the rift within the Church, levelling criticism in moral rather than doctrinal terms. Indeed, he censored his text carefully so as not to arouse the suspicion of the ecclesiastical authorities, and it is significant that the *Cosmopoeia*, his subsequent work written in a similar tone, was prohibited *donec corrigatur* (until corrected) in 1596.

The preface to the orations of Themistius took shape as a short treatise, *De successione doctrinae ab origine mundi* (*On the Continuity of Doctrine since the Origin of the World*), a history of the wisdom (*sapientia*) granted by God since creation.[76] Safeguarded and handed down from one civilisation to another, this wisdom was embodied by the most important thinkers from antiquity to the early modern age and was expressed through their philosophies. The *docta religio* was its most valuable element and Hermes Trismegistus and Philo of Alexandria were its ancient 'supreme masters' ('supremi maestri'). The *doctrine* was embodied in the idea that God, the governor of all things, was 'one, eternal, immobile, immutable, infinite, and omnipotent.'[77] Drawing on the idea of *translatio sapientiae* (transfer of wisdom), Donzellini illustrated that wisdom had been passed on to the Jews, Egyptians, and Greeks from Armenia, Mesopotamia, and Syria. Among the Greeks, Socrates and Plato had been the most notable embodiments of wisdom, paving the way for Christian thought. The former is described by Donzellini as a skilled dissimulator who concealed wisdom behind external ugliness; he secretly safeguarded his wisdom and knowledge of the truth so as not to ignite the envy and hate of the masses against him ('dissimulanter agens […] ac omnino ne gentium odia in se concitaret doctrinam occultavit'). This depiction calls to mind the Nicodemite doctrine, which was certainly familiar to Donzellini from his contact with Valdesian groups, and the portrayal of Socrates in Erasmus's *Sileni Alcibiadis* (*The Sileni of Alcibiades*, which in turn relied on the image painted by Alcibiades in Plato's *Symposium*). According to Erasmus, although Socrates was poor and awkward, and neglected his own appearance, his genuinely philosophical soul made him similar to a god and even comparable to Christ.[78] With regard to Plato and his disciples, Donzellini took his cue from Augustine of Hippo, maintaining that only a few changes were required to become Christian ('paucis mutatis fiunt Christiani'). He reiterated this idea of a congruence between Platonism and Christianity with the modification of a few terms in later writings.

Donzellini outlined that the doctrine was revived in the Roman Empire through Plotinus, Alexander of Aphrodisias, and Themistius, before Christian theologians combined human and divine wisdom to the great benefit of humankind. Then, more recently, the Fall of Constantinople at the hands of the Turks forced learned Greeks into exile, leading them to Italy. At this point, the peninsula became the cultural centre of the Renaissance, the driving force of the revitalised ancient *doctrina*; to this end, Donzellini cited Lorenzo Valla, Marsilio Ficino, and Giovanni Pico della Mirandola as some of its most illustrious exponents. With 'the light of wisdom' ('il lume della sapienza') illuminating Italy, other thinkers who inherited the *docta religio* included the physician Girolamo Fracastoro, the humanist Celio Calcagnini, the Aristotelian Pietro Pomponazzi, whose inclusion is not surprising given the concordist tone of the work, and the Valdesian Marcantonio Flaminio. The doctrine then spread throughout Europe, breaking through confessional barriers. It was adopted by scholars with different theological stances united by the same irenic religious outlook: to name but a few, Erasmus of Rotterdam, Philip Melanchthon, Jacques Lefèvre d'Étaples, Johannes Reuchlin, Heinrich Cornelius Agrippa von Nettesheim, Sebastian Castellio, and Reginald Pole. Neither Luther nor Calvin was included in the ranks of these men, illustrious for their knowledge of languages and their doctrine.

Donzellini's text was the result of his desire to reduce Christianity to the fundamentals of the faith (*fundamentalia fidei*) and his belief in freedom of conscience. There was an ancient precedent to this in the orations that Themistius had addressed to emperors Jovian, Valens, and Theodosius, putting forward reasons for tolerance on the basis of ethics and political expediency. The Byzantine rhetorician rejected the intransigent absolutism employed to coerce consciences at the time. Indeed, he felt that devotion to the Divine was an individual matter that could not be forced and that was above any threat or form of violence: different religious stances had to be respected and reconciled. His aim of creating harmony between Christianity and the ancient religions, and between the different theological positions within the Christian religion was based on the idea that God loved difference and that a good emperor knew how to transform mercy into a virtue for the good of his subjects and to consolidate his power. Replacing sectarianism with humanism would further the supreme good of harmony among men and peace in the empire.

Themistius and Donzellini thus fully shared the same objectives. However, the physician glossed over the part of the discourse on the political and civil utility of tolerance to focus on the religious question, suggesting that dogma should be radically reduced and that the one universal creed should be defined in terms of the *docta religio*. It is likely that Girolamo was inspired to revisit Themistius's work when he saw it included in the historical sources of religious pluralism in Castellio's *De haereticis an sint persequendi* (*Concerning Heretics, whether they are to be persecuted*, Basel, 1554). Donzellini's text provided a militant contribution to the battle waged by the Basel coterie against Calvinist intolerance. However, the reference to the *docta religio* was more than a philosophical guise for expressing an irenic conception of Christianity. The physician's ideal was driven by a spiritualistic fervour that recognised the presence of God with his all-pervasive power and immutable wisdom in every natural, cultural, and historical event. This paved the way for a form of religious individualism that was averse to any kind of orthodoxy.

Through his contact with humanists in Basel, that drew on elements of Neoplatonic philosophy to substantiate their radical spiritualism, Donzellini encountered an esoteric, underground, nicodemitic tradition. While he was familiar with Hermetic ideas from his social circle in Venice, it was in Basel that these influences came to fruition. The Hermetic overtones in the preface to the orations of Themistius establish a link between Donzellini and scholars like Johann Reuchlin, Francesco Giorgio Veneto, and Heinrich Cornelius Agrippa von Nettesheim, as well as humanists with evangelical and irenic – if not openly radical – leanings such as Jacques Lefèvre d'Étaples and Michael Servetus. Over the following years, this spiritual framework guided Donzellini towards absolute inner freedom in his intellectual research and religious experimentation. However, even though he had abandoned the Protestant faith, he was not safe from inquisitorial persecution when he returned to Italy permanently a year after the publication of the orations of Themistius.

Notes

1 Letter quoted in ASV, Sant'Uffizio, *Processi, Contro Girolamo Donzellini*, Bu. 39, 94v.
2 Rita Mazzei, *Per terra e per acqua. Viaggi e viaggiatori nell'Europa moderna* (Rome: Carocci, 2013).
3 The masterpiece on the phenomenon of Italian migration for religious reasons, with a focus on the development of religious affiliation and feeling in changing geographical and historical contexts is Cantimori, *Eretici italiani*. Recently valuable works about religious migration have been published, among which Nicholas Terpstra, *Religious Refugees in the Early Modern World. An Alternative History of The Reformation* (Cambridge: Cambridge University Press, 2013); Lavenia, Zwielein, *Fruits of Migration*; Nicholas Terpstra, *Global Reformations. Transforming Early Modern Religions, Societies, and Cultures* (New York: Routledge, 2019); Peter Burke, *Espatriati ed esuli nella storia della conoscenza* (Bologna: Il Mulino, 2019).
4 Mazzei, *Per terra e per acqua*, 95.
5 Guglielmo Grataroli, *De regimine iter agentium vel equitum, vel peditum, vel navi, vel curru seu rheda* (Basel: 1561 – unknown publisher).
6 Grataroli and his treatise are analysed in detail in Lynn Thorndike, *A History of Magic and Experimental Science*, vol. 5 (New York: Columbia University Press, 1959), 600–16.
7 Mazzei, *Per terra e per acqua*, 131–35.
8 Ibid., 128.
9 Manuela Doni, 'Il '*De incantationibus*' di Pietro Pomponazzi e l'edizione di Guglielmo Gratarolo,' *Rinascimento*, 15 (1975), 183–200; Pietro Pomponazzi, *De incantationibus*, Vittoria Perrone Compagni (ed.) (Florence: Olschki, 2011).

10 On the divine role of the physician, see Guglielmo Grataroli, *De vini natura* (Strasbourg: Theodosius Rihelius, 1565), 284: 'Blessed is the physician to whom God gives knowledge and intelligence, since he is God's ally and assistant' (Felix igitur ille medicus, cui dat Deus scientiam et intelligentiam, quia sit naturae socius et secretarius.' See also the reference to St Luke added by the heterodox physician Girolamo Massari to his *Eusebius Captivus* (*Eusebius the Prisoner*) to justify the publication of the book, a pamphlet against the Inquisition, and his interest in religious matters. As if medicine and religion were two sides of the same coin, Massari reiterated that those who were able to dispense medication that benefitted the health of the body could, in the same way, reveal the true heavenly medicine by following the example of St Luke the apostle, whose involvement in writing his Gospel never overshadowed his medical work. Girolamo Massari, *Eusebius captivus. Sive modus procedendi in Curia Romana contra Luteranos* (Basel: Oporinus, 1553), 7–8. On Massari, see Achille Olivieri, entry 'Massari, Girolamo,' in *Dizionario Biografico degli Italiani*, 71 (2008); idem, 'L'*Eusebius Captivus* (1553) di *Hieronymus Marius* (Massari): sul *De tolerantia* e i movimenti calvinisti del Cinquecento,' in Peyronel Rambaldi, *Giovanni Calvino*, 359–83; Michaela Valente, *Contro l'Inquisizione- Il dibattito europeo, secc. XVI-XVIII,* (Turin: Claudiana, 2009); Lucia Felici, 'Pasquino oltralpe. Gilbert Cousin e un'inedita miscellanea basileese del Cinquecento,' *Rivista storica italiana*, 130, no. 3 (2018), 747–89; Alessandra Celati, 'Heretical Physicians in Sixteenth-Century Italy: The Fortunes of Girolamo Massari, Guglielmo Grataroli, and Teofilo Panarelli,' *Society and Politics*, 12 (2018), 11–31.

11 As medical students, they would embark on a so-called *peregrinatio medica* (medical peregrination) to prestigious European universities (above all in Italy) in order to receive the best teaching and after graduating, they often travelled to take on new professional positions. The phenomenon of religious exile, moving from Italy to Germanic lands, can be considered a sort of inversion of the typical *peregrinatio medica*.

12 On the "Medical Republic," see Ian Maclean, 'The Medical Republic of Letters before the Thirty Years War,' *Intellectual History Review*, 18, no. 1 (2008), 15–30; Siraisi, *Communities*; Suitner, 'Reformation'; Paula Findlen, Suzanne Sutherland (eds.), *The Renaissance of Letters: Knowledge and Community in Italy, 1300–1650* (New York: Routledge, 2020).

13 Around 26% of a sample of two hundred Italian heterodox physicians chose to migrate regardless of whether they were persecuted by the Inquisition. This decision may have been motivated not only by the desire to escape repression but also by the wish to move to tolerant places where they could conduct their own theological research. A survey of the exile destinations suggests a tendency for Calvinist views, with regard to the Magisterial Reformation, and, more generally, the development of alternative ideas to both the Wittenberg and Geneva reformations. While twelve physicians out of forty-nine (the total number of exiles) initially chose to migrate to Geneva, not all settled there for the rest of their lives. Furthermore, 18% of the total (nine physicians out of forty-nine) opted to take refuge – at least temporarily – in Basel, a city known for its broad-minded views, while the tolerant countries of Eastern Europe – Poland, Transylvania, and Moravia – welcomed 20% of the refugees (ten physicians out of forty-nine). See Celati, *Medici*.

14 On Grataroli, see Leandro Perini, 'La *Bibliotheca venalis* di Guglielmo Grataroli,' *Rinascimento*, 7 (1967), 293–308; Alessandro Pastore, entry 'Grataroli, Guglielmo,' in *Dizionario Biografico degli Italiani*, 58 (2002); Ian Maclean, 'Heterodoxy in

Natural Philosophy and Medicine: Pietro Pomponazzi, Guglielmo Gratarolo, Girolamo Cardano,' in Brooke, Maclean, Heterodoxy, 1–29.

15 See the letter that Grataroli wrote to Bullinger on 28 October 1553, the day after the execution of Servetus, in which he defined the Spaniard as a 'pertinacious and proud heresiarch' and reported the first accusations in the city likening Calvin to an executioner. Guglielmo stated that he was ready to defend the good name of Calvin to the death. In fact, although he was aware of the potential adversity that might result from this, he was more careful to 'please God than man.' He expressed an even more extreme position in his letter of 16 November, stressing to Bullinger that Servetus deserved to die not once but twice, as a warning to all those who could not otherwise be persuaded of the absurdity of the views held by the Spaniard, an instrument of the devil. See John Calvin, *Opera quae supersunt omnia*, vol. 14, William Baum, Edward Cunitz, Edward Reuss (eds.) (Brunsvigae: C.A. Schwetschke, 1863–1900), 1840, 1850.

16 The first version of this book was published in Zurich in 1553 by Andreas Gesner, who belonged to the same family of the botanist and physician Konrad Gesner. Grataroli then worked on an updated version of the book, which he published in Basel the following year.

17 'But certainly, those who cannot know, or do not want to know, do not know. God speaks to those to whom he wants to speak.' ('At vero, qui scire nequeunt, aut nolunt, nescinat: cui Deus favere vult, faveat.'); Grataroli, *Verae alchemiae artisque metallicae, citra aenigmata, doctrina, certusque modus* (Basel: Perna, 1561), 2.

18 In the edition of *De incantationibus* edited by Vittoria Perrone Compagni in 2011, she gives detailed account of this influence by focusing on Grataroli's naturalistic works, see Pomponazzi, *De incantazionibus*, 2011.

19 In Geneva, he started his controversy by asking Calvin astute theological questions about the mystery of the incarnation of the Word, the relationship between God the Father and the Son, and the meaning of terms such as *persona, essentia*, and *substantia* (person, essence, and substance) with their underlying implications of anti-Trinitarianism; Caccamo, *Eretici italiani*, 14–15.

20 The cultural relationships between Italy and Poland are also documented by the exceptional case of the female apothecarist Camilla Erculani, who published her *Letters on Natural Phylosophy* in Krakow in 1584 (and was put on trial by the Inquisition as a result). See Camilla Erculani, *Letters on Natural Phylosophy*, Eleonora Carinci (ed.), (Chicago: Chicago University Press, 2019).

21 On the presence of Italian (in particular Tuscan) merchants in Poland in the early modern period see Rita Mazzei, Itinera mercatorum. *Circolazione di uomini e beni nell'Europa centro-orientale (1550–1650)* (Lucca: Pacini Fazzi, 1999).

22 The Polish-Lithuanian Commonwealth was created in 1569. The Voivode of Transylvania, Stephen Báthory, married the Polish princess Anna Jagiellon in 1576 and ascended to the throne of the Commonwealth, assuming the title of Prince of Transylvania, King of Poland, and Grand Duke of Lithuania. On Polish and Transylvanian political history, see Caccamo, *Eretici italiani.*

23 See the letter of 9 April 1559 sent by Vermigli to Calvin to expose and condemn Biandrata's 'poison' ('venenum'); Calvin, *Opera,* vol. 17, letter no. 3042. Lismanini was Minister Provincial of the Franciscans and the Poor Clares in Poland, Secretary to Queen Bona Sforza, and the driving force behind the humanist circle that gathered at court. He formally severed ties with Catholicism in 1553 during a trip to Geneva and became Superintendent of Evangelical Churches in Lesser Poland; see Mazzei, *Per terra e per acqua*, 160.

24 See in particular the dedication to the King of Hungary at the beginning of the *De falsa et vera unius Dei, Filii et Spiritus Sancti cognition*, quoted here from the

English translation: 'We may say that we must refrain to the greatest possible extent from using alien terms and from deviating even to the slightest extent from God's holy pronouncements since it is a dangerous thing to speak even the truth about God if it is not based on His word, and everything that is from outside that Source is cursed.' See Antal Pirnát (ed.), *De falsa et vera unius Dei, Filii et Spiritus Sancti cognitione*, (Utrecht: Bibliotheca Unitariorum, 1988), 49.

25 See Antonio Rotondò, entry 'Biandrata, Giorgio,' *Dizionario Biografico degli Italiani*, 10 (1968); the work included the first ever publication of Lelio Sozzini's *Brevis explicatio in primum Ioannis caput* (*A Brief Explication of the First Chapter of John*).

26 Dainora Pociute, 'Eterodossia e medicina nella prima età moderna. I "medici ariani" alla corte di Stefano Báthory,' *Rivista di storia del Cristianesimo*, 16, no. 1 (2019), 45. On the theological results achieved by Italian exiles in Central and Eastern European countries, see also Caccamo, *Eretici italiani*; Massimo Firpo, *Antitrinitari*. In this context Biandrata also curbed the spread of non-adorantist beliefs (which rejected the veneration of Christ, seen as a mere man) that were endorsed by David, his former collaborator. After a long, futile debate in which he was accused of blasphemy by Biandrata, David was imprisoned in the Fortress of Deva, where he died of cold and malnutrition in 1579. In Biandrata and Sozzini's view, the denial of the Trinitarian dogma and the assertion of the human nature of Christ paved the way for a form of Christianity combining the Erasmian, rational humanistic, and Anabaptist anti-authoritarian traditions. They felt that David's demands were extreme enough to weaken the newly established Unitarian Church, depriving it of the king's support. Biandrata acknowledged this danger as an astute politician and sacrificed his friendship with David for the sake of the unity of the new Church. See Caccamo, *Eretici italiani*, 29.

27 Vincenzo Malacarne notes the following works that earned Biandrata his place at court and were thus drafted before 1540 (publication details are not provided): *Gynaeceorum ex Aristotele et Bonaciolo a Georgio Blandrata medico subalpino noviter excerpta de fecundatione, gravitate, partu et puerperio*; *Cimelia muliebria*; *Aenneas Bonacioli compendiata a Georgio Blandrata*; *De promovenda foecunditate, et de cura graviditatis, puerperii, et primae natorum infantiae; Quae cur quando non sunt agenda in gestatione in partu post partum eodem Giorgio Blandrata auctore*; Vincenzo Malacarne, *Commentario alle opere e alle vicende di Giorgio Biandrata nobile saluzzese archiatro in Transilvania e in Polonia* (Padua: Tipografia Bettoni, 1814), 22–27. See also Michele Buniva, *Biografia medica piemontese* (Turin: Tipografia Bianco, 1824), 201–03.

28 ASV, Sant'Uffizio, *Processi, Contro Niccolò Buccella*, Bu. 36, deposition of 31 July 1574 by Yacopo de Gattis.

29 Ivi, *Contro Giovan Battista Ballarin*, Bu. 38, deposition of 4 November 1574 by Giovan Lippona. On Prospero Provana, see Rita Mazzei, *La trama nascosta: storie di mercanti e altro (secoli XVI-XVII)* (Viterbo: Sette città, 2006), 98, 100.

30 Tedeschi, *Intellettuali in esilio*, 166.

31 Ochino, *Prediche* (1542), 8r-8v. See also the letter from Ochino in the collection of writings that belonged to Vittore Soranzo (Rome: Biblioteca Apostolica Vaticana, *Vat. Lat.* 10755) edited by Benedetto Nicolini, *Ai margini dell'epistolario ochiniano*, now in Nicolini's volume, *Studi cinquecenteschi. Aspetti della vita religiosa, politica e letteraria,* vol. 2 (Bologna: Tamara Editori, 1968), 103–17.

32 Tedeschi, *Intellettuali in esilio*, 166.

33 Ibid., 167.

34 Arturo Pascal, 'Da Lucca a Ginevra. Studi sulla emigrazione religiosa lucchese a Ginevra nel secolo XVI,' *Rivista storica italiana*, 51 (1934), 473. On Giovanni

Valentino Gentile, see Luca Addante, *Valentino Gentile e il dissenso religioso nel Cinquecento. Dalla Riforma italiana al radicalismo europeo* (Pisa: Scuola Normale Superiore, 2014).

35 On Nicola Gallo see Guido Dall'Olio, entry 'Gallo, Nicola,' in *Dizionario Biografico degli Italiani*, 51 (1998).

36 Valerio Marchetti, entry 'Cattani, Francesco,' in *Dizionario Biografico degli Italiani*, 22 (1979).

37 Filippo Rustici, *Lettera ai principi e repubbliche d'Italia che si debben leggere le Sante scritture in lingua volgare*, which introduces *La Bibia, che si chiama il vecchio Testamento, nuovamente tradutto in lingua volgare secondo la verità del testo Hebreo, con molte et utili annotationi e figure e carte per più ampia dichiaratione di molti luoghi, edifici, e supputationi* (Geneva: Francesco Durone, 1562), 2. On the phenomenon of vernacular versions of the Bible, see also Gigliola Fragnito, *La Bibbia al rogo, La censura ecclesiastica e i volgarizzamenti della Scrittura: 1471–1605* (Bologna: Il Mulino, 1997), in particular on Rustici see p. 39. Adorni Braccesi, 'Le "Nazioni" lucchesi nell'Europa della Riforma,' *Critica storica*, 28, 3 (1991), 363–426, refers to Rustici on pp. 380–81, 383, 398–99, 402, 420.

38 'Un'esaltazione della parola divina e una critica aspra di tutte le scuole filosofiche, fomiti di conflitti,' Perini, *La vita e i tempi*, 19.

39 Servetus had also produced another edition of Pagnini's Bible. See Manzoni, *Umanesimo ed eresia*, 40–41.

40 Rustici, *Lettera*, 1.

41 Ibid., 6; See also Addante, *Valentino Gentile*, 176.

42 'Heed well, you [...] who do not allow those that follow the true doctrine and religion of Jesus Christ to stay in your cities and their houses, against all justice and civil and divine law. Indeed, it can be seen that you persecute them, imprison them, torture them cruelly, burn them, banish them, make them outlaws and confiscate their property and put a price on their head for whomever kills them, against every human law and civil decency. [...] In which book of canon or civil law or of your statutes it has ever been stated that heretics must be burned in effigy, made outlaws, and then persecuted to death with a reward given to whomever kills them [...] only to eradicate, if you could, the members of Jesus Christ and suppress his Gospel?' ('Considerate bene voi [...] che non permettete che quelli i quali seguitano la vera dottrina e religione di Giesu Cristo stieno nelle vostre città e case loro, contro ogni giustizia e legge tanto civile quanto divina, anzi come pure si vede gli perseguitate, gli imprigionate, gli tormentate crudelmente, gli abbrusciate, gli bandite, gli fate ribelli e consifscate i beni loro e mettete taglia sopra di essi a chi gli ammazza, contro ogni humana legge e honestà civile. [...] In qual libro di leggi o canoniche o civili o dei vostri statuti ancora s'è giamai letto che gli heretici dopo havergli in statue abbrusciati e fatti ribelli debbino essere perseguitati a morte co' dar premio a chi gli ammazza [...] solo per estirpare, se voi poteste, i membri di Giesu Christo e suffocare il suo Evangelio?'); Rustici, *Lettera*, 7.

43 Pascal, *Da Lucca a Ginevra*, 478. Three reprints – in Venice in 1566, in Lyon in 1596, and in Geneva in 1599 – show that the text was received favourably. Nevertheless, it fell into oblivion in the following century.

44 Ibid., 475.

45 Addante, *Valentino Gentile,* 141–43. For the Italian context, see below, the case of Panarelli.

46 On Simoni see Delio Cantimori, 'Un italiano contemporaneo di Bruno a Lipsia,' *Studi Germanici,* 3 (1938), 446–66; Massimo Firpo, 'Alcuni documenti sulla conversione al cattolicesimo dell'eretico lucchese Simone Simoni,' in *Annali della Scuola normale superiore di Pisa. Classe di lettere e filosofia*, 3, 4, no. 4 (1974),

1479–1502; Caccamo, *Eretici italiani*, 131–45; Claudio Madonia, 'Simone Simoni da Lucca,' *Rinascimento,* 20 (1980), 161–97; Nutton, '"It's the Patient's Fault." Simone Simoni and the Plague of Leipzig, 1575,' *Intellectual History Journal,* 18, (2008) 5–13; Alessandra Celati, entry 'Simoni, Simone,' in *Dizionario Biografico degli Italiani*, 92 (2018).

47 Although Cattani never abandoned Calvinism and signed the 1558 profession of faith, he advocated the release of Valentino Gentile and opposed any violent settlement of the doctrinal conflict.

48 While Suda's lexicon described atheists as those who denied the immortality of the soul, Zanobi Acciaiuoli defined them as 'deniers of God' ('Deum negantes'), or 'those who think that no God exists' ('opinatos nullum omnino Deum esse'). Instead, at the Synod of Strasbourg in 1535 they were defined as those who 'believe that this life is not followed by any eternal life, and that there is no judgement or damnation after this life, with no devil or hell' ('croient que cette vie n'est suivie d'acune vie eternelle, ou encore qui'il n'ya a ni jugement, ni damnation après cette vie-ci ni diable, ni enfer') and 'all those who claim that God does not care about our actions ('tous ceux qui prétendent que Dieu ne se soucie pas de nos actes'): see Jean Wirth, '"Libertins" et "epicuriens": aspects de l'irréligion au XVIe siècle,' *Bibliothèque d'humanisme et de renaissance*, 39 (1977), 601–27. On the extensive debate on the subject of atheism/impiety/unbelief in the early modern period, see at least Micheal Hunter, David Wootton (eds.), *Atheism from The Reformation to the Enlightment* (Oxford: Clarendon, Press, 1992); Jean Wirth, *Sainte Anne est une sorcière Sainte Anne est une sorcière: et autre essais* (Geneva: Droz, 2003); Vittorio Frajese, entry 'Ateismo,' in *Dizionario Storico dell'Inquisizione*, vol. 1 (2010), 114–18; Federico Barbierato, *The Inquisitor in the Hat Shop. Inquisition, Forbidden Books and Unbelief in Early Modern Venice* (Farnham: Ashgate, 2012); Jean-Pierre Cavaillé, 'The Italian Atheist Academics: A Myth of the French Pre-Enlightenment?' in Friedrich Vollhardt (ed.), *Religiöser Nonkonformismus Und Frühneuzeitliche Gelehrtenkultur* (Berlin: De Gruyter, 2014), 39–50; idem, *Libertinage, athéisme et incrédulité*, 1–2 (Toulouse: Presses Universitaires du Midi, 2017).

49 'He thinks God should not be seen as soul, mind, or intelligence; not the movement of the soul, as the Peripatetics argue, but precisely warmth. By this, I mean a vitalising warmth' ('Non vult Deum esse animum aut mentem sive intelligentiam, non motorem, uti peripatetici tradunt, sed quendam calorem. Calorem inquam quendam vivificum.' Marcello Squarcialupi, *Simonis Simonii Lucensis, primum Romani, tum Calviniani, deinde Lutherani, denuo Romani, semper autem Athei summa religio* (Kraków: A. Rodecius, 1588), 9–11.

50 In 1572, Simoni developed an idea in the framework of the *De vera nobilitate* (*On True Nobility*), according to which the nobility had a purely materialistic, naturalistic, and genetic origin, conditioning the future of humankind; Caccamo, *Eretici italiani*, 140–44.

51 Cinthya Klestinec, *Theaters of Anatomy*, 66.

52 Pociute, *Eterodossia*, 46.

53 Caccamo, *Eretici italiani*, 94.

54 Squarcialupi, *Summa religio*, 1588. Marcello Squarcialupi was actually born in Piombino in the province of Leghorn. On him, see Amedeo Molnàr, 'Marcello Squarcialupi et l'Unité des frères tchèques,' in *Bollettino della Società di studi valdesi*, 58 (1956), 3–20; Caccamo, *Eretici italiani,* ad indicem; Giampaolo Zucchini, 'Per la ricostruzione dell'epistolario di M. S.: alcune lettere inedite dai Grigioni (1586–1588),' in Robert Dán, Antal Pirnát (eds.), *Antitrinitarianism in the second half of the 16th century* (Budapest Akadémiai Kladó, 1982), 323–40;

Alessandra Celati, entry 'Squarcialupi, Marcello,' in *Dizionario Biografico degli Italiani*, 93 (2018). Squarcialupi, *Simonis Simonii.*

55 Alessandra Quaranta, 'Difficoltà e speranze nell'esilio religionis causa di Marcello Squarcialupi da Piombino (1538–1592),' *Rivista di Storia del Cristianesimo*, 15, no.1 (2018), 107–28.

56 Miklós Kázmér and Gabor Timár, 'The first scientific description of aurora borealis: the 10 September 1580 event in Transylvania, recorded by M. S.,' in *Geoscience letters. Official Journal of the Asia Oceania geosciences Society*, 2016, available online: https://geoscienceletters.springeropen.com/articles/10.1186/s40562-016-0047-2 (3 December 2020).

57 Marcello Squarcialupi, *Difesa contro la peste* (Milan: Francesco Moscheni, 1565), 8–9.

58 ASV, Sant'Uffizio, *Processi, Contro Girolamo Donzellini*, Bu. 39, 10v.

59 Ibid., 98r.

60 Ibid., 52r.

61 Dirk Jacob Jansen, '"A House for All Sorts of People": Jacopo Strada's Contacts with Italian Heterodox Exiles,' in *Fruits of Migration*, 178–231: on his contact with Donzellini, see p. 194.

62 See Vergerio's letter to Bullinger of 6 September 1554 in Calvin, *Opera,* vol. 15, letter no. 43, cited in Perini, *La vita e i tempi*, 242.

63 ASV, Sant'Uffizio, *Processi, Contro Girolamo Donzellini*, Bu. 39, 101r.

64 Ibid., 100r.

65 Ibid., 50v–51v; 55r.

66 'How can you call those who were directly against your faith dear friends? As you were Lutheran, as you have confessed, and they were Catholic, how can there not have been religious discord? He replies: I had friendships with Catholics and others besides and did not break off friendships with those who were also my friends before' ('Come potete chiamare cari amici quelli che erano de diretto contra la vostra fede essendo voi allora come havete confessato luterano confessionista essendo loro cattolici non potendo essere se non discordia di religione? Respondit: io teneva amicitia e con cattolici e con altri ancora e non mi separai dall'amicitia di quelli che anco prima mi erano amici'); ASV, Sant'Uffizio, *Processi, Contro Girolamo Donzellini*, Bu. 39, 113v–14r.

67 On sixteenth-century Basel and the role of the city in the religious debate see also Hans R. Guggisberg, Peter Rotach, *Ecclesia semper reformanda* (Basel: Reinhardt, 1980); Hans R. Guggisberg, *Basel in the Sixteenth Century. Aspects of the City Republic before, during, and after the Reformation* (St. Louis: Center for Reformation Research, 1982); Alfred Berchtold, *Bale et l'Europe: une histoire culturelle* (Lausanne: Payot, 1990); Amy Nelson Burnett, *Teaching the Reformation: Ministers and Their Message in Basel, 1529–1629* (Oxford: Oxford University Press, 2006); Felici, *Senza frontiere.*

68 Lucia Felici, *Senza frontiere. L'Europa di Erasmo (1538–1600)* (Rome: Carocci, 2021), 95. The concept of "world city" is put forward in Antonella Romano, Stéphan Van Damme, 'Sicence and World Cities', *Itineario*, 33 (2009), 79–96, quoted in Felici, *Senza frontiere*, 96, note 6.

69 Lucia Felici, Mario Biagioni, *La riforma radicale nell'Europa del Cinquecento* (Rome – Bari: Laterza, 2012), 90.

70 Felici 2021, p. 100. Oporinus published all the writings by Castellion until the latter's death in 1563, including the De haereticis an sint persequendi. He also distinguished himself for his scientific publications, such as the *De humani corporis fabirca* by Vesalius, Guggisberg, *Basel*, 43. As for Perna, notwithstanding the city's tolerant climate, he was imprisoned in 1578 for having published some original works of Castellion, with the collaboration of the anti-trinitarian Fausto

Sozzini – which shows that even in Basel tensions existed with respect to the ongoing religious controversy.

71 Felici, Biagioni, La Riforma, 94. On Basel, see also Cantimori, *Eretici italiani*, Rotondò, *Pietro Perna*. On Castellio see Stefania Salvadori, *Sebastiano Castellione e la ragione della tolleranza. L'ars dubitandi fra conoscenza umana e veritas divina* (Milan: Mimesis, 2009); Hans Guggisberg, *Sebastien Castellio: Humanist and Defender of Religious Toleration in a Confessional Age* (Routledge: London – New York, 2017).

72 Cantimori, *Eretici italiani*, 124. The publication of many neoplatonic, hermetic and cabalistic texts in Basel has been defined as 'the Basel Renaissance of the Italian Renaissance', Guggisberg, Basel, 43; Felici, Senza frontiere, 101. See also Peter Bietenholz, *Der italienische Humanismus und die Blütezeit des Buchdrucks in Basel* (Basel: Helbing & Lichtenhahn, 1959).

73 Girolamo Donzellini, *Themisti Euphradae philosophi peripatetici orationes octo elegantissimae, ac eruditione varia refertissimae* (Basel: Perna, 1559).

74 See Muccillo, *Platonismo, ermetismo e* Prisca theologia. *Ricerche di storiografia filosofica rinascimentale* (Florence: Olschki, 1996); Cesare Vasoli, '*Prisca theologia* e scienze occulte nell'umanesimo fiorentino,' in Gian Mario Cazzaniga (ed.), *Storia d'Italia. Annali 25: Esoterismo* (Turin: Einaudi, 2010), 175–205.

75 Perini, *La vita e i tempi*, 69.

76 On this text, see Gregorio Piaia, 'Il "medioevo" e le età della filosofia (Postille a un'allegoria di Albrecht Dürer),' in Burkhard Mojsisch and Olaf Pluta (eds.), *Historia Philosophiae Medii Aevii. Studien zer Geschichte der Philosophie des Mittelalters*, vols. 2 (Amsterdam and Philadelphia: Benjamins, 1991).

77 Donzellini, *Themistii Euphradae*, 16.

78 Lynda Gregorian Christian, 'The Figure of Socrates in Erasmus' Works,' *The Sixteenth Century Journal* 3, no. 2 (1972), 8.

4 Heterodox physicians in front of the Inquisition, 1560s–1570s

Donzellini left Venice at the height of the spread of heresy. By the time he returned, however, the religious climate had changed significantly. As the Counter-Reformation took full effect, there was also an escalation of repression in Venice from the early 1560s onwards.

The Holy Office records from this period effectively outline both the repressive measures taken and the structure and development of the heretical movement in the city, including the role played by physicians in a climate less conducive to the dissemination of dissent than twenty or thirty years previously. The heterodox physicians Teofilo Panarelli and Decio Bellebuono are especially significant in this respect; with their eminent religious, intellectual, and professional profiles, they were the lynchpins of a dense network. This chapter will reconstruct their experiences before returning to Donzellini (who was in Verona rather than Venice between 1560 and 1573) in Chapter 5. The final chapter will investigate the intersection between their and Donzellini's networks, adopting a social perspective to highlight the relationship between medical theory and practice, religious thought, and philosophical elaboration in the late Venetian Renaissance. Before that, though, the heretical movement between 1553 and 1576 needs to be contextualised within the vast underground world of contacts, complicities, mutual support, and betrayal which emerges from the sources.

4.1 Venetian heretical networks in the Counter-Reformation, 1560–1575

The Council of Trent concluded in 1563 with the rejection of any potential doctrinal openness to Protestantism and the formalisation of new measures of discipline and control. The Tridentine Index was issued in 1564 and enforced throughout Catholic Europe, imposing censorship on texts whether or not they were religious. Seven years later, a new congregation of cardinals was established alongside the Congregation of the Holy Office with the purpose of updating and distributing the Index. In this way, the Catholic Church implemented a single, far-reaching framework to monitor – and

DOI: 10.4324/9781003218852-5

penalise if necessary – books and ideas, practices and relations, religious and intellectual perceptions, personal experiences, and rites of passage.

The wave of Counter-Reformation repression struck Venice in the second half of the 1560s at the same time as a serious economic crisis and growing frustration at the gradual erosion of the Republic's *Domini da mar* (Domains of the Sea) by the Turks (as well as the ever more costly war effort). Against this backdrop, the population closed ranks and adopted a 'spectacular and monumental' ('spettacolare e monumentale') form of religiosity that became increasingly intolerant of religious dissent.[1] The level of repression in the city had already increased under Pope Paul IV. Then, in the 1560s, even the local nobility were affected for the first time. In 1567, Paolo Moscardo, who had ties with Teofilo Panarelli's heterodox group, maintained that an Inquisition managed only by lay patricians 'as it used to be, would be a delight' ('com'era una volta, saria una dolcezza').[2] Active heterodox dissenters in the 1560s must therefore have developed an even greater sense of being in the "minority" than their counterparts twenty years previously.[3] Isolated and hounded by repression, heterodox networks implemented strategies of solidarity and resistance until the movement was wiped out in the early 1580s. This does not mean, however, as the conclusions will highlight, that the cause was abandoned completely. In fact, there was more of a transformation; by drawing on notions that had developed gradually during the Italian Reformation, the networks continued to operate, adopting updated aspirations and watchwords, and responding to the trend of repression[4] (Figure 4.1).

In this context, physicians were affected by repressive measures both as individual members of heterodox networks and as a professional category. In the second half of the century, the Catholic authorities took steps to protect the medical profession against the intrusion of heresy by tightening their control over physicians, their professional conduct, and their collegial norms. It was not simply a question of image and decorum to identify heterodox practitioners and banish them from the sector but a matter of necessity. Indeed, the role of the physician was too delicate to be entrusted to those involved in religious dissent; the control of consciences, which was the main aim of the Catholic establishment, included the supervision of medical practice. Although such monitoring work was conducted with the complicity of the local medical college in many Italian cities, it led to considerable conflict in Venice. This development can be understood by reconstructing the experiences of heterodox physicians and their associates, analysing the repression they suffered and the resistance they offered. We will start with the members of Donzellini's network and then outline the broader framework.

As we know, Donzellini and the Maggi spouses fled when the proceedings against them were launched. While Donzellini went to Ferrara and then escaped to German soil, Vincenzo Maggi took refuge in Switzerland, first in Chur and subsequently in Basel and Geneva. Lucrezia joined her husband

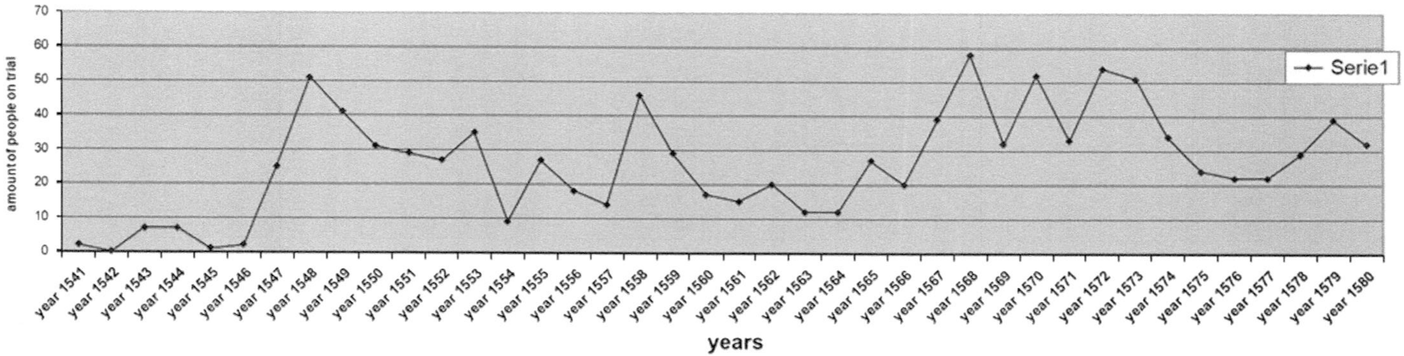

Figure 4.1 Number of prosecutions by year for the period 1541-1580.

Source: Inventario fondo Savi sopra l eresia, ASV.

sometime after he took flight; the couple probably thought that he should check the lie of the land first as the journey was extremely dangerous for a woman. Lucrezia was accompanied by Gian Battista Michiel, a diplomat who probably worked with Vincenzo and was definitely a close friend of Caterina Colbertalda, Donzellini's and Lucrezia's former housekeeper.[5] In the years to come, he became the godfather to Caterina's daughters.[6] Although Caterina had testified against her employers in 1553, it seems that there were still elements of collaboration and support in Donzellini's network. In the 1560s, Caterina also forged a close friendship with Publio Francesco Spinola, who played a crucial role in her conversion and had known Donzellini since their youth.[7] In 1562 Spinola dedicated a poem to the physician's 'excellent' library, before he was executed by the Inquisition five years later.[8]

Gian Battista, Lucrezia Maggi's "bodyguard," was the natural son of an unknown patrician in the Michiel family. He had been a suspect in the trials against Anabaptists in early 1550s Venice. His position as a diplomat, however, allowed him to travel frequently and he managed to evade the Inquisition by leaving with Lucrezia. He was brave enough to return to Venice, though, along with some heterodox books (by Pier Paolo Vergerio and Francesco Negri). Partly because of his Nicodemite stance, he continued to act undisturbed as a heretical broker for at least twenty years.

Michiel's story takes us to the heart of the 1560s and the heretical narratives played out in the city at the time. Aware of the danger hanging over them, the members of the different heterodox networks were increasingly forced to adopt clandestine strategies. In this climate, Gian Battista Michiel organised a secret propaganda campaign by sending a series of anonymous letters to Celestino, the preacher at the church of San Polo and at the *Ospedale degli Incurabili*. The missives took issue with the content of his sermons, specifically the way he addressed the matter of the Eucharist ('de sacramento') and the cult of images.[9] Michiel implemented the plan at night by hiding in the shadows disguised as a friar and approaching passers-by (such as Michael della Pieve da Bon) to ask them to deliver the letters to the preacher.

When the episode came to the attention of the Inquisition judges, they launched a manhunt that ended in the arrest of Vincenzo Negroni. This Venetian physician had studied in Padua and graduated in Venice in 1547; here, in the 1560s, he lived at the *Nunciaria* apothecary shop, in Campo dei Frari, and had strong ties with heterodox circles. He was tried in 1567 on the strength of some significant evidence: in San Polo, he had been seen 'contradicting and challenging' ('contraddire e impugnare') certain sermons, speaking badly of the Church, and making 'gestures that seemed as if he were mocking' ('gesti che pareva chel se burlasse') the preacher's comments on the intercession of the saints during Lent that year. Furthermore, on St Gregory's Day he had turned his back on the preacher when the latter encouraged good works (an episode which is underlined in the trial records).[10] A few apothecaries came to his defence at the trial, but the physician was unable to present a convincing defence and was subjected to torture. In the end, he admitted that he did not believe in the value of works 'without the grace of God' ('senza la grazia di Dio'). He also offered an unsolicited excuse in reference to the anonymous letters that made the judges even more suspicious. This was a sign that even though he was innocent, as it later became apparent, he was connected to or perhaps even part of the network responsible for the initiative.[11]

On 10 October, the physician admitted that he had denied the existence of purgatory and the saints, the need for prayers for the dead, and the authority of the pope. He also confessed to having believed that 'predestination is because of Christ, that is to say that everyone who was redeemed through his blood was predestined because of the merits of Christ without our works, and that we are justified through the merits of Christ' ('la predestinazione sia per Cristo cioé che tutti che erano redenti per il suo sangue erano predestinati per i meriti di Cristo senza le nostre opere, e che siamo giustificati per li meriti di Cristo').[12] When pressed on the doctrinal details of his beliefs, he added: 'to tell you the truth I do not consider it to be such an important matter [...] I erred in speaking, but I do not understand these errors as I am ignorant in this field' ('a dirvi la verità mi nun la intendo per esser cosa di tanta importanza [...] ho detto questi errori ma non li intendo per essere ignorante in questa professione').[13] This form of religiosity recalls the *Beneficio di Cristo* both in its use of language to underline the importance of the merits of Christ and in its perception of doctrinal subtleties as adiaphora. Exhausted after months of questioning, Negroni agreed to recant and was sentenced to public repentance. He had to wear a yellow tunic for three consecutive Sundays in the church of San Trovaso and submit to spiritual penalties for the following two years. In 1568, the case was mentioned by Paolo Moscardo, who was himself on the run from the Inquisition; in a letter to his siblings explaining why he had taken flight, he praised the physician's skill in escaping punishment.[14]

The judges were sure that the mystery of the letters had been solved when they convicted Negroni. However, it was all a terrible mistake, emblematic of the Church authorities' deep-rooted suspicion of the medical environment. Just four years later, in 1571, the Inquisition investigated the entire medical community because of their reluctance to apply the directives on confession in the *Super gregem dominicum*, a papal bull issued in 1566. This established that physicians could only continue treatment if patients confessed within three days of their first medical examination.[15] Physicians' reluctance to comply with this ordinance reveals some level of involvement with heterodoxy or at least their exasperation with the interference of the Catholic Church. The proceedings *Contra medicos* (against physicians) were launched after a medical practitioner from Cremona, Antonio Secco, a member of the College of Venice, disregarded the bull and let a patient die without confessing. The local parish priest of San Marziale, Antonio Rocha, was outraged and filed a complaint, arguing that 'physicians are not concerned about persuading the sick that they have to confess and take communion, under the pretext that the sick do not want to or for another particular physicians' interest' ('li medici sotto pretesto di non voler gli infermi, o per qualche altro suo particolare interesse non si cureno di persuader li infermi a dover confessarsi et comunicarsi').[16] As a result, parish priests were instructed to disseminate the new measures in the city: patients would not be examined more than once if they had not confessed.

On this occasion and during subsequent disputes on the matter between the College and the Inquisition, physicians showed collective solidarity in resisting ecclesiastical meddling.[17] The renewed emphasis on a rule dating back to the thirteenth century stemmed from the Church's desire to increase the number of confessions. The sacrament of confession had always played a fundamental role in monitoring behaviour, 'religious preparation, and the ideas of the faithful,' taking shape as a valuable auxiliary tool of repression in the Counter-Reformation climate.[18] It is possible that physicians in Venice really did attempt to limit encounters between patients and their confessors; after all, many were active members of the movement who resented ecclesiastical interference in their profession and displayed group solidarity. The latter came to the fore during numerous other trials. During the proceedings against Negroni, for example, the defendant was warned about the impending court case by Lelio Rama, a fellow member of the College.[19]

Various trials held at this time show that failure to confess on a sickbed was an expression of adherence to Protestant doctrines or was in any case seen as proof of such by judges. One of the most sensational cases involved Francesco Franco, the son-in-law of Giulio di Stan, a goldsmith in the heterodox group of jewellers in the Ruga dei Oresi (the main street for his profession) and an associate of Teofilo Panarelli. When Franco died without having confessed at Giulio's house in 1564, the family hid his body for sixteen days.[20] Another significant case features two physicians. When Giuseppe Moscardo, who fled Venice to escape the Inquisition, was on his deathbed, he was joined in Trieste by Panarelli, also on the run. Panarelli exhorted him not to reconsider, encouraging him to refuse confession until the very end.[21] After Moscardo died as a Protestant, the episode became a serious accusation in the trial against Panarelli in 1571, which ended in a death sentence even though he was not a relapsed heretic. To use Roger French's words, physicians aspired to become 'the faithful companion*s* of the body of *their* patient': they had to build a sympathetic relationship with the invalid that combined deontological ethics and successful treatment.[22] In sickness, physical and psychological defences were weakened, and the fear of impending death forced the sick to confront the destiny of their souls. It was therefore a situation that could easily develop into forms of collusion and protection.[23] At his trial, Vincenzo Negroni also admitted that Pasqualino Boccalier, described as a 'heretic' ('eretico'), had served ('servito') him during 'sickness' ('infermità') and shared 'bad opinions' ('cattive opinioni').[24] Negroni was so grateful for his help that he continued the friendship despite its potentially damaging consequences, of which he was fully aware. Bonds forged at sickbeds could thus strengthen heterodox relations even when the patient was a physician.

It was not until 1572 that Vincenzo Negroni was fully exonerated during the trial against Girolamo Parto, Gian Battista Michiel's half-brother. After he was denounced by the cloth merchant Domenico di Steffani, Parto stated in his first deposition that the physician could not have written the letters as his level of theological knowledge was too rudimentary. When pressed by his judges, he was forced to admit Michiel's involvement in the matter. He must have made the tip-off with a heavy heart as at the end of his confession he asked somewhat pointlessly: 'Gentlemen, do you not think that being an accuser is the worst role?' ('Signori non pensi esser il pezor officio questo esser accusador?').[25] The trial of Parto triggered proceedings against Michiel, who confirmed his role in writing the letters together with Antonio Diedo, a lawyer, and Parto, who contributed by suggesting a quotation from Jeremiah. In this way, Michiel's heterodox network was disbanded between 1574 and 1575. As Parto was a relapsed heretic, he was sentenced to death, while Michiel recanted. The *Due colombine* apothecary shop, one of Michiel's regular haunts, became the subject of an investigation. Every member of the Gemma family, who owned it, was interrogated, but the proceedings mostly focused on the apothecary and physician Gian Battista.[26] He had already been tried with his brother in 1565, two years after graduating from Padua University, and both had been forced to recant;[27] another conviction would mean the death sentence. When Gian Battista reappeared on the Inquisition's radar less than ten years later, he first stayed hidden and then fled with the help of his family (they presented his brother Marcantonio to the Inquisition officers, thereby giving him time to escape). From Venice, he travelled to Florence, Friuli and finally Poland, where he took the place of Niccolò Buccella as court physician. Alongside the trial against 'those at the Colombine apothecary shop' ('quelli delle Colombine'), 1574 also saw proceedings against Caterina Colbertalda, who was cousin to Marita (Marcantonio Gemma's wife). Now known as La Sartora, she was tried together with her husband.[28] She was accused of heterodox practices and comments, and her position was compromised above all by the support that, with her husband's approval, she had given to the prisoner Publio Francesco Spinola. Through a chain of solidarity, she made soup for Spinola, arranging for it to be delivered to his cell in secret, along with a bed sheet, by a boy called Menego, who was in turn instructed by Iacopo Baldassarre, Menego's father and Spinola's father-in-law.[29]

Before all this, however, an initial round of investigations and arrests in 1567 dealt a harsh blow to the heretical movement, revealing the involvement of physicians often in a leadership capacity. Teofilo Panarelli was denounced on 10 January 1567 and the Moscardo brothers were investigated four months later. A year later, in September 1568, the inquiries extended to others associated with the same group including the patricians Andrea Dandolo and Giacomo Malipiero, old childhood friends of Gian Battista Gemma.

4.2 Teofilo Panarelli and his sect: A secret sociality

Even though Teofilo Panarelli belonged to the generation after Girolamo Donzellini, there are many similarities between their stories.[30] Both were instructed in heresy by their fathers at an early age (Panarelli's father was also a physician) and studied in Padua, where they further explored heterodoxy and added to their intellectual and heretical contacts. They were also key players in the Venetian heterodox network and eventually received death sentences for their crimes against the faith. Furthermore, they both had wide spheres of action: although Panarelli never left Italy, he lived in many different cities in the Republic of Venice and the rest of the peninsula. His father, Nicola Antonio, was a district physician in various places – Venice, the Padua area, Veglia, and Cres – and frequently took his children back to his childhood home in Monopoli (in Apulia). Then, after graduating, Teofilo worked in Istria and Venice before escaping first to Trieste and then to Ancona, the probable place of his capture. From there he was transferred to papal lands, investigated by the Roman judges, and burned at the stake.[31]

Finally, just as the young Donzellini benefitted from an exceptional teacher, Michelangelo Florio, Panarelli was tutored by the 'most excellent' and 'Lutheran' ('excellentissimo [...] luterano') preacher Bartolomeo Fonzio in the 1550s. Fonzio was known for his particularly subversive proselytism with concepts such as the ideal of poverty, no need for baptism, and a non-hierarchical Church: members of the invisible, hidden Church were united by their faith in Christ.[32] They later met up again in Venice, where the preacher had a sizeable following among the Germans at the Fondaco, and in 1562 the pupil witnessed the execution of his master, 'that truly great man' ('quel grandissimo huomo').[33] The young Panarelli was given the *Catechismo* (*Catechism*) by Fonzio and continued to appreciate it in adulthood. He distributed the work among his circle and encouraged them to attend Fonzio's sermons. The trial records make particular reference to Giulio di Stan, a goldsmith, and the Galli brothers, who were active members of the heretical network of jewellers in the Ruga dei Oresi. Through them, Panarelli swapped his *Catechismo* for a *Beneficio di Cristo*, describing the latter as the 'most salvific thing for human redemption' ('cosa più salvifera alla redenzione umana').[34] Friendship and complicity in Venice were consolidated through pro-Reformation publications, which were often specially designed to be passed around and hidden easily. For example, Fonzio's 'creed' ('credo') was drafted 'by hand and was extremely small, written on not even half a sheet of paper' ('a penna et era cosa picciola scritta in manco de mezzo foglio di carta').[35]

As we have seen, Panarelli explored Reformed ideas during his university days in Padua, exchanging heterodox books with his fellow students and building friendships based on common interest in the new religious ideas. He lived at Giordano Trivisano's house in the city, sharing his room with a soldier from Belluno named Antonio Paulino, who 'had brought with him an *Institutes* [*of the Christian Religion*] by Calvin from the borders of Germany and [...] a German Bible' ('aveva portato con sé dai confini dell'Alemagna un'istituzione di Calvino, e [...] una Bibbia d'Alemagna').[36] The soldier listened to Panarelli's 'reasoning' ('ragionamenti') and let him use these texts to 'study them' ('studiarli'), as it was natural for a medical student to apply the tools of philological criticism in both the medical and religious fields.[37] In this way, when Virginia Panarelli testified about her brother's religious outlook, she was able to claim that he had 'denied purgatory as a philosopher' ('negato il purgatorio come filosofo').[38]

After graduating in the late 1550s, Panarelli worked as a district physician in Sacile (in Friuli) and Pirano, where Lutheran ideas had circulated since the 1540s thanks to Gian Battista Goineo. He subsequently returned to Monopoli before moving to Venice in the first half of the 1560s. He lived there first with his sisters, Virginia and Flaminia, and then shared a house in San Luca with the polygraph Girolamo Ruscelli for eight months between 1566 and the beginning of 1567, when he met Caterina Guarniera, with whom he had two daughters. Panarelli and Ruscelli became close friends, and the latter married the former's sister, Virginia.[39] It is probable that Panarelli introduced Virginia to Girolamo. Indeed, now the head of his family, Panarelli might have wanted to use the marriage to cement his relationship with a well-known and respected figure in the Italian intellectual and scientific panorama. Although Ruscelli had not been to university, he forged many intellectual relations during his career, lived in various Italian cities, and focused on a variety of different subjects (from mathematics to cartography), specialising in the pharmacopoeia of 'secrets' ('segreti').[40] While living with his brother-in-law, Panarelli acquired innovative techniques for manipulating nature and expanded the boundaries of his expertise. For example, two of Ruscelli's engineer friends ('meccanici') from Apulia that lived in the same house taught him about their subject, a form of practical and collaborative knowledge that would have flowed into the broader scientific revolution.[41] In this way, exploiting interests and skills connected to the increasing importance that practical knowledge assumed in Venice (spreading out from the Arsenal and from the artisan shops in the city) he developed a passion for applied knowledge and worked on engineering projects himself. He created a 'permanent screw' ('vite perenne') to operate mills and a hydraulic system to 'dig canals' ('cavare li canali'). These inventions must have been a source of income as he left the sales revenue to his daughters in a will written before his execution.[42] Although practical knowledge was not always quietly accepted by members of the academic professions like physicians, its influence enriched modern science and Panarelli made a significant contribution in this respect. His interests extended beyond medicine to astronomy, geography, and the anthropology of peoples and lands all over the world including those recently discovered. He procured an astrolabe through his friend Giulio di Stan and a *Cosmographia* (*Cosmography*), probably the one by the Lutheran Sebastian Münster, whose 1550 edition also included the entry *Sardiniae brevis historia et descriptio* (*Brief History and Description of Sardinia*) by Sigismondo Arquer (a jurist from Cagliari who was executed for heresy by the Spanish Inquisition in 1571).[43]

When the young physician lived in San Luca, his life was punctuated by heterodoxy, barely legal behaviour, and sexual licentiousness: he stole (mostly prohibited) books from Arrivabene's bookshop, visited prostitutes, and played an active role in the city's heteroox circles. His point of reference was the *Castello* apothecary shop near San Domenico, where he hid his copy of the *Beneficio di Cristo* with the collusion of the owner, Carlo, who protected members of the group whenever necessary. Teofilo was most active in the Rialto area, where he regularly visited the Ruga dei Oresi and the numerous local bookshops, other than, as already noted, the *Spinon* and *Due colombine* apothecary shops.

He probably kept his friendships with jewellers separate from the rest of his group, which consisted of the apothecaries Marcantonio and, above all, Gian Battista Gemma at the *Due colombine*, members of the liberal professions such as Paolo and Antonio Moscardo, various patricians, a German named Angelo Noise, a musician named Giacomo Negron, and three other physicians: Francesco Pegolotto, Giovanni Gatta, and Giuseppe Moscardo. The latter is an interesting case of a heterodox district physician as he used his profession to leave Venice and move to a Reformed country in the 1550s. In addition, at the end of his life in the late 1560s, he sheltered Panarelli on the run from the Holy Office. In a letter to his siblings on 28 May 1568 (after the family had suffered a year of repression), Moscardo explained that he had been 'out of the country' ('fuori dal dominio') for eleven years in Carinthia and avoided contact with anyone except them to prevent unnecessary risks. Nevertheless, the Inquisition intercepted their correspondence. In the letter in question, Giuseppe suggested exonerating himself and his family from the most serious accusations, mentioning that he had previously 'offended the judges' ('offeso i giudici') by writing that 'he was about to partake of the holy supper' ('stava per fare la santa cena'). He attributed this and other religious habits acquired abroad to the need 'for physicians, especially those of us who are poor, to travel around when they are young so that they can then return to their homelands and provide for themselves' ('che noi medici massime quelli che sono poveri bisogna mentre sono giovani vadano in su e in giu et havere delle condotte per poter andare poi alle loro patrie e poter stare su le spese').[44] Apart from financial reasons, however, Moscardo's friendships (like Panarelli and an unnamed 'agent of the king of Transylvania' ['agente del re di Transilvania'], the land of heretics) show that he embraced Protestant religious customs more for spiritual reasons than for opportunism, moving away to escape the persecution that soon affected the rest of the group.

Along with Panarelli, the lifeblood of the Venetian heretical group was Ludovico Abioso, son of the physician Agostino Abioso, a member of Donzellini's network in the 1540s. Ludovico's brother Girolamo was also a physician; in 1589, when he was Prior of the College, he had to face a fresh wave of controversy about the failure of physicians to comply with the directives on treatment and confession.[45] Tried immediately before Panarelli, Ludovico mounted an effective defence, presenting the image of a slightly naive young man misguided by his older friends, above all Panarelli and Paolo Moscardo, his 'preceptors of the devil' ('precettori del diavolo').[46] However, if we compare Ludovico's testimony with the comments made about him during other trials, it is clear that his role in the group was anything but secondary. Indeed, he procured numerous prohibited texts for Panarelli together with the German Noise, who was able to obtain supplies of heterodox books with ease thanks to his contacts at the Fondaco. The texts circulating among the group (some of which were bequeathed to Panarelli by his father) included Ochino's *Prediche* (*Sermons*), Calvin's *Institutio*, a letter written by Giulio da Milano to Italian prisoners, the '*Commonplaces* by Philip Melanchthon' ('*Luochi comuni* di Filippo Melantone'), 'a tome by Erasmus' ('un tomo di Erasmo'), 'a [work by] Oecolampadius about the Eucharist, and a piece by Martin Luther' ('un Ecolampadio che trattava di eucarestia, et un pezzo di Martino Lutero'), a book by Wycliffe, a 'Bible from Germany' ('Bibbia di Alemagna') and a New Testament. Non-religious volumes included Baldassarre Castiglione's *Il cortegiano* (*The Book of the Courtier*, Venice, 1528) and a text by Marcus Aurelius. In addition to the aforementioned *Beneficio di Cristo*, there was also 'a copy of Savonarola's *Miserere*' (*An Exposition of the Psalm Miserere Mei Deus*) at the *Colombine* apothecary shop. Panarelli was the main reader and commentator of these texts. One witness stated that 'he read matters of God' ('lezzeva cose da Dio'), also at a neighbour's house, and encouraged discussions about original works such as 'a text that he hid up his sleeve that [...] he had written about the Gospel of St John [...] about "In the beginning was the Word"' ('una scrittura che nascondeva nella manica che [...] aveva fatto sopra l'evangelo di San Zuanne [...] sopra l'"in principio era il verbo"').[47] The conclusions drawn by Panarelli's group on the verse from John are not known, but it is extremely significant that the passage was debated as it was liable to give rise to Neoplatonic tendencies with anti-Trinitarian implications, as had happened in the case of Servetus and the Sozzinis.[48] In the 1580s, one of Panarelli's friends, Grazioso Percacino, published a *foglio volante* (broadside) offering an emanationist interpretation of the verse, for which he had to answer to the Holy Office.[49]

The conventicle also listened to Panarelli reading from Marcantonio Flaminio's version of the Psalms and discussed the option of fleeing for religious reasons. This was prompted by a letter printed in Basel in which Francesco Betti, a heterodox Roman, explained the reasons for his voluntary exile to his former employer, the Marquis of Pescara. A second letter along the same lines circulated in the group, written by Andrea Da Ponte, an aristocratic relative of the doge, who had brought disgrace to his family by leaving Italy for Reformed soil. The letter was sent to Francesco Emo, Da Ponte's *nipote* (nephew or grandson), through Paolo Moscardo; Emo first feigned a scandalised reaction but then asked his friend to deliver it in private.

For the noblemen in Panarelli's heretical circle (Marcantonio Canal, Alvise Mocenigo, Andrea Dandolo, and Giacomo Malipiero, as well as Emo), fear of loss of freedom was combined with anxiety about loss of social privilege. However, the matter did not only affect patricians. In Panarelli's experience, the problematic nature of living on Catholic soil as a minority must have been a constant issue. He was jeopardised by life-threatening dangers but could not bring himself to leave the country, where he not only had a successful career and an affluent lifestyle (as his will illustrates) but also played a pivotal role in a network of protection, religious and intellectual debate, and friendship.

Panarelli adopted Nicodemite positions knowingly, both in practical and theoretical terms. While he admitted to his judges that he had suggested attending Mass 'by simulation' ('per simulazione'), his Nicodemism was not limited to opportunism. The apothecary Bernardo Vergolino testified that Panarelli had reproached his superstitious behaviour on seeing that he had bought 'one of the coins that are made on Good Friday' ('uno di quei denari che si battono il Venerdì santo'). He had added, however, that 'you who know the truth can also use it for worship' ('voi che conoscete la verità potete prenderlo anche per devozione').[50] This was a clear statement about the irrelevance of rituals, ceremonies, and any external form of religiosity, key elements in the Nicodemite doctrine. Vergolino's awareness of the truth thus justified the superstitious purchase of the coin. In another instance, Panarelli showed that he had assimilated one of the central features of Nicodemism, namely the need to conduct propaganda gradually in stages on a case-by-case basis according to the level of theological knowledge. He admitted discussing delicate theological matters such as justification in *spezierie* with his colleague Francesco Pegolotto but stressed that he had been careful not to involve the pharmacists. With them, he had only addressed less controversial issues like the abuses of the clergy.[51]

In light of the above, the reading of texts written by Valdesians (like Ochino's *Prediche* (*Sermons*), Flaminio's *Parafrasi* (*Paraphrase*), and above all the *Beneficio di Cristo*) assumes a precise meaning in defining Panarelli's doctrinal approach, which also included the Calvinist rite of Holy Communion. The cornerstones of Valdesian beliefs were Nicodemism, gradualism, and the primacy of the internal forum, teachings which seem to have been partly absorbed and reworked by Panarelli. The necessary secrecy and lack of strong theological guidance undermined any concrete possibility of a Reformation in the Italian peninsula. However, at the same time, these aspects helped educated heterodox dissenters like Panarelli to develop their own independent theological visions, which must have been a common occurrence in the group. The expertise of certain members like Panarelli was employed to address complex matters such as the real presence of Christ's body in the Eucharist, on which there was not always common consensus; the debate was ongoing, with frequent fresh input.

One of the places where the group met for debates and reading was the Fondaco dei Tedeschi, to which they were granted access by Angelo Noise. They also carried out the same activities on islands in the lagoon, reached by gondola after meeting opposite the *Due colombine* apothecary shop on the *Rio terà della Maddalena*, clearly a place safe from prying eyes. Panarelli also often visited the printing house at the Santi Apostoli owned by his friend Grazioso Percacino, who he had known since university. The future imperial physician Giulio Alessandrini had been a habitué of Percacino's shop in Padua, where he 'spoke for my [Panarelli's] benefit on matters of faith' ('parlava a favor mio delle cose della religione').[52] After meeting up again in Venice, Panarelli indulged in frequent anti-Catholic outbursts in Percacino's *bottega*. The latter was summoned by the judges for the trial against Panarelli at precisely the same time that he was hiding his friend in his early days as a fugitive. In this way, Teofilo was informed about what they had been told and warned about the answers he should give. When Virginia Panarelli was also arrested in January 1572 and placed under house arrest on bail of two hundred ducats, Percacino stepped in to pay the required amount.[53]

Secrecy, reciprocal support, and collusion were essential ingredients in the day-to-day lives of group members. For instance, when Panarelli needed money to escape, he received a ruby ring from Isabella, Paolo Moscardo's partner (which he returned to her in his will). In a similar episode, Gian Battista Gemma was asked to vouch for the trustworthiness of Andrea Dandolo, a young patrician, when he first attended a group meeting on the Giudecca. As Dandolo later testified, his friend was more than happy to oblige as they had known each other since their schooldays, becoming firm friends, nurturing a mutual passion for poetry, and learning 'the ways of love' ('a fare l'amore').[54] Heresy was more than a theoretical abstraction in the lives of these individuals. Indeed, it permeated every aspect of their existence, playing an integral role in their work (first and foremost the medical profession), social relations, and daily habits. As their network was confined to the peninsula, they missed out on the opportunities for intellectual, philosophical, and doctrinal exploration that were available to, say, Donzellini in Basel. However, their experience provides an excellent case study for exploring the element of *secret sociality* in the lives of heterodox dissenters. In addition to reading and discussing religious texts, they celebrated the Eucharist together following the rite of the Supper, praised the Huguenots, and drank and sang with musical accompaniment by Negron, thereby seamlessly blending coarseness and holiness. Panarelli also often promoted heterodox ideas while practising as a physician. There is more than one case in which he derided the supposedly thaumaturgical value of sacred images or criticised the habit of calling for a priest when an illness was so serious that a miracle was the only hope, deeming it to be an act against 'the honour of God' ('all'honor di Dio').[55]

Panarelli's heterodox network fell apart in the late 1560s following the arrest and trial of those who met at the Fondaco and on the Giudecca, the goldsmiths, and Virginia Panarelli. Several of them, including Panarelli, were subsequently banished from Venice in May 1567. Teofilo went into hiding for some time (first protected by Percacino and then by his sister) before deciding to flee. After several years on the run, he made the mistake of entering papal territory, which was probably when he was captured by the Holy Office (the last record of his movements in sources is in Ancona). He remained in the papal prison in Torre di Nona for nearly a year and was subjected to torture. Isolated from his network and his family, he was broken by his experience of jail and agreed to repent. He accepted full responsibility for his 'errors' ('errori') before dying; his will asks for 'many Masses' ('tante messe') to be said in his name. He also wrote to his sister and wife, telling them to follow him down the path of reconciliation with the Holy Mother Church. This created problems with the Inquisition for Virginia, who was tried in 1572. In addition, his former fellow lodger at Ruscelli's house, Gelli, an engineer from Monopoli, became embroiled in an Inquisition trial in Apulia because of their close friendship. Caterina Guarnera, on the other hand, escaped with a single interrogation in which she managed to convince the judges that she was not involved in any heresy even though her partner had exposed her to heterodox views, such as the idea that praying in church was pointless as God could be addressed anywhere. Teofilo had also dismissed the vows she made to saints while in labour as superstitious.[56] Unlike Virginia, who read Latin and was familiar with Ochino's works, Caterina's illiteracy was enough to divert any suspicion away from her.

Although he repented and was not a relapsed heretic, Panarelli was burned at the stake on 23 February 1572. When Virginia drew up her will in 1606, she left her few possessions to her niece, Marina, who she had raised like a daughter.[57] Just before his death, her brother entrusted his daughters to her care should anything happen to their mother, Caterina (the fact that the couple were not married is another sign of a non-conformist lifestyle). Therefore, even though the final letters between Virginia and Teofilo contained harsh reciprocal accusations, fraternal love and family ties proved to be stronger than repression in the long term.

4.3 Heresy and alchemy at the *Frari* apothecary shop: Antonino Volpe and Decio Bellebuono

Many ecclesiastics who cast off their habits during the sixteenth-century Italian religious crisis embarked on a medical career. One such man was Antonino Volpe from Ferrandina (in the region of Lucania), a former Dominican friar turned empirical physician, who became the protagonist of a long and complex Inquisition trial held between Padua and Venice in the late 1560s.

Volpe's professional path was rather common. Since the Middle Ages, the charitable, compassionate, and salvific aspects of medical work had led to an overlap between carers of souls and healthcare workers. This became appealing during the Reformation for those who abandoned Catholicism in search of a religion with renewed theological foundations and ethical aspirations. Apostates such as Ortensio Lando, Ludovico Manna, Girolamo Massari, and Lorenzo Tizzano, to mention but a few, shared an interest in medical matters and were frequently involved in alchemy and astrology. A passion for medicine was also cultivated by some members of the clergy that were active in the Italian Reformed movement, as shown by the medical and anatomical texts in their libraries. One such individual was Giulio Della Rovere, a Hermit of St Augustine with Protestant sympathies who studied medicine in Padua between 1527 and 1528. When Della Rovere was tried in Venice, the inquisitors highlighted his friendship with the physician Melchiorre de Cirono, 'a sincere and ingenious man' ('uomo sincero e di cervello') who was wont to speak 'about predestination' ('di predestinazione'). By contrast, his correspondence showed an emphasis on matters relating to medicine and alchemy.[58] Even more significantly, the Inquisition discovered numerous 'books of medicine and the humanities' ('libri di medicina e di humanità') at the house of Francesco Scudieri, a heretical former Canon Regular from Cremona. These works included two volumes 'written in pen with Andreas Vesalius's plates' ('scritti a penna con le tavole di Andrea Vesalio'), works by Girolamo Cardano, a 'handwritten book about medicine' ('libro scritto a mano de medicina'), and works by Jacques Dubois, Leonhart Fuchs, and Galen.[59]

In the case of Volpe, there was a more matter-of-fact explanation for his apostasy and interest in the Reformation: his love for Camilla, a widow from Padua, and his desire to acquire wealth and leave together for the lands of prosperity and freedom over the Alps. Although he lived in Padua, Volpe spent most of his time in Venice, where he treated patients in their homes and prepared his remedies at the Frari *spezieria*. He built his reputation in the city thanks to a powerful medicine of his own creation which he administered so effectively to cancer sufferers that he earned the nickname of the 'canker friar' ('frate del cancaro'). This professional success also ensured a certain level of financial wellbeing, and he acquired the *spezieria*, where he had worked since 1564, from Paolo Antonieli della Cava. He also lent forty-four ducats to a certain Antonio Vincenzino and one hundred ducats to Properzio Bellebuono, a matter which we shall return to shortly. His contacts in Venice included physicians, apothecaries, surgeons, distillers, and glassblowers, who were essential figures in the production of the ampoules required to practise alchemy. This network extended northwards from the south of Italy to Padua and Venice, and was used to exchange secrets, know-how, materials (such as oils and ointments), and money. Most notably, it established connections between natives of the south of the peninsula (one of Volpe's friends was Dionora Calia from Apulia, the former housekeeper in the Ruscelli-Panarelli household). Volpe worked above all with the physician Decio Bellebuono, originally from the Kingdom of Naples, who lived in Venice with his father, Prudenzio, and two brothers: Galeno, who was also a physician (enrolled at the College of Physicists since 1568) and Properzio, Volpe's debtor.[60] In 1565, Volpe agreed to accompany the youngest brother to Apulia to teach him 'to make acqua vitae' ('a fare acquavita'), a trip that marked the beginning of all his troubles.

Decio Bellebuono, formerly called Giacomo da Campagna, had fled Naples with his family following a murder. He changed his surname to Bellebuono to ward off suspicion and offer an impression of honesty and respectability. The family moved to Venice, and Decio started to work as a medical practitioner, cultivating friendships with members of the College of Medicine (such as the aforementioned Antonio Secco, who was accused of letting a patient die without confessing in 1571) and Venetian aristocrats like Pellegrino Bragadin.[61] He took over the Frari *spezieria* from Volpe, running the business in his brother's name to bypass the law that forbade physicians from making medicinal remedies. The funds for this purchase were borrowed from the 'canker friar.' After Volpe went into business with Bellebuono, however, he was 'destroyed' ('assassinato') by his partner and his family. He was denounced to the Inquisition for his religious views and arrested by the Holy Office while crossing Campo San Lio one day in January 1567 with no respect for the priestly robes he was still wearing.[62] While the Inquisition was busy investigating Panarelli's network at the time, the judges also had to contend with this case, which soon took shape as a real conundrum.

Defendants were usually summoned by the court in an inquisitorial process; only in extreme cases did the judges order the arrest of the suspect. The charges against the charlatan physician were therefore particularly serious. In addition to apostasy, Volpe was accused of denying the existence of purgatory, claiming that the Madonna of Loreto was the 'pope's whore' ('putana del papa'), and stating that the popes were doing 'terrible work' ('pessimo officio'). His position was further exacerbated by the fact that he lived as man and wife with Camilla. Michele Cantrana, a barber-surgeon, testified during the trial that Volpe had told him about the lands of 'Germany' ('Alemania') where people 'lived in a community' ('si vive*va* in comun') during a home visit to a sick patient. He had also revealed 'that a certain extremely capable barber-surgeon had moved to the Grisons and made a fortune' ('che un certo cerusico valentissimo era andato in terra di Grisoni et si era fatto ricco').[63] Volpe's way of thinking blended desire for religious freedom with thirst for social equality, ambition for wealth (reinforced by stories about Italian exiles with well-paid medical positions abroad), and the dream of no longer needing to hide his relationship. It is possible that the barber-surgeon in question was Niccolò Buccella, whose story was certainly well known in Padua. As one of the Buccella brothers acted as Volpe's lawyer (until he received threats from the Bellebuono family and stepped aside), Antonino was probably party to first-hand knowledge of the case or might even have met Niccolò.[64] Rumours and stories circulated between countries and cities and from person to person, thereby influencing choices and experiences.

The evidence against Volpe indicates a level of radical thinking common to other medical practitioners that were not learned physicians. Like all such individuals, Volpe did not enjoy the social and financial status of his educated colleagues.[65] However, his opinions were based on a theoretical as well as a socio-economic framework. Although he was an unpopular figure among surgeons in Padua, who felt that his reputation was undeserved as he had not graduated, he had spent time at the university, where he developed an interest in theological matters and engaged with heterodox ideas.[66] He attended Fra Adriano's lectures 'on the Holy Scripture' ('sulla sacra Scrittura')[67] and studied medicine and philosophy as an autodidact, reading texts by Alessandro Piccolomini and the Valdesian physician Donato Antonio Altomare. The latter's work had been recommended by another Neapolitan physician, Domenico de Juniis, who worked at the *Aquila* apothecary shop in Venice. De Juniis had known Volpe since their days in Padua (when they attended Fra Adriano's lectures together) and confirmed Bellebuono's damaging stories about his friend at the trial. The bond between the two is also shown by the fact that Volpe entrusted De Juniis with several books before travelling to Apulia: a text by Altomare, an edition of *Dioscorides*, Piccolomini's *Filosofia* (*Philosophy*), and an exposition of the Psalms.

Volpe's library also contained a book of pharmaceutical and therapeutic techniques by Leonardo Fioravanti, the empirical physician par excellence.[68] The latter knew the 'canker friar' personally and testified in his favour during the investigation.[69] The fact that Fioravanti stepped forward to help Volpe underlines that even a charlatan physician could build an illustrious relational network in sixteenth-century Venice. Fioravanti also showed his admiration for Bellebuono (after his death), describing him as a 'highly experienced physician' ('fisico di tanta esperienza') in his *Dello specchio di scienza universale* (*The Mirror of Universal Knowledge*, Venice, 1567).[70] In the game of intellectual accolades and compliments played by writers to pander to readerships and celebrate professional achievements, Fioravanti praised a physician that had successfully overcome the boundaries between medical science and the pharmaceutical art. Fioravanti's comment also highlights the professional standing that Decio Bellebuono must have enjoyed in the late sixteenth century. Indeed, his professional reputation remained intact despite accusations of murder, chicanery and, as we will see shortly, heresy. While Bellebuono's therapeutic experimentation led to a long, messy dispute with Volpe, it also earned him everlasting fame in the work of a well-known figure in the medical world at the end of the sixteenth century. The balance of power was certainly in Bellebuono's favour and Volpe's counteraccusations were no more than a minor setback to his thriving career. In 1569, the heterodox Paduan Marziale Clemente sent a letter from his Venetian prison cell to Volpe, who was also imprisoned in Padua. He warned him about Bellebuono's power and influential contacts (including a 'monsignor reverend legate' ['monsignor reverendo legato']), explaining that these factors would allow Decio to plead his case and consolidate his reputation.[71] Volpe was thus advised to walk the path of reconciliation for his own present and future good.

Volpe stated, as did several other witnesses, that Bellebuono had made the first approach to learn how 'to make soap' ('a fare de' savoni') and receive training in the art of distillation, in which Volpe was a leading expert. He came to consider Bellebuono as a close friend as their professional relationship developed, lending him two hundred ducats and revealing his most valuable secret (his remedy for cancer). When he explained his religious views, however, the Neapolitan denounced him to the Holy Office to destroy his rival, drawing on his reputation as an apostate. What Bellebuono failed to consider, though, was the level of support enjoyed by Volpe. The judges were also less gullible than he had hoped. His denunciation thus backfired rapidly, triggering an investigation against him that led to his arrest. Not only did Volpe counter-denounce Bellebuono as a fraud, murderer, and thief, but the magistrates also deemed the latter's version of events to be dubious and implausible. After all, this was not the first time that Bellebuono's name had been mentioned in an Inquisition trial. In 1566, the aforementioned humanist Publio Francesco Spinola had denounced Bellebuono as one of his accomplices, explaining that he was wont to speak of 'German matters' ('delle cose di Alemagna')[72] and was hostile to the clergy and the authority of the Church. Furthermore, the lawyer Matteo Avogari, under investigation in 1567, had described Decio Bellebuono as a skilled dissimulator whose real opinions were hard to decipher as 'he preferred to ask questions rather than let himself be understood' ('preferiva interrogare che lasciarsi intendere').[73] All the same, he was a regular member of Avogari's heretical group, who had devised 'a way of praying covertly against the directive of the Holy Catholic Church' ('un modo di far oratione copertamente contra l'ordine della santa Chiesa cattolica').[74] In a network of shrewd Nicodemites, the Neapolitan must have surpassed everyone in terms of simulation skills.

At the same time that he created legal problems with the ecclesiastical authorities for Antonino Volpe, Bellebuono also denounced a 'Frenchman named Claudio' ('Claudio francese'). This figure can be identified as Claudio Textor, a French alchemist who was sentenced to death by the Holy Office in 1587 as a relapsed heretic. This illustrates the breadth of his heretical and professional network. It is also known that the physician was in contact with Textor's good friend Cornelio Sozzini, an alchemist, inventor, and the brother of Lelio Sozzini.[75] Indeed, during a trial against Cornelio in 1577, a year after Decio had died, his son Lelio Bellebuono was cited as a witness in possession of the facts.[76] It is highly probable that Bellebuono shared the same dogmaless religious inclinations as Textor and Sozzini, as well as a passion for the secrets of alchemy.[77] Bellebuono's affinity with these figures and his tendency to question theological doctrine rather than work out effective dogmatic solutions suggests that he was one of the many heterodox physicians reluctant to identify with any of the new Reformed orthodoxies. Also significant is his intermediary role in sharing out the money sent home by Italian exiles at the behest of Giorgio Biandrata and Prospero Provana.[78] Both this element and his contact with Cornelio Sozzini account for his association with the most radical fringes of Italian heretics in exile.

The complexity of Bellebuono and Volpe's professional relationship also shows that the boundary between scholarly medicine and empirical healing was sometimes extremely blurred. Physicians bridged the two largely incompatible worlds of the nobility and the popular classes, encouraging the circulation of ideas in different contexts and through different channels. There was still, however, a certain distance and mistrust between learned physicians from the liberal professions and their colleagues from humbler social ranks. It is definitely true to say that the two groups were not on equal footing. Although Volpe proved better qualified to defend himself than Bellebuono had imagined, he was effectively deceived by his colleague. The Neapolitan expected to emerge from the matter unscathed, and this is indeed what came to pass. With the judges failing to untangle the mess, both defendants were eventually acquitted after a long trial.

Chapter 5 will show that empirical physicians and alchemists also featured in Donzellini's professional and religious network on his return to the Republic of Venice. Even though there is no evidence that Donzellini had any direct contact with Panarelli and Bellebuono, their destinies were certainly united in terms of feelings, practices, and social relations.

Notes

1 Paolo Ulvioni, 'Cultura Politica e cultura religiosa a Venezia nel secondo Cinquecento. Un bilancio,' in *Archivio Storico Italiano* 141, no. 4 (1983): 591–651. On religiosity in Venice, see also Zorzi, *La vita quotidiana a Venezia*, 254–87.

2 ASV, Sant'Uffizio, *Processi, Contro Paolo Moscardo*, Bu. 23, letter from Paolo Moscardo, 12 May 1568.

3 This term referes to a residual group structured around 'an alternative project to the dominant or prevalent one' ('a un progetto alternativo a quello dominante o prevalente'); see Franco Motta, *Elogio delle minoranze. Le occasioni mancate dell'Italia* (Venice: Marsilio, 2012), 1.

4 On the escalating repression in the second half of the century, see Andrea Del Col, 'La repressione della Riforma in Italia durante il Cinquecento,' in *La Réforme en France et en Italie: contacts, comparaisons et contrastes* (Rome: École Française de Rome, 2007), 481–98.

5 ASV, Sant'Uffizio, *Processi, Fascicolo 3,* deposition by a man identified only as Raphael of 4 November 1553.

6 Ivi, *Contro Girolamo Parto nodaro, Contro Gianbattista Michiel fratrem eius uterinum*, Bu. 37, 33 v.

7 Ibid., *Denuncia contra Caterina 1574* [in *Contro Gian Battista Gemma*], deposition of Caterina Sartora of 15 October 1575.

8 On Spinola, see Pio Paschini, 'Un umanista disgraziato nel Cinquecento: Publio Francesco Spinola,' in *Nuovo archivio veneto*, 37 (1919): 65–189, Marion Leathers Kuntz, *The Anoitment of Dionisio. Prophecy and Politics in Renaissance Italy* (University Park: The Pennsylvania State University Press, 2001), 177–186. Archival information about Spinola can be found above all in ASV, Sant'Uffizio, *Processi*, *Contro Andrea di Ugoni*, Bu. 11, passim. For other sources and a bibliography, see Giovanna Paolin, 'Spinola, Publio Francesco,' in *Dizionario Biografico degli italiani*, 93 (2018). See also Publio Francesco Spinola, 'De Hieronimo Dongellini, Brixiani, Medici philosophique, singularis bibliotheca, Elegia V,' in *Francisci Spinulae mediolanensis elegorum de variis argumentis, liber tertium* (Venice: Ziletti, 1562).

9 ASV, Sant'Uffizio, *Processi, Contro Girolamo Parto nodaro, Contro Gianbattista Michiel fratrem eius uterinum*, Bu. 37. On Parto, see Seidel Menchi, *Erasmo in Italia*, 132–33.

10 ASV, Sant'Uffizio, *Processi, Contro Vincenzo Negroni*, Bu. 22, deposition by Giovanni Antonio "mercadante" of 22 March 1567.

11 I briefly addressed the case of Negroni in my *Contra medicos*, erroneously holding him responsible for the letters on the basis of the interpretation of the Holy Office and the subsequent conviction. I realised my mistake by examining the trials of Michiel and Parto. The correct sequence of events can therefore be found in this book, which in this respect updates my previous article.

12 ASV, Sant'Uffizio, *Processi, Contro Vincenzo Negroni*, Bu. 22, deposition by Negroni of 10 October 1567.

13 Ibid., deposition by Negroni of 9 December 1567.

14 Ivi, *Contro Paolo Moscardo,* Bu. 23, letter from Paolo Moscardo, 12 May 1568.

15 Ivi, *Processi, Contra medicos*, Bu. 35. On this episode see Palmer, 'Physicians and the Inquisition,' 120–21; Celati, 'Contra Medicos,' 76–79.

16 ASV, Sant'Uffizio, *Processi, Contra medicos*, Bu. 35, complaint by pre' Antonio Rocha.

17 In 1557, the medical authorities warned physicians to 'remind the sick to confess' ('ricordino agli amalati il confessarsi'): Venice, Biblioteca marciana, Ms Ital VII (2342=9695), *Notizie cavate dai libri dei priori*, 8v. In 1579, 'The four Savi [wise men or senators] of the Order of the Inquisition told the College that physicians must not examine sick people who do not confess. The College replied that this could not be carried out for five reasons' ('I 4 savi ordine dell'inquisizione al collegio che li medici non visitino li infermi che non si confessano. Risposta del collegio non potervisi questo eseguire per cinque ragioni'); ibid., 17v; while ten years later, once again 'the prior was called by the Inquisition to make physicians comply with Pius V's bull about examining those who do not confess. The

College responded, explaining the difficulties' ('chiamato il priore dall'inquisizione perché faci osservare da medici la bulla di Pio V circa il visitar chi non si confessa. Risulse il collegio rispondere et addir le difficoltà'); ibid., 21r.

18 The twenty-second canon of the Fourth Council of the Lateran issued by Innocent III in 1215 required physicians treating seriously ill patients to ensure that they had spoken to a confessor before starting medical treatment. The decree reads as follows: 'The infirmity of the body sometimes results from sin, as in Christ's words when he healed a sick man: "Go and sin no more, lest a worse thing come unto thee." By this decree, it is therefore established and strictly ordered that physicians of bodies who are called to the sick must first warn and encourage them to call physicians of souls. In this way, after the spiritual health of the sick has been provided for, the remedy of the medicine for the body can be carried out more effectively, since when the cause ceases, the effect also ceases.' ('L'infermità del corpo dipende talora dal peccato, come disse il Signore all'ammalato che aveva sanato: "Va e non voler più peccare, perché non debba accaderti di peggio." Col presente decreto pertanto stabiliamo e comandiamo severamente ai medici dei corpi che quando sono chiamati presso gli infermi, prima di tutto li ammoniscano e li inducano a chiamare i medici delle anime, cosicché dopo che è stato provvisto alla salute spirituale degli infermi, si proceda al rimedio della medicina corporale con maggior efficacia: cessando infatti la causa, cessa anche l'effetto.') The quotation is taken from Decree 22 of the Fourth Lateran Council. See also Norman Tanner, *I concili della Chiesa* (Milan: Jaca Book, 2007), 68–69. On the importance and applications of the bull *Super gregem dominicum* in some Italian cities, see Giovanni Romeo, *Ricerche su confessione dei peccati e Inquisizione nell'Italia del Cinquecento* (Reggio Calabria: La Città del Sole, 1997), 107–14; on the relationship between physicians and ecclesiastical institutions in the late sixteenth century, see Adriano Prosperi, *Tribunali della coscienza. Inquisitori, confessori, missionari* (Turin: Einaudi, 1996), 469–70. See also ibid., 220–23 on the importance of confession for the populace and for the Catholic authorities, and on the 'strategy of kindness' ('strategia della dolcezza') adopted by Julius III. On the exploitation of confession to acquire information on the heretical movement and to repress it see: Elena Brambilla, *Alle origini del Sant'Uffizio. Penitenza, confessione e giustizia spirituale dal medioevo al XVI secolo* (Bologna: Il Mulino, 2000), 347–379.

19 On the reasons for opposing the ecclesiastical norms that attempted to control medical staff in contexts strongly influenced by heresy, see Celati, 'Contra Medicos,' 81–82; Domizia Weber, *Sanare e maleficiare: Guaritrici, streghe e medicina a Modena nel XVI secolo* (Rome, Carocci: 2011), 97–121.

20 ASV, Sant'Uffizio, *Processi, Contro Ludovico Abioso e Teofilo Panarelli*, Bu. 32, testimony by Giovanni Catena, 26 January 1572.

21 Palmer, 'Physicians and the Inquisition,' 121; Celati, 'Contra medicos,' 91. ASV, Sant'Uffizio, *Processi: Contro Ludovico Abioso e Teofilo Panarelli*, Bu. 32, deposition by Panarelli of 6 December 1571.

22 Roger French, 'The Medical Ethics of Gabriele de Zerbi,' in Andrew Wear, Johanna Geyer-Kordesch, Roger French eds., *Doctors and Ethics: The Earlier Historical Setting of Medical Ethics* (Amsterdam: Rodopi, 1993), 84.

23 See, for example, the case of Donzellini and the nuns who escaped from the convent of Santa Lucia in 1551. The key role played by physicians in maintaining the physical and spiritual health of their patients is shown among other things by the fact that the Dutch Reformed Church established special figures, *zie-kentroosters*, who were entrusted with comforting invalids, praying with them at their sickbed, helping them to accept their sickness, and as a result deriving reasons for coming closer to God, as well as providing medical opinions. See Mary Lindemann,

Medicine and Society in Early Modern Europe (Cambridge, Cambridge University Press, 1999), 210. On the matter of propaganda conducted at the sickbed and for some case studies, see Celati, '*Contra medicos*,' 2018, 89–98.

24 ASV, Sant'Uffizio, *Processi*, *Contro Vincenzo Negroni*, Bu. 22, depositions of 10 April and 21 June 1567.

25 ASV, Sant'Uffizio, *Processi*, *Contro Hieronimo Parto nodaro 1572 et Joannem Baptistam Michiel fratrem uterinum 1573*, Bu. 37, 8r.

26 ASV, Sant'Uffizio, *Processi, Contro Gian Battista Gemma*, Bu. 37.

27 Ivi, *Contro speziali delle Colombine*, Bu. 20. Gian Battista was the only member of the family with the title of doctor: Elisabetta Della Francesca, Emilia Veronese (eds.), *Acta graduum academicorum Gymnasii Patavini, ab anno 1551 ad annum 1565* (Padua: Antenore, 2001), 506–07. On Gian Battista Gemma and his family, see Joanna Kostylo, 'Contested Devotions: Space, Identities and Religious Dissent in the Apothecary's Home,' in Maya Corry, Marco Faini, and Alessia Meneghin (eds.), *Domestic Devotions in Early Modern Italy* (Leiden – Boston: Brill, 2019), 408–36; *Eadem*, 'Pharmacy.'

28 ASV, Sant'Uffizio, *Processi, Denuncia contra Caterina 1574* [in *Contro Gian Battista Gemma*], Bu. 37. On her case see also Federica Ambrosini, "El cervel intrigà nelle cose della fede': donne e Riforma a Venezia (secoli XVI-XVII), in Anna Bellavitis, Nadia Maria Filippini and Tiziana Plebani (eds.), *Spazi, poteri, diritti delle donne a Venezia in età moderna* (Verona: Qui Edit, 2021), 166–70.

29 ASV, Sant'Uffizio, *Processi, Denuncia contra Caterina 1574* [in *Contro Gian Battista Gemma*], Bu. 37, passim.

30 There is an initial exploration of Panarelli's story in Celati, 'Heretical Physicians in Sixteenth-Century Italy,' 18–23. Among other things, the article presents and discusses a digital visualisation of Panarelli's ego-network.

31 Teofilo was the fourth and last child of Nicola Antonio and Marina Sardini, a Venetian. His parents probably met at some point between his father's university studies in Padua and his first job as a physician in Venice. His siblings were Agostino, Flaminia, and Virginia. Agostino died in Padua after being educated in Germany in the retinue of Melanchthon, while his father died in Monopoli during one of his visits. The family then met up again in Venice, where Teofilo lived with Virginia and Flaminia for two years (the sisters lived upstairs while he resided downstairs). See ASV, *Sant'Uffizio, Processi, Contro Teofilo Panarelli e Ludovico Abioso*, Bu. 32, deposition by Virginia Panarelli, 24 January 1572.

32 Fragnito, 'Fonzio, Bartolomeo.'

33 ASV, *Sant'Uffizio, Processi, Panarelli Teofilo* [e suoi complici] 1572, Bu. 32, 4r.

34 Ibid., *Contro Teofilo Panarelli e Ludovico Abioso 1568*, Bu. 32, deposition by Panarelli of 23 November 1571.

35 Ibid., *Panarelli Teofilo* [e suoi complici] 1572, Bu. 32, 4r.

36 Ibid., *Contro Teofilo Panarelli e Ludovico Abioso 1568*, Bu. 32, deposition by Panarelli of 16 November 1571.

37 Ibid., deposition by Panarelli of 6 December 1571.

38 Ibid., *Panarelli Teofilo* [e suoi complici] 1572, Bu. 32, 7r.

39 In addition to the references made in the first chapter, see Virginia's second testament in 1587, when she stated that she was the 'widow of Mr Girolamo Ruscelli' ('relitta del q. ms Hieronimo Ruscelli'), Paolo Procaccioli, entry 'Ruscelli, Girolamo,' in *Dizionario Biografico degli italiani*, 89 (2018).

40 On Ruscelli, see ibid.

41 Edgar Zilsel, 'The Sociological Roots of Science,' *Social Studies of Science* 30/6 (2000), 935–949; Matteo Valleriani, *Galileo Engineer* (Berlin: Springer, 2010); Pamela O. Long, *Artisan/Practitioners and the Rise of the New Sciences, 1400–1600* (Corvallis: Oregon State University Press, 2011).

42 Panarelli's will is published in Domenico Orano, *Liberi pensatori bruciati in Roma dal XVI al XVIII secolo* (Rome: Tipografia dell'unione cooperativa editrice, 1904), 45–49.
43 Panarelli received this astrolabe from the goldsmith Vittor da Gallo through the intermediation of Giulio di Stan; see ASV, *Sant'Uffizio*, *Panarelli Teofilo* [e suoi complici] 1572, Bu. 32, 21r; On Arquer, see Firpo, *Dal sacco di Roma all'Inquisizione*, 161–220.
44 ASV, Sant'Uffizio, *Processi, Contro Paolo Moscardo*, Bu. 23, letter from Giuseppe Moscardo.
45 Ivi, *Relatio circa visitationem et confessionem infirmorum* (loose leaf), Bu. 65.
46 Ivi, *Contro Teofilo Panarelli e Ludovico Abioso 1568*, Bu. 32, 16v.
47 Ibid., 6v.
48 Lelio and Fausto Sozzini, *Le* Explicationes *Giovannee*, Mario Biagioni (ed.) (Rome: Edizioni di Storia e Letteratura, 2020).
49 See infra Chapter 7.
50 Ibid., 3r.
51 'We did not go beyond a certain limit with apothecaries. Needless to say, I had one of St Augustine's letters [...] and this letter speaks about justification, and we read it many times' ('Non ci allargavamo con speziali. È beninteso che io havevo una lettera di s. Augustino ... la quale lettera parla de Justificatione et quella legessimo molte volte'). Pegolotto, from Reggio Emilia, was in the city to 'sell velvet' ('vendere dei velluti') in 1567, when Panarelli was a regular visitor to the *Spezieria dell'Elmo*. Teofilo passed some books on to Pegolotto (whose titles are unknown) and gave the apothecary a copy of the *Beneficio di Cristo*. ASV, Sant'Uffizio, *Processi*, *Contro Teofilo Panarelli e Ludovico Abioso 1568*, Bu. 32, deposition by Panarelli of 23 November 1571.
52 Ivi, deposition by Panarelli of 20 November 1571.
53 ASV, *Sant'Uffizio*, *Processi*, *Panarelli Teofilo* [e suoi complici] 1572, Bu. 32, 30v.
54 Ivi, *Contro Alvise Mocenigo, Contro Marcantonio Canale, Contro Andrea Dandolo*, Bu. 23, deposition by Andrea Dandolo of 2 September 1568.
55 Ibid., *Contro Teofilo Panarelli e Ludovico Abioso*, Bu. 32, 18 June, 1568.
56 ASV, Sant'Uffizio, *Processi*, *Panarelli Teofilo* [e suoi complici] 1572, Bu. 32, deposition by Caterina Guarnera of 19 February 1572.
57 ASV, *Notarile, Testamenti*, Bu. 49, 4 June 1606. This was her third will after those in 1582 and 1586; see ibid, Bb. 1266 and 583, cited in Procaccioli, 'Ruscelli, Girolamo.'
58 ASV, Sant'Uffizio, *Processi*, *Processus magistri Iuli Mediolanensis*, Bu. 41, 38r-38v and fascicolo 2, enclosed letters. Della Rovere's enthusiasm had grown stronger over time: in 1543, Bassiano Lando, a physician with connections to heterodox circles, explained in his *Iatrologia* (*Dialogues on the Art of Medicine*, Basel, 1543) that Giulio often discussed medical matters with Ortensio Lando.
59 'A book entitled *Contradicendium medicorum*, a handwritten book about medicine, a medicine black book, an anatomy book' ('un libro intitolato 'Contradicendium medicorum,' un libro scrito a mano de medicina, un libro in medicina negro, un libro di notomia'); ibid., *Francesco Scudieri*, Bu. 15, inventory of his books. See also Ferretto, *Il 'caso' Pomponio Algieri*, 73. See also the case of Seripando, the General of the Augustinian Order with connections to Valdesian circles and a devoted Neoplatonist: in establishing a religious and personal relationship with his physician, the Valdesian Donato Antonio Altomare, he developed his passion for medicine, which led him to collect books about medical practice and focus on healthcare structures; Maria Conforti, 'Girolamo Seripando e Donato Antonio Altomare: note sulla medicina a Napoli a metà Cinquecento,' in Marco Santoro (ed.), *Pomeriggi rinascimentali* (Rome-Pisa: Fabrizio Serra, 2008), 1332.

60 Galeno Bellebuono spent a few years abroad, but there are records that he was a member of the College between 1575 and 1578. It is possible that his decision to leave Venice was in some way connected to the Inquisition proceedings involving his brother and the chicanery against Volpe, in which he was also involved; Venice, Biblioteca Marciana, Ms It VII 2329 (=9723), *Libro dei priori D, Collegio medico fisico,* passim.

61 Both testified in his favour in July 1567 when the judges started to investigate Bellebuono as part of the inquiry against Antonino Volpe, who had in turn accused the physician; ASV, Sant'Uffizio, *Processi, Ad defensam Antonii Volpe de Ferrandina*, Bu. 23, depositions of 17 July 1567.

62 On this episode, see ibid. Many details, especially regarding Decio Bellebuono, can also be found in ASV, Sant'Uffizio, *Processi, Contro Francesco Anovacii*, Bu. 27; see also William Eamon, 'The Canker Friar. Piety and Intrigue in an Era of New Disease,' in *Piety and Plague. From Byzantium to the Baroque*, Franco Mormando and Thomas Worcester eds. (Kirksville: Truman State University Press, 2007), 156–76; Elizabeth Horodowich, *Language and Statecraft in Early Modern Venice* (Cambridge: Cambridge University Press, 2011), 126–27.

63 ASV, Sant'Uffizio, *Processi, Ad defensam Antonii Volpe de Ferrandina*, testimony by Michele Cantrana, 20 July 1568, Bu. 23

64 On the heretical Buccella brothers, see Ambrosini, *L'eresia di Isabella*, 70–71.

65 See the case of Zanetto Barberotto, the barber at the *Ospedale degli Incurabili* referred to in Chapter 3. Such grievances were also common among district physicians, who did not share the wellbeing of their colleagues in the College or in cities. To this end, see the cases of Agostino Vanzo, on whom see Celati, 'Il caso di Agostino Vanzo,' and Stefano de Giusti, a district physician in Gardone with Anabaptist tendencies, who complained that there was no difference between weekdays and feast days for those who were forced to work in order to eat. De Giusti had also taken steps to feed the sick in his district by buying beef at his own expense; ASV, Sant'Uffizio, *Processi, Contro Stefano di Gardone*, Bu. 4, deposition by Stefano de Giusti of 17 November 1550.

66 ASV, Sant'Uffizio, *Processi, Ad defensam Antonii Volpe de Ferrandina*, Bu. 23, testimony by Nicola Quirini of 18 March 1568.

67 Ibid., see the testimony of 6 May 1567 by a Neapolitan physician referred to as Dominicus De Juniis Cavensis.

68 He also had a text by Dioscorides and an exposition of the Psalms; see ibid., the testimony by the physician Domenico de Iunis of 25 May 1568. On the life and medical work of Leonardo Fioravanti from Bologna, see Pietro Camporesi, *Camminare il mondo: vita e avventure di Leonardo Fioravanti medico del Cinquecento* (Milan: Garzanti, 1997); William Eamon, *The Professor Of Secrets: Mystery, Medicine, And Alchemy In Renaissance Italy* (Washington D.C: National Geographic Society, 2010).

69 ASV, Sant'Uffizio, *Processi, Ad defensam Antonii Volpe de Ferrandina*, Bu. 23, testimony by Leonardo Fioravanti of 6 May 1567.

70 Fioravanti, *Dello specchio di scienza universale* (Venice: Eredi di Marchio Sessa, 1583), 13 (first edition 1567). Fioravanti also dedicated his *Della fisica divisa in quattro libri* (*On Physics Divided into Four Books*, Venice: Eredi di Marchio Sessa, 1582) to Bellebuono, a 'dear fellow, who died some time ago' ('compar carissimo, qual è morto già molti giorni sono'). There are also references to the Neapolitan physician in the *Tesoro della vita umana* (*Treasury of Human Life*), Venice: Eredi di Marchio Sessa, 1582), in which Fioravanti praises Bellebuono as one of 'the men of greatest authority in their abilities' ('gli uomini di grandissima autorità nelle facoltà loro') in a list that also includes Agostino Gadaldino.

71 ASV, Sant'Uffizio, *Processi, Contro Francesco Anovacio (Campagna Giacomo o Bellebuono Decio)*, 32 v.

72 The dossier on Volpe's defence contains a file – 'Contra Decio Bellimboni medico' – that includes extracts from depositions made by other heretics active in Venice. In this case, Publio Francesco Spinola was interrogated 'in the place of torture on 10 October 1566' ('in loco tortura sub die 10 octobris 1566'); ASV, Sant'Uffizio, *Processi, Ad defensam Antonii Volpe de Ferrandina*, Bu. 23.

73 Ibid., deposition of Avogari of 19 April 1567.

74 Ivi, *Contro Matteo Avogari*, Bu. 22, complaint of 31 March 1567.

75 Cornelio Sozzini had submitted a project to the Provveditori alle acque (Superintendents of the Water) for draining rainwater that created 'extremely harmful sticky and putrid mud hated by everyone' ('fango attaccatizzo e putrido tanto dannoso e odiato da tutti') and for cleaning and draining canals in Venice. It was designed to improve levels of hygiene in the city and to help women and elderly people cross bridges. ASV, *Esecutori alle acque*, Bu. 270, 11v-12v.

76 Stella, *Dall'anabattismo al socinianesimo*, 153.

77 Ibid., 144. We will return to Textor in the final chapter.

78 ASV, Sant'Uffizio, *Processi, Contro Nicolò Buccella*, Bu. 36, testimony by Iacopo de Gattis of 31 July 1574: 'And he said: I retrieved five hundred ducats of those belonging to Lippino and another five hundred were retrieved by the most illustrious physician Decio Bellebuono, who still has the remainder [of this money]. And I believe that the money is Biandrata's because he wrote several times about its recovery. He was asked: to whom was this money given? He replied: to various people in the order that I was given by Mr Prospero [Provana], but I do not remember the names of the people.' ('Et adducit ex se: Io recuperai 500 ducati de questi del detto Lippino et 500 ne furono recuperati per opera del ecc.mo medico Decio Bellebuono et il resto sta ancora appresso quel gentiluomo. Et credo che siano del Brandata perche lui scriveva et ha scritto piu vote per la recuperatione di detti danari. Fuit ei dictum: a chi sono sta' distribuiti questi danari da voi? Respondit: A diverse persone secondo l'ordine che io ho avuto dal signor Prospero sopradetto ma non mi ricordo el nome delle persone.').

5 Donzellini's return to the Republic of Venice, 1560–1587

During the Counter-Reformation, when Panarelli's group, Bellebuono, and Volpe all fell afoul of the repression raging in Venice, Donzellini was also targeted by the Inquisition on four occasions (in 1560, 1574, 1578, and 1587). However, Girolamo now had a different religious profile. This change resulted from the new historical context and his personal experiences: in particular, his first-hand contact with the Holy Office (which started in 1553) and his freshly acquired philosophical and intellectual maturity. While Donzellini had been a driving force in the group fighting to establish the Reformation in Italy in the 1540s and early 1550s, such aspirations seemed fanciful in the second half of the century, even in Venice. In this context, there was a significant shift in his religious outlook, his approach to relations, and more generally the objectives of his militancy. As this chapter narrates, the second part of his life (1560–1586) was characterised by Nicodemism, tolerant non-confessional spiritualism, interest in Hermeticism and alchemy, and efforts to distribute books and knowledge across the confessional divide.

5.1 Venice – Verona, 1560–1573

After seven years abroad, Donzellini had grown tired of the destructive doctrinal controversies in the new Reformed Churches. The fact that religious repression in Geneva was just as harsh as its Roman equivalent was also a great source of disappointment. His homeland thus offered a more attractive alternative: as well as practising as a physician exploiting his Italian network, he would come into the rich inheritance that his uncle had left for him. He thus appeared voluntarily before the Venetian Holy Office on 12 November 1560 to settle his debt with the religious legal system. At this stage, he was investigated as 'strongly suspected' ('vehementemente suspetto') of heresy: the judges focused on his friendships and the books he had read in the 1540s without examining the more profound aspect of his religious beliefs and affiliation.

To allay suspicions and justify his behaviour, Donzellini produced an *apologia* that emphasised his status as a learned medical professional.

DOI: 10.4324/9781003218852-6

As a physician, he was required to treat all patients, including the heterodox ones, and as a man of letters he was naturally interested in the new cultural ideas stirring the consciences of humanists, theologians, and scholars from Wittenberg to Naples. It should not have been surprising then that he read texts and debated with numerous other physicians. For instance, he had corresponded with Giovan Battista Pigafetta, a physician and surgeon from Vicenza to whom he had also sent prohibited books. Moreover, he had exchanged views on ecclesiological and doctrinal matters with doctors of medicine 'since it was necessary to practise together as physicians every day' ('poiché bisognava ogni giorno praticare insieme come medici'): these medical practitioners included Giambattista Canova, Ludovico Manna, Giambattista Susio, Marcantonio Passeri, Angelo Odoni, Matteo Fabbri, Agostino Gadaldino, and a man referred to simply as Agacio.[1] With the connections between medical practice and religious debate, it would have been both undesirable and impossible for him to opt out; after all, he was a brilliant man of culture with extensive professional and intellectual networks. His occasional interest in theology had been limited to condemning the abuses of the clergy in public and indulging his literary passion by reading a few heterodox books. He acknowledged that his reputation had been tarnished most seriously by his associations with 'unfrocked friars' ('sfratati'). However, he refused to betray friends or purported fellow believers and did not denounce those seemingly overlooked by the legal authorities.

Donzellini deployed a successful defensive strategy that was a masterpiece of religious simulation.[2] Despite the inconsistencies highlighted by the judges when they read the apologia (their marginal notes stress the contradictory nature of many of its defensive justifications), the physician emerged from the trial virtually unscathed. Although he was sentenced to a year's confinement at the convent of Santi Giovanni e Paolo, he only served part of his punishment and regained his freedom in 1561. This was partly thanks to intervention on his behalf by Mocenigo, his patron, and partly because he petitioned for release on several occasions. His pleas focused on urgent family matters that required his attention and the importance of not blotting his professional record with the indignity of a prison sentence, one of the reasons that had prompted him to flee in 1553. As he was eager to move to Verona and start a new life, he implored the inquisitors not to cause 'considerable damage' ('tanto danno') to his reputation by making him 'enter another city, where I am held in high esteem, with a shameful beginning' ('intrar in una tal città dove che sono in bona consideratione con un principio infame')[3].

His worries were well founded, as the stain of his religious crime damaged his medical career significantly over the following decade. In the short term, though, the clemency of the judges enabled him to settle in Verona, where he stayed for twelve years. During this period he married Lucrezia, who came from an illustrious local family, and together they had a son, Virgilio, in 1566.[4] While in Verona, he focused on his family and medicine, built a new network of professional and personal contacts, became a citizen of the *Respublica literaria* (Republic of Letters), and reduced his involvement in the Venetian heretical movement.[5] He also worked with a pharmacist known for his experimentation – Giovanni Andrea Bellicocchi, the apothecary at the hospital of San Giacomo – just as he had in Venice. Donzellini sent Bellicocchi's remedies to his non-Italian friends and recommended them in his book on treating the plague, published in 1576. He was welcomed into the Veronese College of Physicians on 30 July 1561 and served as *inquisitor* and Prior during some of their sessions in 1568.[6]

The College in Verona was decidedly more conservative than its Venetian counterpart in religious and social terms.[7] Whereas members of the latter came from all over the peninsula, and indeed Europe, Veronese collegians were required to have original citizenship.[8] Moreover, Veronese physicians were particularly receptive to the new direction sparked by the Counter-Reformation, through which they became increasingly involved in the post-Tridentine redefinition of the religious life of the city in the second half of the century. The measure that obliged physicians to stop treating patients who avoided the Catholic sacraments was unconditionally approved in Verona (as well as in Brescia, Piacenza, and Reggio Emilia).[9] One article in the College statutes of 1580 sidelined physicians 'known for heretical depravity' ('haeretica pravitate notati'), as well as religious defectors and physicians of Jewish origin. Furthermore, religious control and repression in Verona extended to the whole medical world, just as in Venice, affecting pharmacies, hospitals, and colleges alike. In 1569, Giovan Francesco Manfredi, the Prior of the hospital of Sant'Antonio and the former physician to Pope Pius IV, was tried by the Veronese Holy Office and transferred to Venice, accused of abstaining from liturgical fasting and attempting to seduce his young servant.[10] Donzellini blended into this milieu for around ten years without any difficulty, strengthened by the Nicodemite approach he had learned during his religious training and perfected in exile. When the local physicians took part in the processions honouring the city's patron saint as a compact group, Donzellini took centre stage, carrying the baldachin with the statue of St Zeno on his shoulders.

During this period, he became friends with Bishop Agostino Valier, who often spoke out in his favour when he was on trial in the following decade. This friendship should not come as a surprise, and it would be a mistake to class it as purely tactical. Valier had been educated at the school of Gian Matteo Giberti, a bishop interested in religious renewal and reform, and his episcopate implemented the idea of 'transferring the essence of practical theology to concrete pastoral practice.'[11] Like Donzellini, he also had a humanist mindset and was driven by philosophical interests. It was therefore undoubtedly a genuine friendship. Indeed, when Donzellini was sentenced to life imprisonment in 1575, his wife Lucrezia appealed to the Holy Office in the vain hope that he would be able to serve out his punishment in Valier's custody, benefitting from his financial and material support.

Girolamo also forged friendships with members of the wealthy Serego family in Verona between 1560 and 1573: he was close to the brothers Antonio Maria and Federico (now best known for commissioning work from the architect Andrea Palladio), and Alessandro, a physician.[12] A letter of June 1577 from Antonio Maria to Federico mentioned Donzellini, who had been pardoned by the Holy Office two months previously after his third trial had ended in a conviction.[13] Antonio Maria warned his brother about the potential danger of returning from Venice after his involvement in the expulsion and imprisonment of men in Verona 'at the behest' ('a istanza') of Donzellini. The news was the talk of the town, tarnishing the aristocrat's reputation for assisting a man guilty of religious crimes. Indeed, Donzellini's name was besmirched after his imprisonment, and he was also expelled from the College of Physicians in 1575 when his surname was emphatically crossed off the register. This might have been the episode that prompted the College to establish the official exclusion of physicians tainted by heterodoxy in the statutes of 1580.[14] As a result, Antonio Maria Serego advised Federico to keep his return from Venice a secret and 'be on guard for his life' ('aver cura della vita sua'), also by procuring arms.

No details are known about the friendship between Donzellini and Federico Serego, but it must have been solid if a member of the powerful family was prepared to risk his own wellbeing to help a man that had clearly made enemies in Verona. They were probably first introduced by Alessandro Serego, Girolamo's medical colleague. When he graduated in Venice in 1551, Alessandro first became a reader in surgery at Padua University and subsequently concentrated on anatomy at the University of Florence. He was also passionate about botany and collecting, interests he shared with his correspondent Ulisse Aldrovandi, who visited him in 1571. In the 1560s, in the same period as Donzellini, Alessandro became a member of the Veronese College of Physicians. However, he had turbulent relations with his colleagues because of his insistence on practising 'manual' ('manualiter') surgery, which damaged the dignity of the whole body, and on 'doing experiments and work in the art of surgery' ('fare qualche esperimento et opera nell'arte chirurgica') in order to 'make [medicine] greater and more fruitful' ('fare più grande e fruttuosa').[15] When Alessandro had to justify himself officially to this end in 1562, he promised to practise surgery 'in the most honourable manner' ('nella più onorata maniera'), making sure that he was always accompanied by 'a servant or external minister for the most wretched operations' ('un domestico o estraneo ministro per le operazioni più abiete').[16] His reasoning did not convince the other collegians, though, and they threatened to remove his name from the register and exclude him 'from this and the other College' ('de dicto et altro Collegio'). In 1563, the College even appointed two procurators to defend their interests in the case against Serego, who was persuaded to do penance and comply with the College statutes in May. The dispute dragged on for years, but the tables were turned in 1575 when Alessandro earned public recognition for the treatment that he had given during the plague that ravaged the Republic. Before this outcome, Donzellini had attempted to mediate between Serego and the College in December 1562, appealing to the group spirit that was supposed to unite all members.[17] Serego's bond with Donzellini was probably strengthened by their common penchant for medical experimentation and their questioning of the College regulations. Indeed, when Donzellini received a *damnatio memoriae* and was expelled from the College in 1575, the accusation against him was *eleutherania*, in the sense of intellectual and religious freedom, a quality that was unacceptable to the Veronese College.

The Serego brothers and Donzellini had another friend in common: the Veronese empirical physician Tommaso Zefiriele Bovio. Donzellini was cited in several of his texts and, as we shall see, they were both collaborators and rivals. Marcantonio Serego (the founder of the Serego-Alighieri dynasty) was Bovio's patron, and the empiric's work *Melampigo* is dedicated to his son Giordano.[18] This friendship not only partly reflects Donzellini's medical approach but also confirms his reluctance to comply with the College regulations; many rulings endeavoured to exclude empirics from medical practice in the city and prohibit any form of collaboration between learned physicians and the so-called charlatan physicians who 'made medicinal preparations of no benefit for financial gain at a high price.'[19]

Tommaso Zefiriele Bovio came from an impoverished noble family that sent him to study law in Padua, Bologna, and Ferrara. He never completed his studies, though, and after a failed military career he decided to practise as an itinerant physician, also acquiring a reputation as an astrologer and an alchemist. His operative and theoretical framework always bordered on heterodoxy for several reasons: his passion and support for judicial astrology (condemned outright by Sixtus V in the 1586 bull *Coeli et terrae creator*);[20] his ostentatious knowledge of the magical arts;[21] his endorsement of religious concord; and his polemic against the temporal claims of Rome. Following the Venetian Interdict, Bovio sent the pope a letter in which he took sides with Venice.[22] He underlined that Christ had never meddled in political matters or claimed to have the power of princes, and even denied it to his apostles. In the same way, he felt that His Holiness should acknowledge the rationale of the Republic and stop interfering in the governance of the temporal domain.[23] In a similar vein, Bovio had encouraged interreligious dialogue some years before by sending letters to Philip II and Clement VIII that urged the Catholic authorities to reconcile with Henry of Navarre.

Bovio's religious inclination was a perfect match for his philosophical outlook. Like Donzellini, he was fascinated by the concept of *prisca theologia*; he saw Plato as the 'lynchpin' ('chiave di volta') joining the Hermetic and Judeo-Christian worlds, and his thinking was influenced by Neoplatonism, which is apparent in his *Theatro dell'infinito* (*Theatre of the Infinite*).[24]

His approach blended empiricism, esotericism, alchemy, and philanthropy.[25] He was also highly critical of scholarly medicine. Bovio wrote three works in the controversy against 'rational physicians' ('medici razionali'): the *Flagello de' medici rationali* (*The Scourge of Rational Physicians*, Venice 1583), the *Melampigo, ovvero confusione de medici sofisti che s'intitolano rationali* (*Melampigo, or The Confusion of Sophist Physicians Who Are Called Rational*, Verona 1585), and the *Fulmine contro de' medici putatitii rationali* (*Invective Against Those Considered Rational Physicians*, Verona 1592). The relative success of these texts led to several reprints during the seventeenth century (in 1601, 1626, and 1676). His points of reference in the medical world were Arnaldus de Villa Nova, Leonardo Fioravanti, whom he had written to asking for advice about some challenging cases, and Paracelsus, 'a great man among the greats' ('huomo grande tra i grandi'). As we will see more thoroughly in Chapter 6, these works reveal important details about Bovio and Donzellini's relationship and are useful for outlining the latter's medical approach, especially with regard to Paracelsianism.

Despite the inclusive and dissimulative nature of his attitude, it cannot have been easy for a cosmopolitan, intellectually restless physician like Donzellini, who was reluctant to embrace religious dogma, to live in Verona during the Counter-Reformation. In the early 1570s medical controversies put an end to the period of calm. These new problems were triggered by Donzellini's close collaboration with Giuseppe Valdagno, a physician, astrologer, and philosopher also driven by pharmacological interests.

Like Donzellini, Valdagno worked between Verona and Brescia and is best known for his contribution to the extensive debate on the 'new star' ('nuova stella,' or *nova*) that appeared in European night skies between 2 and 6 November 1572.[26] He also edited an edition of *De motu* (*On Motion*) by Proclus – the last great Neoplatonist, a commentator on Plato, mathematician, and astronomer –, published by Pietro Perna in 1562. The fact that a work by a Veronese physician was printed by Perna when Donzellini was in Verona and corresponding with his friends in Basel suggests that Girolamo played a role in the undertaking (although this is never mentioned in the sources consulted for the present volume). In 1581, Valdagno was responsible for the first pharmacopoeia compiled for the medical college in Verona. His interest in medicinal remedies can also be seen in the long and bitter polemic with the Brescian Vincenzo Calzaveglia between 1570 and 1573. The controversy was about the use of theriac – a potent and mysterious antidote made with viper flesh – in the treatment of pestilential fever. Donzellini also became involved in the dispute, a move which had fatal consequences for him.

There was renewed enthusiasm for theriac in the sixteenth century, partly as a result of the rediscovery of Galen, who had deemed it an infallible remedy against countless diseases.[27] The medication became so popular during the Renaissance that it was often prepared in public ceremonies in accordance with astral influences. As a marvel of alchemy, it acted through the mechanism of "sympathies" between substances and the notion of treating like with like. Viper poison was said to attract any impure elements in the patient's body to one place; they were then attacked and removed by the other beneficial properties of the medicine. In the dispute with Calzaveglia, Donzellini and Valdagno endorsed the value of theriac in treating pestilential fever, a position in line with the thinking of the great Veronese physician Girolamo Fracastoro. This shared opinion was probably due to a broader intellectual convergence. Indeed, Donzellini and Fracastoro both held the Neoplatonic view that the cosmos was an animate organism imbued with divine energy and intersected by sympathetic processes; it was the duty of the physician-philosopher to learn about these and adapt them to therapeutic and cognitive needs.[28] While the fascination with theriac was certainly widespread in the sixteenth century, it is particularly significant that it united physicians with a common interest in Hermetic knowledge and practices. Like Donzellini, some of these individuals were influenced in religious terms by their encounter with spiritual and/or radical doctrines and fell afoul of inquisitorial repression. For instance, Ulisse Aldrovandi, who since the 1560s was professor and chief physician in Bologna, had been influenced by Camillo Renato's radical spiritualism and was arrested by the Inquisition in 1549. Aldrovandi was an acquaintance and correspondent of Donzellini, who provided him with simples for his museum.[29] He also engaged in a bitter quarrel with the College of Physicians and Apothecaries in Bologna about the preparation of theriac.[30] Another case in point is the Neapolitan physician and botanist Bartolomeo Maranta, who associated with Valdesian groups, studied poisons, and wrote a work on mithridate in 1572; he was tried in 1562 but acquitted.[31] Two of Donzellini's correspondents, Theodor Zwinger and Joaquim Camerarius (one of Aldrovandi's pupils), were also enthusiastic users of theriac. These Protestants with an interest in Hermetic ideas traded viper pills (*trocisci*) with Donzellini from 1560 onwards.[32]

When Valdagno prescribed theriac to petechial typhus patients in Brescia in 1570, he was criticised by the local College of Physicians; he responded by defending the use of the medicament in a volume entitled *De theriacae usu in febribus pestilentialibus* (*On the Use of Theriac in Pestilential Fevers*, Brescia, 1570).[33] Vincenzo Calzaveglia intervened at this point to support the stance of the College, of which he was a member, maintaining that there was a difference between pestilential fever and malignant fever: theriac was useless against the latter, which was the disease afflicting Brescia at the time (his work was entitled *De theriaca abusu in febribus pestilentibus* [*On the Abuse of Theriac in Malignant Fevers*], Brescia, 1570). When Donzellini entered the debate, he defended Valdagno by endorsing Galen's theories.[34] Calzaveglia responded with a series of polemical pamphlets and an acrimonious 'letter in Latin' ('lettera in latino') which, alongside medical arguments, attempted to discredit his rival by criticising his track record with the Inquisition and his exile for religious reasons.[35] The controversy dragged on for three years with further scathing publications until Donzellini and Valdagno were both banished from Brescia. Girolamo's enemies even made an attempt on his life, and he was only saved when the crowd stepped in to help, as he informed Zwinger in a letter in 1573.[36] The repercussions of the polemic had now spread well beyond the borders of the Republic, and Donzellini was adept at finding support. One of his allies was Marsilio Cagnati, a young Veronese graduate of Padua University; in a letter written to his older friend in 1571, Cagnati described the Hippocratic manuscripts he had found in the Vatican Library and asked if he could read Donzellini's and Valdagno's books about pestilential fever.[37]

As Donzellini's enemies had failed to undermine his reputation by drawing on his unorthodox past and had botched their assassination attempt, they decided to denounce him to the Holy Office in Verona.

5.2 The trials in the 1570s

When Donzellini was again summoned before the Inquisition judges in 1573, the resulting trial lasted more than two years. The fact that his 1560 abjuration was deemed to have been insincere posed a major risk to the defendant. He was thus transferred to Venice, where the investigations used lengthy, detailed interrogations and torture to focus on his religious ideas, behaviour, reading, heretical relations, and years spent abroad.

At the beginning of the trial, Donzellini was interrogated about his religious views prior to 1560. The discovery of certain letters written to family members during his exile allowed the judges to establish that Girolamo had been involved in heretical circles in the north of Italy. The missives also enabled them to ascertain that his escape in 1553 had not only been prompted by the 'ignominy' ('ignominia') that would have resulted from imprisonment, as he had stated in his 1560 apologia.[38] He had taken flight because of reluctance to renounce his faith. There was therefore enough evidence to step up the pressure in gruelling interrogations, focusing on why he had not admitted his errors during the previous trial and why he had not reported them in confession. The inquisitors' strategy alternated between attempting to lead him into self-contradiction, appealing to his 'intelligence' ('intelligenza'), and encouraging him to reveal his sins 'naively' ('ingenuamente'). This tug-of-war between the physician and the inquisitors lasted for months. Donzellini explained when and how he had first encountered heterodox ideas, blaming his long-dead brother Cornelio for leading him astray. He then provided further details about his sojourn in Rome and his years away from the peninsula, claiming that he had recanted his heresies on German soil. The strategy of accusing his brother and stressing his reformed character did not produce the desired effect, however. It was felt that as he had lied during the previous trial, he was probably still doing so. While Rome recommended torture by strappado, the Venetian approach focused on questioning witnesses and obtaining further information in collaboration with the court of Padua.

This cooperation between two branches of the Holy Office in the Republic was particularly effective. Donzellini's old friend Gaspare Parma, Paola Marcello, the former nun who had also been his patient, and Marchetta Schiavona, his friend and accomplice, were brought to the stand and interrogated as part of an inquiry into the network they had been part of twenty-five years previously. The other witnesses included the Parmas' former landlord, the head of the convent of Santa Lucia, and Marietta Cagnon, who as we know attended the group's heretical meetings before repenting, frightened by the prospect of being denied absolution if she did not denounce her heretical acquaintances. It was Cagnon's testimony that launched the parallel investigation in Padua. Adopting a particularly fierce and resentful tone, she confirmed that Donzellini had been part of the heretical group that met at Gaspare and Pantasilea Parma's house in Venice in the early 1550s. She also highlighted his involvement in the escape of the two nuns – his patient Cecilia Morosini and Paola Marcello – from the convent of Santa Lucia, claiming that he had caused 'their downfall' ('la rovina'). The judges could never have imagined anything so serious and extended their investigation, questioning Paola Marcello and the nuns that were still alive and potentially remembered the event. Witnesses that had been active in the heretical movement in the 1540s and 1550s joined the sisters in attempting to play down Donzellini's role, sometimes hiding behind memory lapses and female naivety. Nevertheless, Girolamo's position worsened significantly as a result of these parallel investigations. Not only had he lied in his first recantation, but the crimes he had committed before the 1553 trial were far greater than the judges had imagined both at the time and during the 1560 proceedings.

As the months passed, Donzellini was assailed by increasingly pressing questions and cornered by overwhelming evidence. He was thus forced to admit his former heterodox opinions, reveal the books he had read, and name the dissenters he had associated with; although he provided a more detailed list than in 1560, all the individuals in question were either dead, in exile, or had already confessed. He maintained, however, that he had been an impeccable Catholic since his 1560 recantation; as confirmation, he cited testimonies by the archpriest of his local church, San Paolo in Verona, and the bishop of the city, Agostino Valier. He also endured torture with great dignity, limiting himself to praying 'to Jesus' and crying out in pain; he did not confess to crimes for which he felt no responsibility and did not mention his ongoing contact (not yet suspected by the judges) with Perna and the Protestant humanists Zwinger and Camerarius, or name any other accomplices.[39] He solemnly recanted his heresies on 9 June 1575 and was sentenced to life imprisonment. In the meantime, as we have already seen, he was expelled from the College of Physicians in Verona, and his name was removed from the register.

With the death sentence established for relapsed heretics, it is surprising that it was not handed down to a known heterodox dissenter involved in heretical networks stretching from Rome to the north of Italy and in contact with Italian dissidents and scholars of Germanic origin abroad. His avoidance of capital punishment might have been due to the esteem he enjoyed among Veronese prelates, his willingness to collaborate, his reputation as a physician and humanist, and the protection of influential Venetian patricians, most notably Leonardo Mocenigo (who had already intervened in his favour in 1560 so that he could be discharged from house arrest and move to Verona). They were powerless, however, to persuade the judges to remit a sentence that imposed appalling living conditions.

Humiliated by his colleagues, far from the comfort of his loved ones, and exhausted by the harshness of prison, Donzellini was plagued by agonising physical and psychological suffering over the following two years. As is apparent in his petitions to the judges, he believed that his physical health was a consequence of his spiritual wellbeing, a perspective in line with the sixteenth-century dictates of his profession. Both, however, degenerated to a state of total collapse. Girolamo lacked the strength to live in a dark, cramped cell without his books or the comfort of 'teachings of good authors' ('letione de' boni autori') and was forced to live with coarse and unreasonable men (in particular, he mentioned a German clockmaker whose snoring inflicted additional torment).[40] He therefore offered to pay a substantial bail so that he could be transferred to another prison or placed in the custody of Bishop Valier. His wife attempted to move the inquisitors to pity by explaining that she and her son were living in poverty and that they would soon have to 'beg for a living' ('mendicare il vivere') if her husband were not moved. Nevertheless, the petitions all fell on deaf ears.[41]

Paradoxically, the drama of the plague that afflicted Venice between 1575 and 1577 proved timely for Donzellini. On 12 December 1576, the Patriarch of the city authorised his temporary release so that he could treat victims. He then received a pardon when the epidemic ended the following April, probably for services rendered to the city during one of the darkest episodes in its history, in which about a third of the population (around fifty thousand people) died.[42] Working in close contact with their patients, physicians were extremely vulnerable to infection. Indeed, after a year of the epidemic almost all medical practitioners had either died or escaped to the rural hinterland.[43] For a prisoner like Girolamo Donzellini, this was the perfect opportunity to serve the community and redeem himself in the eyes of the judges – especially since imprisonment in times of plague would entail certain death. To this end, Donzellini drafted a series of 'chapters' ('capitoli') and sent them to the judges, providing a dramatic account of the plague in the prison in the *sestiere* of Castello and highlighting his behaviour as a model prisoner. This account now constitutes an excellent source for studying everyday prison life at the time of the plague.[44]

Donzellini explained that the disease first spread to houses near the *cason* (prison) where he was serving his sentence between late August and the beginning of September 1576 and entered the jail a few days later.

The building was sequestered, and no further access was allowed: the physician and his fellow inmates were left to fend for themselves. There was no longer anyone to 'dispense everyday things, meals, wine, water' ('sumministrare le cose quotidiane, pasti, vino, acqua') to the prisoners or remove 'the daily rubbish' ('le immondizie quotidiane').[45] These conditions of extreme danger and hardship prompted Donzellini to channel all his physical and mental energy into writing a *Discorso nobilissimo e dottissimo preservativo et curativo della peste* (*Very Noble and Most Learned Discourse on Protection against and Treatment of the Plague*, Venice 1577), which offered the Venetian authorities a series of theoretical notions and concrete means for eradicating the epidemic. At this time of 'high mortality' ('grande mortalità') and 'terrible calamity' ('grandissima sciagura'), Donzellini concentrated on his medical vocation and his 'reasoning' ('ragione') so as not to be overwhelmed by fear of death or the wrath of the disease. We will return to this text in Chapter 6, reiterating for now that his medical work led to his permanent release on 19 April 1577. This enabled him to return to Venice and practise his profession.

Unfortunately for Donzellini, though, his troubles with the religious court were far from over. He was summoned back by the Holy Office only a year later and interrogated about the escape of Nascimbene Nascimbeni, an elderly grammarian from Ferrara who had been sentenced to life imprisonment in 1571 as a follower of Giorgio Siculo and became Donzellini's cellmate. The pair developed a firm friendship strengthened by their shared experiences of the rigours of prison and the plague.[46] Donzellini was even prepared to jeopardise his own liberty by coming to Nascimbeni's defence; it was therefore an important relationship that also casts light on Girolamo's religious profile. During his trials, while he strongly denied accusations of collusion with any form of sectarian group, the judges seemed reluctant to explore this line of inquiry (just as they did not follow up Marchetta's statements that she had been rebaptised by the physician). On the other hand, it is possible that Donzellini's core subjectivist and spiritualist imprinting prompted him to associate with radicals both during his early years in Venice, when his heretical outlook was reinforced by a variety of heretical environments – he might have had access to Siculo's *Libro Grande* (*Great Book*) at the Maggis' house for example –, and above all after his return from Basel. At this point, when he had abandoned Protestant doctrines, his preferred form of spiritualism followed a path that might have nurtured interest in extreme doctrines like anti-Trinitarianism (which will be explored in Chapter 6) and the teachings of Giorgio Siculo. However, Donzellini never became a member of any of these groups and always retained his spiritual independence. Indeed, his inclusive, open concept of religion rejected individual confessions and sects as he felt that he was only accountable to his own conscience and to God, who was alone in being able to 'see into hearts' ('cognoscere i cuori'); everything else was a matter of indifference (*adiaphora*).[47] This doctrinal fluidity and interest in religious experimentation made him more likely to bond with others with similar heterodox profiles. Giorgio Siculo's theology, embraced by Nascimbeni, might have reverberated with Donzellini's religious sensibilities; it was hostile to both Catholicism and the Reformation, had strong spiritual overtones, and was of an initiatory nature. Furthermore, both prisoners shared a strong humanist propensity.

As a loyal friend, Donzellini continued to visit the prison after Nascimbeni's release to check on his health, urging the magistrates to allow him to serve out his sentence in conditions better suited to his ailing condition. The judges obliged by releasing him into the care of the physician, who thus became responsible for his friend and his medical treatment, acting as the guarantor of compliance with the measure.

Nevertheless, after regaining his health, on 10 July 1578 Nascimbeni left a letter of regret and thanks for Donzellini and his family and absconded without saying goodbye. He was concerned by a fresh summons from the Inquisition, which he saw as potentially perilous given the apparent hostility of the patriarch towards him. As Donzellini had already been tried three times by the Holy Office and was considered an 'astute person' ('persona astuta') that was 'familiar with worldly matters' ('pratica delle cose del mondo'), he was deemed an accomplice in Nascimbeni's escape. He justified himself and numerous Venetian patricians spoke out in his favour but to no avail.[48] Just as the 1577 decision to pardon the physician had been made in Rome and disclosed to Venice by Cardinal Rebiba, the same court now ordered that Donzellini be placed under house arrest and forced to stop his medical work.[49] The fact that the Roman Congregation had been monitoring Donzellini since his 1574 trial demonstrates that he was considered a major figure in the Italian heterodox world, and that his case was deemed worthy of the attention of the Roman court.

Despite this new conviction, Donzellini was soon able to resume his career. In the summer of 1579, the medical reputation he had earned during the plague helped him to obtain the support of the Venetian Senate, which even petitioned the pope for his release, asking for him to be allowed to practise as a physician.[50] This turnaround was occasioned by his friends in high places as well as his practical merits: by his own admission, he enjoyed the backing 'of one of the most influential men' ('di uno degli uomini più influenti') in the city. Thanks to a generous guarantor who undertook to pay the court two thousand crowns as security against a potential escape, Donzellini was released and reinstated as a medical practitioner a year after his fourth trial.[51]

In this respect, Donzellini's case was only partly exceptional. Intervention by local aristocrats often hindered the plans and actions of the Catholic authorities in the first half of the sixteenth century, allowing heterodox physicians to escape the worst-case scenario. As medical practitioners encountered many kinds of people and played a respected role in the social hierarchy of *ancien régime* society, they were able to forge valuable relationships that could be used to fight inquisitorial repression. A case in point occurred in the State of Milan in 1552. Girolamo Maccagno was a physician and an active member of the heretical movement in Cremona; he even stated that 'all physicians in Cremona are heretics' ('a Cremona tutti i medici sono eretici').[52] He was released following pressure from eminent local supporters who claimed that his medical services were essential to the community.[53] The same agreeable fate befell Calisto Villani from Lodi, who was arrested in 1548 and released on bail soon afterwards, and Girolamo Cardano's cellmate Lucillo Filalteo (aka Lucillo Maggi), a physician, philosopher, and classicist.[54] In the 1570s, however, the ecclesiastical authorities were less willing to accept that those guilty of religious crimes could emerge from their judicial proceedings (almost) unscathed thanks to influential patrons. The trial of Francesco Severi, for instance, ended quite dramatically. This physician from Argenta, who had been a member of Giorgio Siculo's sect with Nascimbene Nascimbeni, was executed as a relapsed heretic in 1570. He had been sentenced to life imprisonment in 1568 but was released soon afterwards so that he could minister to the Duke of d'Este's health. He had avoided the death penalty in court thanks to a Nicodemite recantation and the false claim that he had never been tried by the Inquisition before. However, when he approached the pope to denounce the friars that had 'done [him] wrong' ('fatto torto'), the brothers sealed his downfall by retrieving his previous recantation, driven by hostility and the desire to counter his political protection at court.

After Donzellini was released from house arrest and reinstated in the medical profession, he had no further legal troubles for the following eight years. He focused on medicine and philosophy and cultivated a network of scholars with common humanist and scientific interests stretching from Venice to German lands. It was this undertaking that led to his last, fatal encounter with the Inquisition.

5.3 Donzellini in the *Respublica medicorum*

With the increase in Inquisitorial repression, the ageing Donzellini's dissident efforts became increasingly focused on promoting the free circulation of knowledge and defending religious and intellectual freedom. He studied theology through the works of the Fathers of the Church and contemporary religious books and developed his interest in Hermeticism.

He built a network that reflected his outlook.[55] From the 1560s onwards, when he was a member of the College of Physicians in Verona and came into contact with people with different social and religious backgrounds, he increasingly identified with what he defined as the *Respublica medicorum*.[56] This was an international "republic" of physicians and humanists that aimed to spread knowledge across the confessional divide by fostering religious debate grounded in rationality and mutual understanding, and promoting scientific discussion and progress. With its Erasmian influence, this cosmopolitan, irenic, and interconfessional network has been seen as one of the cultural forerunners to the development of the Enlightenment. Although contrasting scientific leanings and rivalries sometimes triggered internal controversies, the *Respublica medicorum* was undoubtedly a remarkable achievement in a century ravaged by religious wars.[57]

Donzellini contributed to the network through his intense letter writing. His Italian correspondents included physicians like Girolamo Mercuriale, Ulisse Aldrovandi, and Marsilio Cagnati.[58] Together they exchanged medical information and opinions, and searched libraries in the peninsula for Hippocratic manuscripts to publish. His most significant correspondence, though, was with German-speaking humanists, above all Theodor Zwinger and Joachim Camerarius the Younger, who were both around twenty years younger than him and exchanged letters for about thirty years. A scientist, physician, and humanist, endowed with great culture and involved in a dense network of correspondence (which included scholars from all Europe and of all denominations), Zwinger was one of the most important sixteenth-century European men of culture and the main driving force in Basel's cultural life between the 1560s and the 1580s.[59] After receiving his education in Paris (where he was a pupil of Peter Ramus) and Italy, where he graduated from Padua University, he returned to Basel in 1559, where Donzellini probably befriended him through Pietro Perna. Zwinger's studies at Paris and Padua had a crucial impact on his thought. The antidogmatic teaching of Ramus was combined with the fresh Aristotelianism which he met in Veneto, while the Paduan experience also allowed him (like many other German students) to develop intense scholarly relationships with prominent Catholic colleagues, such as Mercuriale. Zwinger's education thought and network thus represent a living testimony of resistance against confessionalism. Zwinger's most notable traits were the openness and tolerance of his religious and intellectual outlook, his committed defence of freedom of research (he was one of the first German physicians to show interest in the thought of Paracelsus), and his generosity in protecting exiles and victims of religious persecution.[60] He developed a great passion for Neoplatonic works and philosophy, collaborated with Perna, and was the author, among other things, of a *Teatro della vita umana* (*Theatre of Human Life*). With its four thousand pages, this work reflected the encyclopaedic ambitions of sixteenth-century humanism to capture the totality of knowledge (with no qualitative boundery between theoretical and practical knowledge) and make it accessible to the human mind. For his part, Joachim Camerarius the Younger – son of the great humanist of the same name (known as the Elder) – was a member of the networks of medical culture and Protestant humanism. Born in 1534, he received his initial education from Melanchthon in Wittenberg and in Breslau (Wroclaw), where he was an apprentice to the powerful imperial physician Johannes Crato von Krafftheim (also one of Donzellini's contacts, perhaps through Camerarius). After this, he moved to Italy, where he completed his studies in

Padua and Bologna, and worked with Ulisse Aldrovandi before finally settling in Nuremberg. There is evidence that he was in Verona to purchase theriac in the 1560s, which is probably when he and Donzellini cemented their lasting friendship.

Donzellini and Camerarius focused on medical and therapeutic issues in their correspondence, also bequeathing a wealth of useful information for reconstructing biographical details.[61] Donzellini's exchange of letters with Theodor Zwinger instead casts light on the scope of his action within the cultural and religious framework of Basel, with its ties to the Venetian Republic, in the second half of the sixteenth century. They collaborated to find, restore, publish, and distribute many different texts – Zwinger was Perna's 'editorial consultant'[62] – and their correspondence highlights Donzellini's commitment to a publishing network in which Castellio's ideas of tolerance and anti-dogmatism still exerted a strong influence. From the 1560s onwards, Perna's printing house became the centre of production, collection, and distribution of pioneering scientific literature. His publications blended philosophical and scientific experimentation, radical freedom of research, and spiritual reform, and adopted approaches deemed dangerous in both Rome and Geneva. Zwinger was the driving force behind this publishing programme; under his influence and thanks to the collaboration of consultants and mediators like Donzellini, Perna's printing house published works about magic, alchemy, and Hermeticism. These included the *Enneads* by Plotinus; the works of Proclus; an anthology of medieval alchemy texts edited by Guglielmo Grataroli; the *Arbatel* on the magic of the ancients; and the works of Paracelsus, who was condemned by exponents of Protestant medicine like like Crato Von Krafftheim and Thomas Erastus (their respective irenism and religious radicalism did not affect their medical conservatorism).[63] The underlying cultural premise of this undertaking was philosophical study; philosophy was seen as an insight into the ultimate laws of nature and a tool for worshipping God, who had granted creative and cognitive human potential.

Donzellini's correspondence with Zwinger also reveals his involvement in the publication of Neoplatonic texts that were 'subversive of every philosophical and scientific position based on the authority of Aristotle.'[64] As we will see in more detail in the final chapter, these included works by Franciscus Patricius, whose *Discussiones peripateticae* (*Peripatetic Discussions*) Perna also published in 1581. Furthermore, between the 1570s and 1580s Donzellini promoted the circulation of a *Theatro* (*Theatre*) by Alessandro Citolini, a member of his Venetian heterodox network in the 1540s and the author of a treatise on the art of memory – the *Tipocosmia* – published by Valgrisi in Venice in 1561. Clearly modelled on the *Tipocosmia* (and the work of Delminio, Citolini's master), the *Theatro* had never been published. Ludovico Perez, son of Marco Perez, a Spanish merchant in Basel, visited Donzellini in Venice and acted as an intermediary to deliver the *Theatro* to Zwinger and the physician's other friends in the Swiss city.

Donzellini praised the work, underlining the importance of its subject matter (the art of memory), and asked for it to be returned between 1585 and 1586 following a request by Teofilo Citolini, the author's son.[65]

The bulk of Donzellini's correspondence naturally reflects his professional experiences and medical interests. Many of his letters address his efforts to find and distribute manuscripts and Hippocratic commentaries between Italy and Basel. He also introduced Zwinger to Mercuriale's *De arte gymnastica* (*On the Art of Gymnastics*, Venice, 1569) and requested forbidden medicine and philosophy texts for his studies. The works in question, which were in the first class of prohibited books, included the *Ratio inveniendi medium terminum in Syllogismo Categorico* (*Explication of the Method to Discover the Middle Term of a Categorical Syllogism*, Basel, 1549) by Cristoph Cornerus.[66] In addition, Donzellini provided his correspondent with general information on the Italian medical context. In his letter of 10 August 1577, written during the plague, he explained about the situation regarding the disease and the concerns raised in Rome following Girolamo Cardano's ominous prophecies. He also referred to Cardano's *De rerum varietate* (*On the Variety of Things*) and the process against the author in the Inquisition court (described by Donzellini as 'rapacious Dominican wolves' ['domenicani lupi rapaci']).[67]

In addition, Donzellini's correspondence makes frequent reference to theological works. In 1583, he informed Zwinger that Alessandro Giustinian, a Greek living in Genoa, had given him access to numerous patristic manuscripts. He suggested publishing an edition of works by Athanasius of Alexandria; Theodoret of Cyrus; John Chrysostom; Gregory of Nyssa; two texts by Origen, the most 'philosophical' of the Fathers of the Church, namely *Contra hereticos* (*Against Heretics*) and *In Ioannem* (*In the Gospel of John*); and two by Basil – his *Opera omnia* (*Complete Works*) and *Commentario sopra i primi 16 capitoli di Isaia* (*Commentary on the First Sixteen Chapters of Isaiah*).[68] This project reiterated Zwinger's desire to return to antiquity and the Fathers of the Church to restore Christ's teachings, which he felt had been damaged by the flood of theological opinions during the century of the Reformation.[69] Although we do not know what was actually published, the episode demonstrates Donzellini's wish to contribute to the religious debate through a measured philological approach, adopting a stance opposed to ideological constriction. From the perspective of Catholic orthodoxy, the desire to retrieve the patrimony of knowledge of the Fathers of the Church revealed an intellectual tendency more dangerous than any defined heresy: a penchant for freedom of inquiry and thought. As a Spanish inquisitor commented in the 1540s, 'he who collects ancient Latin and Greek books is not Catholic' ('chi colleziona libri antichi latini e greci non è cattolico').[70]

This tendency is confirmed by the fact that Donzellini only mentioned two openly Reformed theological texts in his correspondence: *De providentia* (*On

Providence, Zurich, 1530) by Ulrich Zwingli and *De admirabili Dei consilio* by Rivius.[71] Although the references to these works suggest that the ageing physician was still interested in Reformed doctrines, his curiosity should be qualified within a broader perspective. Indeed, these works were part of a longer list of various titles requested from his friend Zwinger in 1583. In his letter, Donzellini stressed that he was aware the Catholic Church saw the books as 'abhorrent' ('esecrabili') as they were on the Index and urged Zwinger to take great care in sending them. He craved fresh copies ('ego illis carere non possum'), though, having lost them during his travails ('naufragium') with the Holy Office.[72] As well as the two volumes of Reformed theology, he also asked for the *De Methodo omnium artium* (*On the Method of All the Arts*, Frankfurt, 1550) by Jodocus Willich – a friend of Melanchthon, humanist, professor of rhetoric, political scientist, and physician – and the *De coelesti agricoltura* (*On Celestial Agriculture*, Augsburg, 1541) by the converted Jew Paulus Ricius. While Willich authored works on a variety of subjects (from cookery to farming techniques) that were placed in the first class of the Index of Prohibited Books, Ricius was a professor of philosophy at Pavia University, an imperial physician, and an expert in astrology and Kabbalah with Protestant connections. He devised a synthesis between the Jewish and Christian religions grounded in Kabbalah, which he saw as the original form of Christianity, having pre-empted some of its most mysterious doctrines (like the Trinity). His religious and philosophical work *De coelesti* collected his most important texts with a preface by Pietro Pomponazzi, his old master.

The variety of books in the list suggests that Donzellini's request was not motivated by confessional affiliation. His main desire was to have physical copies of these works in his library once again. Although the fact that he asked for *De providentia* has been interpreted as a sign of his interest in Calvinist thought and his possible adhesion to the dogma of double predestination,[73] the nature of the text and his intellectual profile at the time suggest that a more cautious approach is required. Zwingli toned down the influence of Reformed dogma in this treatise, interpreting it within the humanist framework of a pantheistic metaphysical doctrine. This was extremely familiar to Donzellini; indeed, in 1586 his *Remedium ferendarum iniuriarum* (which will be examined in Chapter 6, a work that he also discussed in his correspondence with Zwinger) was influenced by the same philosophical and cosmological approach. The impact of pagan philosophy – especially the teachings of Seneca – on Zwingli's work was significant. Considered the most philosophical of the reformer's texts, it even attracted the interest of a radical pantheist like Baruch Spinoza.[74] Donzellini's desire to read (or reread) the text and add it to his library therefore satisfied humanist and philosophical needs as well as religious requisites. Although he certainly considered the cosmos to be preordained and governed by the divine spirit, this was not the reason why, as a good humanist, he was prepared to remove individual freedom (as the analysis of his *Remedium* will show). It is thus more prudent to explain his liking for Reformed texts and themes in the context of a more general, eclectic interest in the theological debate; he was neither an orthodox Catholic nor a Protestant dogmatist. From this point of view, the request for Rivius's *De admirabili* complicates matters even further; as this theological text in the Protestant tradition is a recurring element in Donzellini's life, it must have been one of his major points of reference. He first read the work at the English embassy in Venice at the suggestion of Pietro Vanni and requested it again from the erudite German Friedrich Sylburg in 1587, an episode that partly determined the death sentence handed down by the Inquisition. It should be borne in mind, however, that Rivius was not Calvin. In fact, he was a moderate humanist and theologian, a man of letters and rector of the University of Freiburg; although he was personally acquainted with Luther, he identified with the thinking of Erasmus. In the text in question, Rivius tackled the 'mystery of human redemption' with emphasis on the sacrifice of the cross as an instrument of grace beyond 'human wisdom.'[75] This might well have resonated with Donzellini's religious feelings.

The works that Donzellini discussed and exchanged with his correspondents highlight his complex profile as an active member the European *Respublica litterarum*. Two of these texts deserve a special mention, both by the Veronese papal historian Onofrio Panvinio: the *De comitiis imperatoris* (*On imperial elections*, Basel, 1558) on the history of imperial elections, and the *De primatu Petri (On Peter's supremacy*, Verona, 1589), on the reasons for papal primacy. They are mentioned in various letters written between 1583 and 1586, in which Donzellini explained that he had come across the still unpublished texts through the author's brother, Paolo. The physician was asked to help salvage them or have them published by 'a printing house' ('typographo aliquo') for, respectively, two hundred and five hundred crowns; his role as an intermediary in book circulation must have been well known.[76] Donzellini raised the matter with his friends in Basel, above all Zwinger, but the project was never realised.[77]

It is striking that books written by a Catholic author, including a work that put forward the case for papal supremacy, featured in his correspondence and publishing network. After all, Donzellini had already been subjected to four trials and was about to undergo a fifth. In order to understand his interest in these texts, a more analytical framework is required.

The texts were first and foremost works of ecclesiastical and political history; in an age of confessional dispute, this discipline provided a valuable channel for outlining arguments. The claims of the two conflicting sides were based on their perception and interpretation of the past of Christianity. While one endeavoured to establish how and when the Church had forsaken the purity of the apostolic age, the other attempted to demonstrate the continuity between the Petrine age and the contemporary structure of the Curia and the papacy. The many historical texts generated by the dispute focused on the origins of the Church institution; the relationship between papacy and empire and the reasons for their respective claims of religious and political universalism; the performance of individual popes; and resolutions made at councils. Donzellini was already interested in such issues before his contact with Panvinio's works, having read a *Istoria* (*History*) by Johann Sleidan, a Protestant annalist considered the father of Reformation history; he recalled 'seeing it in everyone's hands' ('vedendola in mano ad ognuno') at the imperial court during his exile.[78] This testimony, with its image of books changing hands, shows the level of interest – more ecclesiological than theological – in the history of Christianity among men of culture during the confessional age.[79] In his mature years, Donzellini was increasingly prone to approach the religious debate from a balanced humanist perspective, paying more attention to concordance between confessions than divergence. Above all, though, he was chiefly driven by the desire to overcome any obstacle that hindered the free circulation of texts and knowledge. It is therefore not surprising that he was attracted by the idea of helping Paolo Panvinio to publish his brother Onofrio's works.

Although the *De primatu Petri* had been written in 1553, it remained unpublished for decades in the hands of inquisitors and pontiffs who were concerned about the free circulation of such delicate subject matter. After the text was initially submitted to the Congregation of the Holy Office for expurgation, it was transferred to the papal chambers in the late 1560s at the behest of Gregory XIII and remained there under Sixtus V.[80] In 1586, the latter granted official permission for publication following censorship even though its author 'had demonstrated little wisdom' ('avesse mostrato poco giudizio')[81] in his writing. Nothing materialised, however, until 1589. Despite the fact that the text, an anthology of sources demonstrating papal primacy, had been written to counter the militant Protestant historiography of the so-called *Magdeburg Centuries*, its philological historiographic approach avoided descending into pure polemics.[82] Positioned on the cusp of the transition between the Renaissance and the Counter-Reformation, Panvinio's writing stemmed from 'creative interaction' between a genuine desire to recount the past from a critical perspective and the Church's attempts to reduce it to their ideological and propaganda needs.[83] According to Panvinio, the task of historians was to narrate what had actually happened rather than what they would have liked to happen,[84] a position which must have encountered various forms of resistance in the confessional age. From the perspective of Roman censorship, the *De primatu Petri* was not sufficiently respectful towards the popes as it dared to question the fact that Peter the Apostle had been Bishop of Antioch and used offensive or excessively critical tones to refer to beloved Catholic figures. By contrast, Donzellini felt that publication would help to consolidate a well-grounded and rigorous ecclesiological debate using the reasoning of humanist historiography.

Girolamo's attempt to help Paolo Panvinio publish the *De comitiis* followed a similar logic. The first books of the work – dedicated to Emperor

Maximilian II, who was known for his irenic mindset – were published in Basel by Heinrich Petri. The intermediary in this operation was Giordano Ziletti, who had been associated with the Reformed movement before he recanted and who, as we have seen, had known Donzellini since his time in Orzi Nuovi. The work was opposed by Protestants as much as Catholics between the 1560s and 1580s: Matthias Flacius Illyricus and Simon Schard attacked the author for his interpretation of the *translatio imperii* (transfer of rule or, literally, translation of empire) in accordance with the Roman tradition and for post-dating the first imperial elections (an accusation also levelled at him by the Roman authorities).[85]

Donzellini's interest in the works of Onofrio Panvinio can partly be explained by the author's life story. Thirteen years younger than Donzellini, he studied at the school run by Gian Matteo Giberti in the 1530s; known for his evangelical leanings, this Veronese bishop also educated Donzellini's friend Agostino Valier. Five years after joining the Hermits of St Augustine in 1541, he was transferred to the Augustinian *Studio Generale* in Naples so that his skills could be put to good use; this relocation came at the behest of Girolamo Seripando, the General of the Order, who was open to ideas of reform and had close ties with many Valdesians. He then moved to the Augustinian *Studio* in Rome, where he became a lecturer (*lector*) in 1553 soon after concluding his theological studies and started his historical research[86]. He drafted the *De primatu Petri* in the same year. After his death in 1568, he was accused of failing to comply with the new Tridentine orthodoxy and omitting the combative spirit of the Counter-Reformation from his historiography. As the resulting ostracism could no longer be directed at him, it targeted his works.

Although there was no shortage of opportunities for direct contact, it is not known whether Donzellini ever met him in person.[87] However, he was certainly acquainted with Onofrio's brother, Paolo, who spent most of his life in Verona. Paolo was the custodian and editor of his brother's unpublished texts together with another of Donzellini's correspondents, Girolamo Mercuriale (who also assisted Panvinio on his deathbed). The fact that the physician collaborated with Paolo Panvinio in the plan, albeit unsuccessful, to publish these works strongly suggests that he was operating in a restructured network and indicates the inclusive and irenic nature of his religious feelings at the time. It is also not insignificant that some of Panvinio's works (*Fasti et triumphi* [*Pomp and Triumphs*, Venice, 1557] and *Epitome Pontificum* [*Epitome of the Popes*, Venice, 1557]) were published by Jacopo Strada, who was known for his 'tolerance and understanding'; in 1558, he had helped Donzellini to obtain his imperial safe conduct.

5.4 The epilogue

While Donzellini's correspondence is certainly useful for reconstructing his intellectual outlook, it should not be forgotten that books and ideas were circulated and discussed by people in the flesh. His book network featured contacts, working practices, and sometimes dramatic personal fates that cast light on the underground reality in which he was involved. Furthermore, his publishing connections were part of an extensive and highly concrete context of "dissidence." This took shape through the tendency to embrace philosophical-religious doctrines regarded as suspect in both Catholic and Reformed countries, and the illegal practice of book smuggling.

Between the 1570s and 1580s, the flow of books between the Protestant north, above all Basel, and Venice was guaranteed by a network whose members were all connected to Girolamo Donzellini. The German hub was naturally Pietro Perna's printing house, which produced original books and collected texts printed elsewhere on Germanic soil. Perna acquired these works personally or through his representatives at the Frankfurt Book Fair. At the other end of the chain were the Venetian bookshops like those managed by Giorgio Valgrisi and Francesco Ziletti, which distributed books either through legitimate channels or clandestinely if the texts were prohibited. Direct contact between printers was required to enable communication between both ends of the network (for example, Francesco Ziletti went to Perna to study the art of the colporteur and learn German), while intermediaries facilitated the transport of books.

The latter included the aforementioned Hispanic-Flemish Calvinist merchant Marco Perez. In his homeland in Flanders, Perez had been involved in the attempt to restore peace between Calvinists and Lutherans. However, he fled to Basel after the arrival of the Duke of Alba, who persecuted the Reformers severely.[88] Despite his Calvinist leanings, Perez's intellectual and religious approach always featured tolerance and cosmopolitanism; during his years in Basel, he sympathised with the religious outlook of the group that included Perna and Zwinger. Donzellini had contact with both him and his son, who he also hosted in Venice, entrusting them with books and manuscripts to deliver to his friends in Basel.

Another fundamental intermediary in the network was Pietro Longo, who is frequently mentioned in Donzellini's correspondence. Grendler uses the general term 'bookman' to describe Longo as he primarily transported books, supplying his personal contacts in Italy upon request, but did not own a bookshop.[89] After abandoning Catholicism, Longo spent some time living with Perna, for whom he had already managed a subsidiary printing press in Strasbourg. He mainly operated, however, as a 'carrier' of books between Germany (Frankfurt and Basel), Venice, and northern Italy, where he worked, for example, for Girolamo Mercuriale and Antonio Riccobono.[90] Girolamo, too, often acquired books that had been transported to Venice in Longo's shipments. Reaching Italian soil presented him with few difficulties. Pietro would set off on a journey after hiding prohibited books in bales below legitimate texts and brought his goods into Venice on a little boat at night to avoid attracting attention and bypass inspections. In any case, searches were often conducted sluggishly and inefficiently; given the huge number of volumes pouring into the city on a daily basis, they were seen as wasted effort.

Pietro Longo was arrested in Venice in August 1587, a few months after Girolamo, because of his involvement in distributing the works of Heinrich Cornelius Agrippa, the ultimate Renaissance occultist. As his depositions have not been preserved, other testimonies must be referenced to reconstruct the trial. The only available document provides an account of an interrogation conducted on 26 January 1588. In this, a Bolognese nobleman who was looking for 'a curious and enjoyable book' ('un libro curioso e di spasso') stated that Longo had supplied him with an unspecified book by Agrippa two years previously. The work in question was 'prohibited in the first class' ('proibito in prima classe').[91] This might well have been the straw that broke the camel's back as Longo was executed for heresy and smuggling prohibited books on 31 January.

Besides the carriers, "cultural mediators" between the Venetian-Italian and Germanic worlds also played an essential role in the network. Donzellini was one such figure. In his letters, he not only asked his Swiss and German friends to supply him with books on his wish list but also gave them information about medical texts published in Italy and the availability of both Hippocratic manuscripts in Italian libraries and other ancient texts awaiting publication (as he did for example with Alessandro Giustinian's manuscripts). Moreover, he attempted to create channels for the publication of works that had fallen afoul of censorship or were difficult to publish in the peninsula like those by Patricius or Panvinio. There was thus a two-way flow of books.

It was probably Donzellini's involvement in smuggling and possessing forbidden books that led him at seventy-four years of age to his final Inquisition trial. He was thrown into the Canal dell'Orfano with a stone around his neck at the beginning of 1587. As his trial dossier does not contain either the final sentence or the records of the last proceedings, other sources must be consulted to reconstruct the final few weeks of his life. One of these is the trial against the bookseller Giorgio Valgrisi, held some months after the execution of Donzellini, in which the defendant's relationship with the physician was presented as evidence of his heterodoxy. The prosecutor, Father Alvise de Ferro, recalled on 28 August 1587 that Donzellini had spoken in a 'scandalous' ('scandaloso') manner in Valgrisi's shop, boasting about his extensive collection of forbidden books. He had also made fun of the censorship rules imposed by 'those friars of St Dominic' ('quei frati di san Domenico'), claiming that he would not part with his precious volumes and wanted to 'keep [them] to spite them' ('tener a suo dispetto').[92] When Valgrisi had then tried to silence his reckless friend, the priest had deduced that they both shared the same heretical views. Another testimony can be found in the trial against the French alchemist Claudio Textor. One of the accusations against him, levelled by his colleague Marcello de Giulii on 28 March 1587, regarded his contact with Donzellini, 'who had been drowned by the Holy Office' ('che era stato annegato dal Santo Officio').[93] Textor was said to be horrified when he learned of the death of the physician, thinking that it foreshadowed his own demise. This fear proved well founded as he too was drowned 'soon afterwards' ('appresso').

Donzellini had been well aware of the potential risks of maintaining friendships and professional relations with Protestant scientists, heterodox printers, and unorthodox alchemists while continuing to smuggle books placed on the Index and possess prohibited volumes. The death penalty for relapsed heretics was a constant threat, and it was not long before he re-appeared on the judges' radar. His letters show that he started 'thinking seriously' about leaving Italy in 1579 to escape the Inquisition once and for all, but this apprehension failed to trigger any concrete action for another eight years.[94]

It was only when the classical scholar Friedrich Sylburg's ill-advised shipment of Rivius's *De admirabili Dei consilio* was intercepted in the winter of 1586–1587 that Donzellini made plans to join his friend Joachim Camerarius in Nuremberg. The project never came to fruition, though. For reasons that are still debated, the temperature at the end of the sixteenth century was four or five degrees lower than it had been in the Middle Ages. This climatic cooling disrupted the cycle of seasons with sudden and unfamiliar extreme weather conditions such as extended freezes, summer hailstorms, and frequent thunderstorms. The disruption inevitably had a knock-on effect on dietary, cultural, and recreational habits, as well as on the lives and plans of those who suffered most as they had been born and raised in a different climate.[95] In a letter of 13 March 1587 addressed to Camerarius, Donzellini wrote that he had not seen a ray of sunshine for weeks and that he would have already set off for Nuremberg if the weather had been more clement;[96] the journey was now even more dangerous than usual because of the snowstorms, cloudbursts, and sheets of ice on the road. But time had run out. With the prospect of escape foundering in the freezing weather of March 1587, the Inquisition was back on Donzellini's trail. There was now sufficient evidence to reopen his case – the delivery of books by Rivius, prohibited books found in a hospital with his name on the cover, and the episode in Valgrisi's shop – and close it in the shortest possible time. On 2 April, Martin Biermann, a medical student, wrote to Theodor Zwinger, telling him that Donzellini had probably been drowned. Shortly afterwards, official notice of the death of the physician was sent to Rome and Florence with a certain satisfaction; at the time, Venice was governed by Doge Pasquale Cicogna, who had temporarily brought the city into line with the strictest Counter-Reformation policies. It was also specified that Donzellini's beloved books had been burned in public a few weeks later.[97]

For Donzellini, membership of a network of religious non-conformists entailed opposing theological struggles and barriers more strongly than Catholicism itself. Indeed, the inquisitors focused on the category of heresy more than Donzellini ever did. Nevertheless, his decidedly marginal ideas in this century of religious wars meant that he always remained a dissident. He followed his humanist vocation and became a champion of religious peace and intellectual freedom, eventually sacrificing his own life for the sake of these ideals. Although his efforts inevitably ended in failure, they constitute a small but important step towards the rise of freedom of thought in the early modern age.

Notes

1 Donzellini gave Pigafetta the *Index bibliorum* (*Index of Books*) by Konrad Pelikan, a humanist, Protestant theologian, and German Hebraist: ASV, Sant'Uffizio, *Processi, Contro Girolamo Donzellini*, Bu. 39, 34v–35r; his son Antonio Francesco was also a physician and became an exile for religious reasons; on him, see Alessandra Celati, entry 'Pigafetta, Antonio Francesco,' in *Dizionario Biografico degli Italiani*, 83 (2015). On Matteo Fabbri, see Eleonora Belligni, *Evangelismo, riforma ginevrina e nicodemismo* (Cosenza: Brenner, 2008), 239.
2 Schutte, 'Donzellini, Girolamo.'
3 ASV, Sant'Uffizio, *Processi, Contro Girolamo Donzellini*, Bu. 39, 72r.
4 Ivi, *Processi, Contro Nascimbene Nascimbeni*, Bu. 30. In 1578, Donzellini was accused of helping in the escape of Nascimbeni, a prisoner of the Holy Office who he was treating: while recounting his version of events in his defence, he mentioned his son, Virgilio, who was twelve years old at the time.
5 The only documented relationship of this kind at the time was with the humanist Publio Francesco Spinola. It was during this period that the latter wrote his aforementioned poem in praise of Donzellini's library after visiting him in Verona. With their friendship dating back to their youth, Donzellini helped Spinola to obtain a job as tutor with Leonardo Mocenigo when he moved to Venice after his first trial.
6 Archivio di stato di Verona (hereinafter ASVr), *Atti del Collegio de' medici, Comune*, 610, 199r. There are references to Donzellini as a member of the Veronese College ibid. and ivi., 611.
7 On the College of physicians in Verona see Alessandro Pastore, 'L'onore della corporazione.'
8 Although Donzellini was born in Orzi Nuovi, he came from a Veronese family.
9 Pastore, *Le regole dei corpi*, 133–34, 137.
10 ASV, Sant'Uffizio, *Processi, Contro Giovan Francesco Manfredi*, Bu. 28.
11 'Trasferire nel concreto esercizio pastorale il succo della teologia pratica'; Elisabetta Patrizi, *Pastoralità e educazione. L'episcopato di Agostino Valier nella Verona post-tridentina (1565–1606). Vol. I Vita e azione pastorale* (Milan: Franco Angeli, 2015). On Giberti, see also Adriano Prosperi, *Tra evangelismo e controriforma. Gian Matteo Giberti (1495–1543)* (Rome: Edizioni di Storia e Letteratura, 2011).
12 Ivano del Prete, *Scienza e società nel Settecento veneto, il caso veronese 1680–1796* (Milan: Franco Angeli, 2008), ad indicem.
13 Verona, Biblioteca civica, carteggio Serego, b. 334, fasc. *Antonio Maria Serego, 18 June 1577*. Thanks to Dr Mattia Corso for bringing this to my attention.
14 Pastore, *l'Onore della corporazione*, 19.
15 Plea by Alessandro Serego to his fellow collegians: ASVr, *Atti del Collegio de' medici, Comune*, 610, 215v–216r. On this matter, see Pastore, *L'onore della corporazione*, 14–16.

16 ASVr, *Atti del Collegio de' medici, Comune*, 610, 211v.
17 Pastore, *L'onore della corporazione*, 14.
18 On the Serego brothers and Bovio, see Del Prete, *Scienza e Società*, 46. The *Melampigo* and the references to Donzellini in this and other texts will be the focus of a separate section in Chapter 6.
19 'Confezionavano a scopo di lucro preparati medicinali ad alto costo e di alcuna utilità'; Pastore, *L'onore della corporazione*, 16.
20 On Tommaso Zefiriele Bovio's involvement in the debate on the comet in 1577 and more generally on the lawfulness of judicial astrology, see Ulvioni, 'Astrologia, astronomia e medicina nella Repubblica Veneta tra Cinque e Settecento,' *Studi trentini di scienze storiche*, 61 (1982), 1–69 15–23. On judicial astrology, see also the *Trialogo sopra l'astrologia giudiziaria* (*Trialogue about Judicial Astrology*), which Bovio claimed to have written in the grip of ecstatic rapture, inspired by the Holy Spirit. He praised 'this subject […] which I value as the finest, the noblest, and the most excellent that we can imagine, given that it deals with the providence, disposition, and order of the interminable and incomprehensible most munificent grace of the perfect and supreme God; and man, created, formed, and constituted from his divine goodness in his image and likeness, was granted the ability to contemplate and understand, gifts which led him to become the secretary of God' ('questa materia […] la quale io stimo la piu bella piu nobile et ecellente che possi cader sotto l'intelletti nostri, trattando ella la providentia dispositione et ordine dell'interminabile et incomprehennsibile munificentissima gratia dell'ottimo et massimo Iddio; dello homo creato formato et constituto di sua divina bontà alla immagine e similitudine sua et fattogli dono di cosi segnalata contemplatione et cognitione, siche mediante questi doni ci ha fatti suoi secretari'). The text also featured a polemic against the Church concession granted to 'seafarers, farmers, and physicians' ('naviganti agricoltori e medici') – the latter were his main target – which meant that they could deal with the discipline without 'understanding it' ('intenderla') and 'with the injury and often the death of the wretched sufferers that trust them' ('con danno et spesso morte de miseri languenti che fidano in loro'); Venice, Biblioteca Marciana, Ms It IV 57, *Trialogo sopra l'astrologia giudiziara.*
21 'I have foretold many things to many, regarding numbers, physiognomy, necromancy, onomancy, chiromancy, astrology, in my capacity as a physician, and with regard to the arts, sciences, and disciplines that divine grace has granted me' ('Ho predetto io molte cose a molti, quando per numeri, quando per fisionomia, quando per neomantia, quando per onomantia, quando per chiromantia, quando per astrologia, quando come medico et quando per quelle arti, scientie et discipline che mi ha concesso la divina gratia.'); Venice, Biblioteca Marciana, ms. it. IV, 57, *Trattato d'astrologia in forma di dialogo*, 75v–76r (the numbering is by Ulvioni, who cites Bovio's work in Ulvioni, *Astrologia, astronomia e medicina*, 15).
22 Ibid., 23.
23 'This focus of Your Holiness against the Venetians and their many subjects is not against one of these humble individuals, but the whole of Christianity and perhaps also the entire world' ('Questa attenzione di Vostra santità contra i veneziani e suoi tanti sudditi non è contra unum de pusillis istis, ma di tutta la Christianità e forse ancora di tutto il Mondo'); Venice, Biblioteca marciana, Ms It IV 57, *Copia di una lettera scritta a nostro Signore Papa Paolo Quinto di Zefiriele Tommaso Bovio veronese, in Padova per Ruberto Meietti.*
24 Ulvioni, *Astrologia, astronomia e medicina*, 22.
25 In this area, the Veronese charlatan earned the respect of the Belgian physician Paulus de Kempenaer, an exponent of a mystical and irenic form of

Protestantism with Erasmian overtones. Kempenaer acknowledged Bovio as a source of medical, cultural, and ethical-religious inspiration. See Alfonso Ingegno, 'Il medico de' disperati e abbandonati: Tomaso Zefiriele Bovio (1521–1609) tra Paracelso e l'alchimia del Seicento,' in Lucilla Borselli, Giancarlo Carabelli, Chiaretta Poli, Paolo Rossi (eds.), *Cultura popolare e cultura dotta nel Seicento* (Milan: Franco Angeli, 1983), 172–73.

26 Dario Tessicini, 'Il dibattito italiano sulla nuova stella del 1572 (con il testo del 'Discorso intorno a la stella' di Giuseppe Valdagno, ms Ambrosiana R 95 sup.),' in Miguel A. Granada (ed.), *Novas y cometas entre 1572 y 1618: revolucion cosmologica y renovacion politica y religiosa* (Barcelona: Universitat de Barcelona, 2012), 43–94.

27 Giuseppe Olmi, 'Farmacopea antica e medicina moderna. La disputa sulla Teriaca nel Cinquecento bolognese,' *Physis*, 19 (1977), 207; Barbara Di Gennaro Splendore, 'The Triumph of Theriac. Print, Apothecary Publications, and the Commodification of Ancient Antidotes (1497–1800),' *Nuncius, Journal of the Material and Visual History of Science*, 2 (2021), Sabrina Minuzzi (ed.), Special issue *Printing Medical Knowledge: Vernacular Genres, Reception, and Dissemination.*

28 As we will see, Donzellini also referred to Fracastoro's work in his 1576 treatise on the genesis and spread of pestilence, citing his notion of the 'seminary of the plague' ('seminario della peste').

29 Biblioteca Universitaria di Bologna, ms Aldrovandi 136 XXIV, 32v.

30 Olmi, 'Farmacopea.'

31 Bartolomeo Maranta, *Della theriaca e del mitridato libri due* (Venice: Marcantonio Olmo, 1572). The text was published a year after the death of Maranta; the publisher dedicated it to Melchiorre Guilandino, the scholar in charge of the botanical gardens in Padua. Maranta had already inserted his own dedication to the Neapolitan apothecary, collector, and naturalist Ferrante Imperato, the curator of one of the most famous natural history museums in Europe and a prominent figure in the *Respublica medica* for the exchange of simples and other natural items. Maranta had learned the secrets for preparing the antidote directly from Imperato. On Maranta's experiences with religion and the Inquisition, see Francesco S. Minervini, *Didattica del linguaggio poetico in un retore del Cinquecento. Bartolomeo Maranta* (Bari: Adriatica, 2004), in particular 16–23.

32 Various letters in the Abteilung Frey-Gryn at the Universitätsbibliothek in Basel, including one dated 10 August 1577, catalogued as G2 8, document this exchange.

33 Vincenzo Calzaveglia, *De theriacae usu in febribus pestilentialibus* (Brescia: Vincenzo Sabbio, 1570).

34 Girolamo Donzellini became involved in the controversy by publishing some short treatises: *De natura, causis et legitima curatione febris pestilentis* (*On the Nature, Causes, and the Legitimate Treatment of Pestilential Fevers*, Venice: C. Borgominieri, 1570); *Libri de natura, causis et legitima curatione febris pestilentis in quibus etiam de theriacae natura ac viribus disputatur apologia per Eudoxum Philalethem edita adversus Thessali Zoili oppugnationes* (*Books on the Nature, Causes, and the Legitimate Treatment of Pestilential Fevers, which also Discuss the Apology on the Nature and Properties of Theriac by Eudoxus Philalethes Published Against the Attacks by Thessalus Zoilus*, Venice: A. Bocchino, 1571; Verona: S. dalle Donne, 1575); *Eudoxi Philalethis adversus calumnias et sophismata cuiusdam personati qui se Evandrophilacten nominavit apologia* (*Apology by Eudoxus Philalethes against the Calumnies and Sophism Pronounced against Evandrophilactes*, Verona: S. dalle Donne, 1573). On this controversy, see Redmond, *Girolamo Donzellino*, 63 et seq.

35 Quaranta, *Medici italiani*, 93.

36 'For two years I have been involved in a medical controversy with an insolent physician from Brescia who, starting from his arguments, launched into clamour and calumny and eventually resorted to weapons. Finding himself rebuffed and no longer in a position to respond, he sent some assassins who almost killed me. However, thanks to the help of God I was freed from their clutches by the crowd and only received a wound, which has already healed.' ('Viget iam biennium quidam medica controversia inter me ac medicum quendam Brixianum insolitissimum, qui a syllogismis ad convicia et calumnias, et ab his ad arma tandem prorupit, cum se videret eo redactum ut amplius respondere non posset, quasi sicarios submisit qui me interficerent, sed dei auxilio ab eorum manibus, populi conditione sum liberatus, unico accepto vulnere quod iam etiam est curatum'); letter written by Girolamo Donzellini to Theodor Zwinger, 18 August 1572, in Universitätsbibliothek, Abteilung Frey-Gryn Mscr II 4.

37 Ibid., letter from Marsilio Cagnati to Girolamo Donzellini dated Rome, 17 November 1571. On Cagnati, see Giorgio Stabile, entry 'Cagnati, Marsilio,' in Dizionario Biografico degli Italiani, 16 (1973).

38 'If I had appeared, I would have been imprisoned. I had lived in in this city with a certain reputation and made a profession out of my art, which lives by honour. Knowing the dishonour that prison entails, I could not go to prison.' ('Appresentandomi sarei stato incarcerato, io che havevo vissuto in questa città con riputatione et fatto professione di mia arte che vive dell'onore, sapendo l'ignominia che seco porta la prigione non potei inchinar l'animo mio alla carcere'); ASV, Sant'Uffizio, *Processi, Contro Girolamo Donzellini*, Bu. 39, 52r.

39 Ibid., 116r.

40 Ibid., 113r.

41 Ibid., 200r.

42 Ibid., *Capitoli della peste.*

43 Venezia, Biblioteca Marciana, Ms Ital VII (2342=9695), *Notizie cavate dai libri dei priori*, 15v–16v.

44 On this episode in Donzellini's life, see Alessandra Celati, 'The Experience of the Physician Girolamo Donzellini in the 1575 Venetian Plague: Between *Scientia* and Heterodoxy,' in Fabrizio Baldassarri, Fabio Zampieri (eds.), *Scientiae in the History of Medicine* (Rome: Erma di Bretschneider, 2021), 189–215. This contribution includes both the original text of the *Capitoli della peste* and an English translation.

45 ASV, Sant'Uffizio, *Processi*, *Contro Girolamo Donzellini*, Bu. 39, 203r.

46 The dossier for this trial can be found ivi*, Contro Nascimbene Nascimbeni*, Bu. 30.

47 Ivi, *Contro Girolamo Donzellini*, 48v.

48 Ivi*, Contro Nascimbene Nascimbeni*, Bu. 30, see the letter of letter of 27 December 1578 sent to Cardinal Savelli by the Venetian authorities, which says that some 'gentlemen made a request at this court for the consignment of Mr Donzellini; they were told that it was not under the jurisdiction of this Holy Office' ('gentiluomini hanno fatto istanzia presso questo tribunale per la ispedizione di messer Donzellino, ai quali è stato detto non appartener ciò a questo Santo Officio').

49 On the Roman interest in Donzellini's trial, see Adriana Buffardi (ed.), *Nunziature di Venezia. 18 giugno 1573–22 dicembre 1576*, 11 (Rome: Istituto Storico per l'Età Moderna e Contemporanea, 1972), no. 166, 214, 227, 232, 243.

50 Quaranta, *Medici italiani*, 96.

51 Ibid., 97.

52 Chabod, *Lo Stato e la vita religiosa,* 357.

53 Archivio di Stato di Milano, *Carteggio cancellerie di Stato*, Bu. 164, petition by Girolamo Bosio of 1 July 1553.

54 On Villani, see ivi., Bu. 88, petition of 1 September 1548. Like Donzellini before him, Filalteo, the former physician to the Marquis of Vasto in Milan, became the envy of his colleagues in 1563. He was reported to the Inquisition and remained in custody for a year before being released; after this, he was soon called by the Duke of Savoy to become a professor at the University of Turin. The president of the Milanese Senate, Pietro Paolo Arrigoni, intervened in his favour, raising the question of the ignominy that the imprisonment of a professor of Filalteo's reputation would cause for the University of Pavia, where he taught: Maria Luisa Baldi, '*Consolatio* e *defensio.* Note su Cardano, Filalteo e Gratarolo,' in Andrea Spiriti (ed.), *Libertinismo erudito: cultura lombarda tra Cinque e Seicento. Atti delle giornate di studio* (Milan: Franco Angeli, 2011) 44–65. On Filalteo, see also Girolamo Tiraboschi, *Storia della letteratura italiana di Girolamo Tiraboschi. Dall'anno millequattrocento al milleseicento,* 3 (Milan: Niccolò Bettoni e comp., 1833 (first edition 1772–1782), 580–82. The bond forged between physicians and their high-ranking patrons in a relationship of protection and defence worked both ways. When Caterina Sauli decided to appear spontaneously before the Holy Office in Mantua in 1567, she consulted the physician Giovan Battista Susio. He helped to organise her defence and drafted a confession for her to present to the judges, allowing her to use his house in Mantua. The fact that Susio had been persecuted by the Inquisition during the previous decade certainly influenced Caterina's decision. Nevertheless, as she asked Susio – rather than her many other heretical contacts – for help at the delicate moment of an inquisitorial interrogation, their friendship must have been characterised by trust and familiarity. Ambrosini, *L'eresia di Isabella*, 175–76; see also the deposition sent to the Venetian judges from Mantua, contained in ASV, *Sant'Uffizio, Processi*, *Contro Isabella Frattina*, Bu. 25, 4/7, 13r–14r. On Giovan Battista Susio, born in Mirandola in 1519, see Pio Paschini, *Tre illustri prelati del Rinascimento. Ermolao Barbaro, Adriano Castellesi, Giovanni Grimani* (Rome: Facultas Theologica Pontificii Athenaei Lateranensis, 1957), 133–39. Donzellini named him as one of the members of the heterodox movement that he had met in Venice and the documentation also shows that Susio was in contact with Pietro Perna: ASV, Sant'Uffizio, *Contro Girolamo Donzellini*, Bu. 39, 1r, 49r.

55 While in the 1560 trial Donzellini mentioned forty-two members of his heterodox network (which was probably actually larger, as he tended to denounce people who were dead or in exile, or those who had already recanted), in 1574 he only named nineteen. More generally speaking, from the early 1560s onwards his heterodox network in the Republic was less dense than in previous decades. There may be multiple reasons for this. Donzellini stated, for example, that during the Venetian plague of 1557, when he was in Germany, many of his former cohorts (most of whom were physicians) had died. It can also be imagined that Inquisitorial repression, which intensified precisely in the mid-1550s, led many to recant or escape. His book smuggling network grew in the same period.

56 Basel, Universitätsbibliothek, Abteilung Frey-Gryn, GII 37, undated.

57 Christoph Lüthy, 'The confessionalization of Physics: Heresies, Facts and Travails of the Republic of Letters,' in Brooke, Maclean, *Heterodoxy*, 81–82.

58 Like Donzellini, Mercuriale was also in contact with Theodor Zwinger. See: Nancy Siraisi, 'Mercuriale's Letters to Zwinger and Humanist Medicine,' in Arcangeli, Nutton, *Girolamo Mercuriale*, 77–95.

59 Gilly, *Theodor Zwinger*; Felici, *Senza Frontiere*, ad indicem and in particular 119–122.

60 Zwinger's relationship with the thought of Paracelsus was ambivalent. In 1564 he authored the first, most solid and longest systematic confutation of Paracelsus' medicine in Basel (within a letter to Gervasus Marstaller), and in the same period

he encouraged the banishment from the university of Basel of the paracelsian alchemist Adam von Bodenstein. However, in the following decade he radically changed his opinion and in 1576 he prefaced Perna's edition of Paracelsus' *Schreiben von den Frantzosen*, praising Paracelsus and his medicine and definig him as the true heir of Ippocrates. Zwinger's letter to Marstaller is published in Gilly, *Theodor Zwinger*, 216–222.

61 The correspondence between Donzellini and Camerarius is the focus of Quaranta, 'Exile Experiences.'

62 Rotondò, *Pietro Perna*, 480.

63 Crato did not oppose chemycal medicine as such. Rather, he condemned Paracelsus for being a «scientifically unsound braggart», a heretic and a black magician, see Tilmann Walter, 'New Light on Antiparacelsianism (c. 1570–1610): The Medical Republic of Letters and the Idea of Progress in Science,' *The Sixteenth Century Journal*, 43 (3), (2012), 701–725, 711. On Crato's irenic approach to the religious controversy see Howard Louthan, *The Quest for Compromise, Peacemakers in Counter-Reformation Vienna* (Cambridge: Cambridge University Press, 1997).

64 Rotondò, *Pietro Perna*, 559.

65 There are many references to Citolini and the exchange of this text in the correspondence with Zwinger. At the Basel Universitätsbibliothek, Abteilung Frey-Gryn, see the letters of: 20 August 1583, Frey Ms II 2; 12 March 1585, Frey MS GII 8; 5 November 1585, Frey Ms II 19; 3 May 1586, 12 May 1586, 28 June 1586, Frey Ms II 23; 3 November 1586, Frey Ms II 4 and, of the same date, Frey MS GII 37; see also the reference in the letter to Camerarius dated 'first day of 1587' ('primo die 1587'), in Erlangen Universitätsbibliothek, Briefsammlung Trew.

66 Corner was a philosopher and theologian who took part in the final meetings to draft the Formula of Concord, the last section of the Lutheran *Corpus doctrinae* (Body of Doctrine), in 1573.

67 Basel, Universitätsbibliothek, Abteilung Frey-Gryn, G2 8, letter of 10 August 1577.

68 Ivi, Frey Ms II, 2, letter to Zwinger of 20 August 1583.

69 Rotondò, 'Pietro Perna,' 495.

70 Jansen, 'A House for All Sorts of People,' 217.

71 The complete title of the book of Zwingli is *Ad illustrissimum Cattorum principem Philippum, sermonis De providentia Dei anamnema* (*Memories of the discourse on the Providence of God dedicated to the very illustrious prince Philip*).

72 Basel, Universitätsbibliothek, Abteilung, Frey Ms II, letter of 2 March 1583, which lists the texts on the physician's wish list; see also Quaranta, *Medici italiani*, 86, whose interpretation of the 'naufragium' as the physician's travails with the Holy Office I endorse.

73 Ibid., 87–88. The author supports this theory, also referring to a letter that Donzellini sent to Camerarius in 1586, in which he uses the term 'reprobates' ('reprobi'); see ibid., 105–06.

74 Carla Gallicet Calvetti, 'Spinoza e il *De Providentia* di Zwingli,' *Rivista Di Filosofia Neo-Scolastica* 61, no. 4/5 (1969), 391. Zwingli claimed that God communicated his perfection to creatures, thereby ennobling them.

75 Johannes Rivius, *De admirabili Dei consilio in celando mysterio redemptione humanae libri tres* (Basel: Oporinus 1545).

76 The *De comitis* was published in 1558, but there was also an expanded version that, according to Donzellini's correspondence, never saw the light of day: only the first two of five books were published. With regard to the *De primatu*, Paolo Panvinio received a printing privilege in 1585, but took no concrete steps towards publication; see Karl A. Gersbach 'Onofrio Panvinio's brother Paolo and His

Role in the Posthumous edition of "De Primatu Petri et Apostolicae Sedis Potestate" and the Purchase of Onofrio's Manuscripts for the Vatican Library,' *Analecta Augustiniana*, 56 (1993), 253. After Panvinio died, the author's manuscripts were seized by the Curia and Paolo Panvinio strove to salvage and publish them for years.

77 The correspondence mentions the *De comitis* between 1583 and 1585, and the *De primatu* between 1585 and 1586. At the Basel Universitätsbibliothek, Abteilung Frey- Gryn see the letters: Fr II 2, 20 August 1583 for the *De Comitis*; ivi, Fr ms II 23, 12 May 1586 for the *De primatu.* In Fr II 19 November 1585, Donzellini refers to both texts.

78 ASV, Sant'Uffizio, *Processi, Contro Girolamo Donzellini*, 48r.

79 On Sleidan, see Alexandra Kess, *Johann Sleidan and the Protestant Vision of History* (Burlington: Ashgate, 2008); Stefan Bauer, *The Invention of Papal History, Onofrio Panvinio Between Renaissance and Catholic Reform* (Oxford: Oxford University Press, 2020), 46–47; on the importance of history in the Reformation era and on Protestant historiography, see Mark A. Lotito, *The Reformation of Historical Thought* (Leiden – Boston: Brill, 2019).

80 Bauer, *The Invention of Papal History*, 85–86.

81 Ibid., 185.

82 Also known as *Historia Ecclesiae Christi* the work covered thirteen hundreds of history and was first published between 1559 and 1574. It was compiled by several Lutheran scholars in Magdeburg, but the editor chief was Matthias Flacius Illyricus.

83 Bauer, *The Invention of Papal History*, 2.

84 Ibid., 140.

85 Ibid., 141.

86 Stephen Bauer, entry 'Panvinio, Onofrio,' in *Dizionario Biografico degli Italiani*, 81 (2014).

87 They both spent time in Augsburg and Verona in overlapping periods. Moreover, from 1571 onwards some of Donzellini's letters were written from Rome on impromptu trips in search of manuscripts in the papal libraries; it is possible that the physician had already been there and met Panvinio.

88 On Perez, see Rotondò, *Pietro Perna*, 496–97.

89 Paul F. Grendler, *The Roman Inquisition and the Venetian Press, 1540–1605* (Princeton: Princeton University Press, 1975), 186–89 and ad indicem.

90 Ibid., 186.

91 'When I was in Venice, I told Pietro Longo that I wanted to obtain a curious and enjoyable book. He said "I'll try to send you one" but he did not say anything about Cornelius Agrippa, whose book he then sent. And I took it as a curiosity, not knowing that it was prohibited.' ('Essendo io in Venetia et ragionando con questo Pietro Longo che io havevo desiderio di haver qualche libro corioso et di spasso, lui disse vedrò di mandarvene qualchuno et non me nominò alhora questo Cornelio Agrippa qual poi ne ha mandato. Et io lo pigliai come libro curioso non sapendo che fosse prohibito.'); ASV, Sant'Uffizio, *Processi, Contro Pietro Longo*, Bu. 61, testimony by Count Antonio Ludovico Isolani, 26 Januray 1588.

92 Ivi, *Contro Giorgio Valgrisi,* Bu. 59, 1v.

93 Ivi, *Contro Claudio Textor Francese*, Bu. 59, 1v.

94 Erlangen, Universitätsbibliothek, Briefsammlung Trew, II, 17, letter to Camerarius dated 5 March 1577, quoted in Quaranta, *Medici italiani*, 100. Donzellini was still under house arrest when he wrote this letter; as we have seen, he was later released.

95 Philip Blom, *Il primo inverno: la piccola era glaciale e l'inizio della modernità europea (1570–1700)*, (Venice: Marsilio, 2018).
96 Quaranta, *Medici italiani*, 100.
97 'In the last few days, the Holy Office of the Inquisition carried out the drowning of the physician Girolamo Donzellini, a relapsed heretic, and soon afterwards [the drowning of] a Frenchman, also a relapsed heretic. The pope was extremely satisfied with this and thanked the Signory, saying that God will always protect this State.' ('In questi giorni il Santo Offizio dell'Inquisizione si mandò annegar Gerolamo Donzellino medico eretico relapso, et appresso un altro francese medesime relapso, di che il papa restò molto soddisfatto e ne ringratiò la Signoria dicendo che Dio sempre proteggerà questo Stato.'); Salvatore Bongi, *Annali di Gabriel Giolito de' Ferrari da Trino di Monferrato stampatore in Venezia,* vol. I (Rome: Ministero Pubblica Istruzione, 1890), 351.

6 'The best physician is a philosopher': The thought of Girolamo Donzellini

This chapter will focus specifically on Girolamo Donzellini's thinking. It will first analyse his interest in Paracelsianism by examining his collaboration with the empiric Tommaso Zefiriele Bovio in the 1570s and 1580s. It will then explore his philosophical and religious stance by examining the final philosophical-medical treatise that he published before his execution – the frequently aforementioned *Remedium ferendarum iniuriarum sive de compescenda ira* – and more generally his profile as a humanist physician.

6.1 Collaboration with the empiric Bovio: Was Donzellini a Paracelsian?

The thinking of the Swiss physician Theophrastus Paracelsus and the resulting medical tradition form a key chapter in sixteenth-century medicine.[1] Paracelsus was a pioneer of the chemical art and a spirited opponent of Galenic medicine who doggedly disputed any form of fixed, purely theoretical knowledge and staunchly attacked all institutions from medical colleges to universities, and from the Catholic authorities to the new Protestant orthodoxies. Furthermore, he made a mission out of studying the hidden properties of nature in a manner akin to other late Renaissance thinkers like Girolamo Cardano and Giordano Bruno, operating within a Hermetic and emanationist philosophical framework. These polymaths envisaged an animated cosmos with multiple interconnections between all natural and supernatural bodies. It is therefore extremely significant, although not surprising, that the sources imply Donzellini's interest in Paracelsian ideas and his involvement in distributing the Swiss author's texts in the Italian peninsula.

Donzellini received the works of Paracelsus from Pietro Perna. As with the distribution of religious and philosophical texts published abroad, the printer relied on the physician for introducing Paracelsus into the Italian market; his works were one of the cornerstones of Perna's pledge to renew scientific knowledge. We have no details of the Italian distribution routes used by Donzellini for these books, but it is known for certain that they were delivered to Tommaso Zefiriele Bovio, the Veronese empiric who had

DOI: 10.4324/9781003218852-7

contact with Donzellini and the Serego family in the 1570s and 1580s. In one of his works, the charlatan claimed to be a close friend of Girolamo, stating that the physician had lent him many books by Paracelsus between 1570 and 1580. Donzellini invited Bovio to his house to show him his collection of Paracelsian works and ask him to share his knowledge of alchemy, which was necessary for a full understanding of the author's thinking.[2]

The situation, however, was more complex than it might first appear.[3] In 1583, Bovio published a polemical booklet in Venice, *Flagello de' medici rationali*, which lambasted learned medical practitioners. The following year, an otherwise unknown Doctor of Arts and medicine named Claudio Gelli responded to the accusations with his own pamphlet (*Risposta dell'eccellente dottor Claudio Gelli ad un certo libro contra medici rationali* [*Reply of the Excellent Doctor Claudio Gelli to a Certain Book against Rational Physicians*], Venice, 1584). In this work, the charlatan was described as an ignorant imposter who was jealous of the class of learned physicians, from which he had been excluded. Then, in a letter written to the imperial physician Johannes Crato von Krafftheim in 1585, Donzellini revealed that Claudio Gelli was nothing more than his pseudonym.[4] The story thus played out on two different levels. On the surface, Bovio and Donzellini had a professional relationship and shared the same philosophical and scientific interests; the learned physician asked the empiric for an overview of alchemical knowledge in order to obtain a greater understanding of unconventional medicine. Underneath, however, they were fierce rivals, with the physician hiding behind a pen name to write a polemical booklet against the charlatan, accusing him of being an incompetent swindler who practised medicine without the necessary qualifications.

On the basis of this episode, historians studying the reception of Paracelsianism in sixteenth-century Italy placed Donzellini in one of two opposing scientific traditions. Some identified him as a pioneer of the spread of Paracelsian ideas in Italy, stressing the connection between religious heterodoxy and "scientific heresy."[5] Others, however, strongly disputed this interpretation, stressing that Paracelsian doctrines were embraced in Catholic contexts like the Medici court and by individuals never involved in religious dissent. These historians also underlined that Donzellini's letter to Crato disproves his affiliation with Paracelsian doctrines.[6] Finally, more recent studies have analysed the strictly medical content of Gelli-Donzellini's pamphlet, highlighting the author's flexibility and open-mindedness when it came to medical treatment.[7] Indeed, Gelli was prepared to use remedies gradually honed by 'experience' ('l'esperienza') and the 'diligence of the art' ('diligenza dell'arte') as well as by 'reason' ('la ragione'), asserting the methodological value of a more daringly experimental form of medicine. At the same time, though, he criticised the 'bad form of empiricism' ('cattiva forma di empirismo') championed by Bovio and expressed a conservative social outlook by defending the integrity of the learned medical class against the pretences of ignorant charlatans.

To make sense of this complex episode, we need to first consider the threat that Paracelsian doctrines posed to Galenism and then link it to the spread of heterodox ideas in sixteenth-century Italy. Initially, indeed, heretical religious tendencies were sometimes accompanied by interest in new medical ideas,[8] and the case of Donzellini illustrates that Paracelsian enthusiasts could also be involved in religious dissent. The physician had repeatedly appeared on the Inquisition's radar and to all intents and purposes "Paracelsian" became a synonym of "heretic" in Counter-Reformation Italy.[9] Girolamo therefore probably felt the need to dissimulate his interest in Paracelsianism by distancing himself from an ambiguous figure like Bovio. Furthermore, the publication of the booklet in the name of the entire order of physicians was his last desperate attempt to win back respect and consideration from a professional body that had expelled him from their ranks (he might have adopted the pen name because he was aware that his conviction for heresy had been a source of embarrassment to the College). It is also conceivable that Donzellini wanted to stress his Galenic credentials in his letter to Crato to please the imperial physician, who was in a position to help him escape from Italy once more.[10] Then again, he admitted in the same missive that he had used chemical remedies in cases of chronic illness, describing their effects as the 'spagyric miracle' ('spagiricum miraculum').[11] He also expressed support for the doctrine of the humanist physician Günther von Andernach, master to Vesalius and Servetus, who had attempted to reconcile Galenism and Paracelsianism.[12]

Any rigid definition of the scientific (and religious) leanings of a figure like Donzellini would thus be ineffective, as would any form of schematism establishing close correlations between Galenism and orthodoxy, and between Paracelsianism and religious reform. In fact, one of the fiercest attacks on Paracelsus was launched by the Reformed physician Thomas Erastus,[13] who was accused of favouring radical religious doctrines. Moreover, the Prior of the highly Catholic College of Physicians in Verona in the 1590s was Vittorio Algarotti,[14] a fearless advocate of spagyric medicine. In the end, despite the prohibition of alchemy and all related practices in 1586, the works of Paracelsus were not fully censored until the 1596 Clementine Index.[15]

As Italy was the birthplace of humanist medicine, it is not surprising that there was opposition to Paracelsianism and its polemical stance towards Galenic thought. Although Italian physicians sometimes observed the effectiveness of chemical remedies and integrated them into their treatments, the influence of Paracelsian philosophy remained marginal. Physicians were primarily interested in the medical benefits of the spagyric method and mostly ignored the philosophical scope of Paracelsian thinking. More debate was triggered in Germany, where, despite their interest in iatrochemistry, many leading Galenic physicians attacked Paracelsus as an atheist who corrupted the younger generation through his rejection of all official ecclesiastical institutions, including the Reformed Church.[16] As such a scenario was inconceivable in Italy, it would be risky to define any sixteenth-century Italian physician as a committed Paracelsian. Even Bovio stated that he did not appreciate the obscure and sometimes incomprehensible style adopted by the Swiss physician to express his ideas.

In addition to the characteristic fluidity of society and culture in the early modern period, we need to consider the specific nature of the late-sixteenth-century Italian historical context, in which the Inquisition and indexes of prohibited books exerted a widespread and profound influence. As mentioned earlier, the reception of innovative scientific and religious ideas in the peninsula was often only partial. In the last few decades of the century, the cultural debate was increasingly curtailed by the secrecy that forced men of science into a form of isolation. This seclusion could only be overcome through learned correspondence, which often piqued the interest of the Inquisition. This backdrop, along with the curiosity and eclecticism typical of exponents of late humanism, led a physician like Donzellini to create a blend of Galenism and Paracelsianism that would have been practically unachievable elsewhere. All in all, Donzellini was probably neither an orthodox Galenian nor a revolutionary Paracelsian. What is certain, however, is that his scientific interests were guided by thirst for knowledge, curiosity about medical innovation, and the notion that medicine was a practical discipline aiming to heal as many people as possible. His humanist approach did not merely recycle classical knowledge or build rigid boundaries between the different medical movements. In fact, it prompted him to seek agreement among them.

More generally, the episode involving Donzellini and Bovio suggests that we should scale down the contrasts drawn between different medical movements, between orthodoxy and heterodoxy, and between learned medicine and empirical medicine. This can be achieved by considering the intellectual journey of versatile and dynamic men of culture like Girolamo Donzellini in fluid terms, focusing on specific contexts and relations.

6.2 The *Remedium ferendarum iniuriarum* between Neoplatonism and radicalism

Donzellini's interest in Paracelsianism needs to be contextualised against the backdrop of the physician's philosophical attitude and his fascination with Hermeticism and emanationism. In this respect, Donzellini's most significant philosophical output is his *Remedium ferendarum iniuriarum, sive de compescenda ira*.[17] Drafted in 1586, only a year before his execution, this tract offers both physical and philosophical analysis of the issue of anger. The stated aim of the work is to promote values of temperance, concord, and love among men by teaching forgiveness and tolerance of offences. To this end, the text blends philosophy, theology, and medicine, with a marked emphasis on the former two. Due to its hybrid nature, the density of its content, and the time of its drafting, the *Remedium* is an excellent anthology of Donzellini's philosophical, religious, and medical ideas. It reveals the extent and manner in which his intellectual profile was influenced by these different aspects. Moreover, it showcases his propensity for a humanist religion that took on potentially subversive overtones in the late Cinquecento. These radical implications and the choice of subject matter suggest that the tract was drafted as a militant work. In this sense, its call to conquer irascibility takes shape as a metaphor for the desire to overcome confessional disputes and the defence of religious tolerance.

The text was published by Francesco Ziletti, a printer who played various roles in Donzellini's network. Francesco was the nephew of the Brescian printer Giordano Ziletti. The latter was a member of the original heretical network in Orzi Nuovi who had supplied Buonamonte Donzellini with forbidden works and, after his book production led to clashes with the Catholic authorities in Rome in the 1540s, had turned informer on Girolamo Donzellini in 1553 at the Venetian Holy Office. In 1570, Francesco Ziletti acquired the bookshop *all'insegna del Pozzo*, formerly owned by the heterodox bookseller Andrea Arrivabene, and in 1579 he married the daughter of Vincenzo Valgrisi (sister of Giorgio, the printer mentioned in relation to the last few months of Donzellini's life and the reasons for his final arrest). Following in the footsteps of his relatives and Arrivabene, he started dealing in prohibited texts (by Vergerio, Brucioli, and Erasmus) as soon as he set up shop. As a result, he occasionally needed to hide them and protect himself during searches by the Holy Office. He printed a new edition of the *Testamento novo* (*New Testament*) by Cornelio Donzellini in 1582, before publishing the *Remedium* in 1586.[18] Girolamo's choice of publisher was therefore far from coincidental.

The *Remedium* was a complex text because it could be used and interpreted on different levels and offered a variety of approaches for analysing the subject of anger and bearing injuries. It joined a series of humanist treatises on wrath, with a flurry of works produced during the sixteenth century: the philosopher Agostino Nifo, the physician Johann Weyer and, later, Justus Lipsius and Michel de Montaigne all wrote on the matter, often absorbing the influence of Plutarch's *De cohibenda ira* (*On the Control of Anger*) and Seneca's *De ira* (*On Anger*).[19] For Girolamo, however, the theme of bearing injustice also struck a personal chord. After all, he had been persecuted, imprisoned, and deprived of the dignity of his profession on two occasions. He explained in the *Remedium* that surrendering to rage – the most dangerous of all passions – could never be justified, even by victims of the worst iniquities. This insight takes on a dramatic significance in the light of his personal experience and, as Alessandro Arcangeli pointed out, it is certainly feasible that the unjustly prosecuted people mentioned in the text, bravely enduring humiliation, were references to his own troubled legal history.[20]

The focal points of the treatise, however, are not of a personal nature. Starting from his dedication to Sisto Visdomini, Bishop of Modena,

Donzellini structures his discourse around the subject of the dignity of man, emphasising above all the value of the word. He sees human beings as superior to other animals because of their use of reason (*ratio*) and discourse (*oratio*), which can also be expressed with the Greek term λόγος (logos). The word is the essential agent of salvation. Indeed, the 'light of the gospel' was revealed to humankind through the *verbum* (word, logos), thereby enabling a new pact with God. The very fact that Christ is referred to as the Logos – 'the word, namely discourse, language' ('verbum scilicet, sermo, oratio') – shows the value of the word, through which man can express his thoughts and thereby prevent discord and violence.[21] The emphasis on the literal meaning of *logos* recalls the teachings of Lorenzo Valla and Erasmus of Rotterdam. The celebration of the word, a gift from God, was widespread in circles that blended humanism, which favoured a philological interpretation of Scripture and valued human reason, with the 'vibrant and mystical religiosity of the Reformation.'[22] In these contexts, which mainly consisted of Italian exiles that Donzellini had encountered in various ways, humanism took shape as the fundamental agent of a form of heterodoxy that could not be reduced to the dictates of Lutheran or Calvinist doctrine.

Besides the general element of continuity with humanist sensibilities and theology, the influence of Platonic thought is apparent throughout the *Remedium*; as the author informed his friend Zwinger, the work was envisaged as a counterpoint to the Aristotelian tradition.[23] Platonism is openly defined in the treatise as 'intellectual religion' ('doctam religionem') and Platonists are classed as those who 'were almost Christians' ('paucis demptis fieri christianos').[24] The philosophy that Donzellini wants to endorse, however, could not be assimilated with 'Gentile' ('gentile') thinking and has to be compatible with the Christian message. Just as the ancient Greeks and Romans absorbed the essential core of Eastern knowledge, above all from Egypt, Christians have to embrace the truths bequeathed by pagan thought: 'I believe, indeed, that there is only one true philosophy, which fully coincides with the true religion, whose end is the truth, pure knowledge, and the worship of God.'[25] Through this statement, Girolamo underlines the harmony of all religious and philosophical systems, and the continuity of doctrine. Acknowledgement of this would enable religious peace, as he had already affirmed in the preface to the orations of Themistius through the concept of the *docta religio*.

Above all, Donzellini draws on the philosophical tradition inaugurated by the Platonic Academy of Florence, founded at the initiative of Marsilio Ficino in 1462. The image of the divine set forth by Donzellini makes explicit reference to the thinking of Ficino, who had also been a physician before he concentrated on teaching *theologia platonica* (Platonic theology).[26] In this perspective, God cannot be seen with the eyes or expressed in words; he can only be approached through regular meditation and the celebration of his mysteries. The contemplation of divine mysteries kindles a light in the human soul, almost like a spark flying off burning wood, which gradually becomes larger and stronger. In addition to its echoes of Neoplatonism, this mystically inclined allusion reflects Girolamo's familiarity with the Valdesian doctrine. Like an 'incorporeal and infinite Sun' ('Sole incorporeo, infinito'), God permeates every aspect of reality.[27] Through a process of emanation, God 'is all in all' ('e*st* omnia in omnibus'). Being present in all men, he shares all good with them. In this process, men become like God and partake of his blessedness.

'If God is an incorporeal and infinite Sun that pervades and inhabits everything, being present in all things; if God is the most loving and eternal light; if, through the communion with his light, man is made similar not only to the angel of God but to God himself, indeed in truth he "becomes" the son of God, like another God inside God, blessed in the most blessed; if this blessedness encompasses, or even amply exceeds, all the joys and pleasures that mankind had and is destined to have from the beginning to the end of the world; if, therefore, God is everything in all things, namely present to such an extent in all individuals that in communicating Himself to them He communicates all good at the same time, what else should one do if not privately concentrating all of one's thought on Him, in order to obtain immense happiness?'[28]

Against the backdrop of the spread of confessional controversy and the Church of Rome's repressive response to the growth of heresy, the revival of a philosophical tradition steeped in Neoplatonism could have implications of heterodoxy.[29] To safeguard Catholic orthodoxy it was essential to maintain a closed, structured cultural system based on the certainties of Scholastic-Aristotelian philosophy. These requirements led, for example, in 1594 to the censorship of the work of Franciscus Patricius, a philosopher that Donzellini knew and admired.[30] This was not a new trend: in the 1530s, Gasparo Contarini, an Aristotelian cardinal, had noted that the 'Arian' ('ariana') theology spreading throughout Italy specifically relied on Platonic doctrines.[31] Moreover, Ficino unwittingly levelled implicit criticism at the Trinitarian dogma in his treatises and Platonic commentaries.[32] Although he always remained within the boundaries of orthodoxy and never directly questioned the Trinity, the Neoplatonic emanationist doctrines that he championed and Donzellini followed featured an underlying immanentist concept of divinity that encouraged a modalist interpretation of the Trinity. According to this, the Son and the Holy Spirit were the "modes" through which God revealed himself in the world: in the shape of the divine spirit and through the example and preaching of Christ. Furthermore, driven by the desire to renew Christianity, Ficino focused on the mystery of the God-Man in order to emphasise man as the 'bond of the world' (*copula mundi*). He thus recommended an irenic religion that coincided with the divine wisdom (*divina sapientia*), which acknowledged humankind as a 'great miracle' ('magnum miraculum').[33] Donzellini's references to Ficino featured the same positive anthropology, which attributed man with divine potential and a central role in God's plan.

In this respect, Donzellini's interest in Paracelsian thought assumes greater significance. Paracelsus had revisited some aspects of Neoplatonism, highlighting their pantheistic repercussions, and his peers had judged that his conception of the cosmos damaged the Trinitarian dogma by viewing the Son as 'a corruptible substance.'[34] The same concepts were also present – through reference to Ficino and the Hermetic tradition – in the work of Servetus, another radical physician whose thinking Donzellini mirrored in many respects. First of all, both referred to the so-called negative theology and the image of an 'invisible and inexpressible' God.[35] Second, they offered identical solutions to the ineffability of God: a 'metaphysics' ('metafisica') of light that mediated 'between the divinity, from whence it emanated, and the world, which it constituted.'[36] Thirdly, they both conceived of the sun as a sign of divinity (*symbolum deitatis*), a visible and 'corporeal' image of the Eternal underpinned by the idea of a God spilling into reality. Finally, the two physicians each adopted the Pauline expression of God as 'all in all' ('omnia in omnibus'). In the wake of the Hermetic tradition, this took on pantheistic overtones that could not be reduced to the original meaning found in the Epistle to the Corinthians.[37] Donzellini, however, also employed an image verging on pantheism when he described the divine nature as 'a sphere whose centre is everywhere.'[38]

The interpretation of the *verbum* as the concrete means through which God had revealed himself to the world (as a "quality" or provision of the divine rather than a *res*, or substance) was also similar in some respects to the theology of Servetus, which in turn drew on Lorenzo Valla. In the works of both Servetus and Donzellini, the humanity of Christ was the fundamental element of mediation between the human and the divine. God had revealed himself through the incarnation of the Son-Logos, thereby redeeming man, his favourite creature.[39] Donzellini used the term θεάνθρωπος (theanthropos) to describe the God-Man 'endowed with divinity' by the Father. On one hand, this emphasised the humanity of Christ, never mortified by his divinity; on the other hand, it highlighted the supremacy of Christ in the eschatological discourse. This notion was consistent with Servetus's anthropocentric and Christocentric vision.

Donzellini also stated that after the creation of the world (*mundo condito*), God decided to make himself visible through the Word (*verbum*); until that moment, he had been 'hidden in the immense and infinite sea of eternity.'[40] Even with the ambiguity of this statement, which glosses over the vexed question of the generation of Christ, he seems to be suggesting that the Son-Word was generated over time, after the creation of the world. This would endorse Servetian Christology, according to which 'the Word was eternal. The son of God was not eternal.'[41] In other words, the Son – the incarnation of the Word – was inferior to God the Father despite being retrospectively endowed with divinity. A further suggestion to this end may lie in the fact that, at the time of writing (1586), radical Christology such as the work of Valentino Gentile had already explored the semantic difference between the terms *aeternum* and *sempiternum*. The former referred to the eternity of life after death, while the latter expressed the timeless time before creation.[42] It was no coincidence that Donzellini only placed God the Father in *sempiternum* and used *aeternus* to define the Son. The intention was not to deny the divine nature of Christ, however, but to emphasise the divine potential of man, which became feasible through the advent of the theanthropos, his sacrifice, his message of salvation, and his word.

While these similarities are not enough to describe Donzellini as an anti-Trinitarian – and there is no intention to do so –, they nevertheless suggest that he was both familiar with and partly inspired by the Spaniard's work. Indeed, it has been established that Girolamo first encountered Servetus's texts before 1554 when he stayed with Pier Paolo Vergerio in Tübingen at the beginning of his exile on Reformed soil. In Vergerio's aforementioned letter to Bullinger, he mentioned that his guest had been 'tempted' towards the Servetian 'plague' ('peste') by the radical jurist Matteo Gribaldi Mofa in Padua. Pietro Perna also provided Donzellini with some of the Spaniard's texts, although we do not know which. It is feasible that they were the *De trinitatis erroribus* and the *Dialogi de trinitate* (*Dialogues on the Trinity*, Hagenau, 1532), which had been available in the Venetian heterodox world since the 1530s. After Servetus was burned at the stake, the Protestant Churches and the Catholic authorities launched such a relentless campaign to eradicate the *Christianismi restitutio* (an anthology of his theological and cosmological ideas in which his debt to the Neoplatonic tradition is apparent) that there are now only three surviving copies. Nevertheless, the *Christianismi restitutio* was distributed in manuscript form, above all in Padua and in academic medical circles. The text might have raised particular interest among Doctor of Arts and medicine because it announced the discovery of the pulmonary circulation of blood and prompted curiosity in new doctrines that were widespread in the medical community.[43] Moreover, Servetian ideas are known to have circulated in Basel since the 1530s. These aspects all strengthen the hypothesis that Donzellini could have read the Spaniard's theological treatises – both his writings from the 1530s and his masterpiece of 1553.

It is likely, however, that the Trinitarian dispute was of no interest to him, a mere adiaphoron that had already caused too much bloodshed and produced schisms that were inevitably negative from his irenic perspective. In this respect, the lack of any attempt to solve the mystery of the generation of Christ or interpret the passage of the Gospel of John ('In the beginning was the Word') is in keeping with the basis of his religiosity.[44] To this end, the references to the nature of the *Verbum* and its importance in practical teaching, despite its divine origin, aimed to establish a form of Christianity reduced to moral law that would focus on the imitation of Christ and the practice of neighbourly charity and love. Donzellini thus joined the tradition of Christian humanism that had moved from Ficino and Erasmus to Valdés and Servetus and culminated in the ethical religiosity of Socinianism.[45]

The essential element of Christ's preaching – of the *verbum* – was the proclamation of eternal blessedness for the humble, the meek, the peace-makers, and the persecuted.[46] In this way, Donzellini combined a mystical and pantheistic approach with a view of Christianity based on the notion of φιλανθρωπία (philanthropy), a 'law of nature' grounded in love, benevolence, charity, and humility whose righteousness could never be repudiated.[47] He explained that this universal law – the 'healthiest' ('saluberrimo') precept for building interpersonal relations – had been established on earth by Christ, the God-Man, through his preaching and exemplary conduct.[48] However, this was a law etched into the human mind in all populations throughout the ages (as Paul had written in Rom 2:15) that had already been effectively interpreted by Gentile philosophers: Plato, Aristotle, and above all Socrates, the first to state that philosophy 'is to become like God.'[49] The nexus between philosophy and religion was thus not only expressed in theological terms but also reiterated in relation to moral doctrinal content.

From this point of view, the proper remedy for dealing with offences is seen as compliance with the evangelical teachings and the law of nature, namely philanthropy. True Christians must be able to tolerate the abuses of others and all forms of insult; only in this way will they be worthy of their nature as God's chosen creatures at the centre of the universe. Therefore, after broaching the main issue of the treatise – the bearing of injuries –, Donzellini continued to embellish his pedagogical and moral intent with theological and philosophical ideas. The key to understanding the *Remedium* lies precisely in this interweaving of cultural motifs, held together by specific notions of the divine and of man and aimed at creating unity among humankind. The concept of 'providence' ('providentia') is also adopted to argue that the right way to address injustices is to use reason and the word, appeal to mutual dialogue, and contextualise the harshness of afflictions. Adversity is indeed part of the divine plan, with God as the 'choreographer' ('choragus') in a world-theatre in which every individual plays a role.[50] God has given a specific task to every person on earth, each of whom is an instrument of his unquestionable will: emperors, kings, and princes just as much as peasants, the crippled, and 'parasites' ('parasiti').[51] In this framework, however, man is not abandoned to his fate or denied the freedom to lead a righteous life. Indeed, God decided to express his will through Christ, who provided a supreme model of virtue and benevolence with his preaching and conduct.[52] In a context where the positions of mutual hostility adopted by the different confessions had become even more rigid, Donzellini launched a heartfelt appeal for the end of discord and persecution, for love among men, and for philanthropy.

As a seasoned Nicodemite, he expressed his religious proposal in the form of a philosophical-medical treatise dedicated to an inquisitor (Sisto Visdomini, also Bishop of Modena) so as not to arouse suspicion. The same dedication, however, also praised the memory of Cardinal Giovanni

Morone, the former Bishop of Modena who had been extremely close to Cardinal Pole and had played an active role in distributing the *Beneficio di Cristo*.[53] Considering that Donzellini had been subjected to several trials and that the cardinal had also fallen afoul of the Inquisition, it seems significant that this reference appeared in a treatise celebrating those who had been unjustly persecuted and suffered trespasses against them with dignity and forbearance.

Donzellini wrote in Latin and ensured that the text was also distributed beyond the Alps (as shown by the frequent mentions of the work in his correspondence with Zwinger). Indeed, his appeal was directed equally at the Catholic and Reformed worlds. It was on Reformed soil that the work was reissued forty years later – in 1635 in Leiden – by the printer Ioannis Maire, known for his editions of Erasmus, Kepler, and Grotius, and for first publishing Descartes's *Discors de la Méthode* (*Discourse on the Method*). This came at the height of the carnage of the Thirty Years' War, a time when Calvinism was convulsed by heated theological debates and fierce clashes.[54] The reissue of the *Remedium* by a printer at the cutting edge of scientific and theological publications cemented Donzellini's intellectual legacy and ensured that his call for harmony among men, religious tolerance, and free scientific research did not completely fall on deaf ears.

6.3 '*Medicus non tantum corporum, sed etiam animorum sit curator*': The medical profile of Girolamo Donzellini

Gary Waite suggested that a religious propensity for irenic, spiritual, and Latitudinarian doctrines often favoured the development of scientific free thinking and an experimental approach that was unlikely to be adopted by uncompromisingly Catholic or Lutheran physicians. By raising the level of credence in personal experience and in the direct inspiration of the divine spirit, a penchant for spiritual doctrines could lead to traditional knowledge being questioned, either consciously or otherwise.[55] The case of Donzellini seems to endorse this hypothesis in many respects. As we have seen, however, it is advisable to avoid overly rigid models when defining the nexus between medicine and the Reformation/heresy, at least with regard to the Italian context. Donzellini's interest in spagyric science and alchemy never undermined his appreciation of Galenic medicine. Indeed, the latter formed the epistemological perspective for transferring experimental and empirical ideas from the medical field to the theological realm. If Waite's theory of 'spiritualism's potential for creativity' is corroborated in Donzellini's theological and scientific method, this is because he employed the Galenic approach. This stance saw medicine as 'philosophy of the body' and encouraged doctors of medicine to address questions regarding the health of the soul. Proficiency in scholarly medicine – a discipline combining care of the body and care of the spirit – was the essential bedrock for integrating medical, philosophical, and religious research into a coherent vision.

Evidence of this position can be found in the *Remedium ferendarum iniuriarum*, where Donzellini also analysed the feeling of anger from a physical point of view. After first pinpointing its location in the heart, 'sparked' (accensus) by the blood and by the 'spirit' (spiritus),[56] he focused on the characteristics of the different humoral temperaments. Indeed, not all types of bile were equal, and the differences between them had an impact on the development and duration of anger, as well as the ability to control it.[57] In this way, the humours were seen as the origin and biological seat of all forms of hatred, deception, enmity, and even war.[58]

In this regard, medical practitioners performed a fundamental dual function. Their first role was to practise evacuation, removing excess bile and its 'highly malignant' ('malignissima') element to restore a healthy balance to the humours. At the same time, they had the less spectacular but decidedly more important task of ensuring that the noxious humour was not regenerated. The knowledge and advice they offered to this end benefitted not only the body but also the soul, making physicians 'teachers of excellent actions' ('optimarum actionum magistr*i*'), just like true philosophers.[59] To prevent bile from heating up and causing new fits of rage, Donzellini recommended eating fresh food like plums and lemons, wearing moderate clothes, and avoiding strong aromatic wines. He also suggested practising music because of its great power to arouse and quell the soul and bring about virtuous actions.[60] Medicine therefore played a vital role in maintaining peace among men by targeting the physical agents responsible for the development and continuation of anger.

There was also another more significant nexus linking medicine to philosophy, religion, and pedagogy. As medicine had the power to cure a bad 'temperament' ('temperamento'), Donzellini highlighted, it could also transform nefarious behaviour into righteous conduct. As Galen had famously put it, the best physician is also a philosopher. Therefore, if 'medicine is the philosophy of the body' ('philosophia corporis'), philosophy 'is the medicine of the soul' ('philosophi*a* vero animi Medicinam [est]'). As physicians were called to take action to aid spiritual as well as physical wellbeing, their fundamental role would be 'glorious [...] for a long time to come.'[61] In this respect, Donzellini felt entitled and indeed duty bound to offer spiritual remedies against the 'plague' ('peste') of anger. In terms of content, the care of souls in the *Remedium* consisted of rediscovering the divine origin of man and affirming the presence of God in all creation. This had to be followed by conduct that was worthy of God's chosen creatures with a philanthropic approach open to dialogue. From an early age, men had to be guided towards 'perfect morals, honest discipline' ('optimi mor*es,* honesta disciplina') and above all the imitation of Christ; in this way, no further care would be required in adulthood.[62]

From a strictly medical point of view, and in terms of the learned influences on Donzellini's conception of medicine, it is worth noting that the doctrine expressed in the *Remedium* can be linked to the thinking of the

French physician Jean Fernel. Among other things, the Frenchman had developed a 'Christian-Platonic' reading of Galenism.[63] It is therefore easy to understand why Donzellini was interested in Fernel's work and included him among the exponents of the *docta religio* in 1559.[64] More specifically, Fernel was one of the first to advocate a new perspective on pathological phenomena. Whilst continuing to work within a Galenic framework, he advanced the idea that disease could be generated regardless of alterations in the humoral balance. Through the concept of *spiritus* (breath of life, spirit), Fernel referred to a reality of divine origin midway between corporeal and immaterial elements – between the earthly and heavenly worlds – that formed the "substance" of any natural object.[65] In his *De abditis rerum causis* (*On the Hidden Causes of Things*, Paris 1548), Fernel developed a complex doctrine based on the notion of *spiritus*. According to this, a material part and a formal part could be distinguished in every body; "occult" illnesses affected the form (*forma*) of a given body and could be eliminated by forces with a diametrically opposed substance (*substantia*).[66] Although Fernel is never directly referenced, Donzellini's ideas are consistent with his thinking. Indeed, Girolamo claims that nature contains properties which come from 'all substance' ('a tota substantia'), previously defined by Galen as 'arcane and recondite.' These affect the body by avoiding the rules of interaction between humours. Then, echoing the *De abditis rerum causis,*[67] he lists a series of phenomena that seemingly go against the manifest qualities of different natural entities such as the lion's inexplicable fear of the cock's crow; the ability of amber to attract straw; the beneficial use of wrens ('uccelli di Troglodite') to break up kidney and bladder stones; the power of green quartz to benefit the human stomach simply through external contact; and the capacity of ostriches to feed on iron, among many others. Donzellini notes that the methods and knowledge of traditional medicine contribute little to an understanding of the forces at work in these natural events. Instead, it is necessary to rely exclusively on the senses and experience, which teach that there is a medicament capable of soothing anger and providing a genuine antidote to fits of rage. The effectiveness of this mineral – carnelian (*corneolus*) – is not based on any specific qualities but on powers that can be ascribed to its entire substance.[68] Besides the treatment itself, it is worth noting that Donzellini was familiar with the latest issues in the medical debate of the time and was receptive to an experimental form of medicine, albeit one within a strong spiritual framework.

Donzellini's treatise on the prevention and treatment of the plague also offers significant insights into his medical views. It can be interpreted as a summary of his ideas on medicine as it was drafted purely on the basis of his knowledge without any help from medical texts or manuals.[69] The physician wrote the work in prison during the tragic summer and autumnal months of 1576, when the horror caused by the plague was only mitigated by his determination to contribute productively to its eradication and his hope of an early release. Published by Oratio dei Gobi of Salò, the *Discorso* opened with a dedication to the *Provveditori alla sanità* (Superintendents of Health) dated 3 December 1576. This direct address to the health authorities was the first indication of Donzellini's thinly disguised polemic with two well-known physicians, Girolamo Mercuriale and Girolamo Capodivacca. At the first signs of the spread of the disease, these illustrious professors at Padua University had been appointed by the Venetian Senate to determine its exact nature and establish whether it was the plague. When they failed to detect a high level of contagion – the fundamental element attributed to pestilence by Galen –, they ruled out a potential epidemic in the city. The municipal authorities were satisfied with these conclusions as they were keen to avoid implementing quarantine measures that would be disastrous for the economy of the Republic. For some time after this, the word plague was banished from the local vocabulary and life returned to normal. Ships docked, goods circulated, and the two physicians (and many of their colleagues) visited the sick without complying with the prophylactic measures adopted in the event of plague.[70] It was not long before the rate of infection soared, and the spread of the disease became uncontainable. Venice subsequently lost a third of its population during the plague of 1575. As a prisoner of the Holy Office who had recently been expelled from the Veronese College of Physicians, Donzellini managed to contribute to the medical debate from his cell by drafting the treatise. In it, he stressed the need to diagnose the plague regardless of the number of cases whenever certain symptoms were found, even if it meant moving away from Galenic thought.[71]

In this case too, Donzellini's approach to the body and the epidemic shows the stirrings of an independent perspective and an attitude that was not entirely deferential to authority. There is a significant example of this is when he describes the most common causes of the plague. He states that there is a 'method or cause not perceived in the ancient writers' ('modo o causa non avvertito negli antichi scrittori'), referring to the innovative theory of contagion advanced by the Veronese physician Girolamo Fracastoro in 1546.[72] In his *De contagione, et contagiosis morbis et eorum curatione* (*On Contagion, Contagious Diseases, and Their Treatment*, introduced by the *De sympathia et antipathia rerum* [*Sympathy and Antipathy of Things*], Venice, 1546), Fracastoro presented a philosophical-scientific vision without any miraculous or prodigious influences, expressed in the 'omnipresent vitalism of the soul of the world.'[73] This vitalism also extended to the most elusive parts of reality, referred to as *seminaria*, imperceptible seedlike entities involved in nature's processes of spontaneous generation and self-destruction, and also responsible for outbreaks of epidemic diseases. Following Fracastoro's teaching, Donzellini identified the basic agent of contagion as 'a filthy body that is called a seed of plague' ('corpo sordidissimo che si chiama seminario della peste') or 'fomite' ('fomite'). This infinitesimally tiny animate particle was said to spread pestilential bacteria by settling on objects, clothing, or the skin of infected people and moving from one subject to another. Given that the disease 'is found in few at the beginning [...] but the term plague can be used wherever its characteristics are found, even if only in a single man' ('da principio si trova in pochi [...] ma ovunque si trova il detto caratterismo della peste quella esser degna di tal nome, anchor che fosse in un sol'uomo'), the physician encouraged the health authorities to employ the utmost 'care and vigilance' ('cura e vigilanza') in order to block the progress of the disease before the rate of infection reached epidemic proportions.[74]

Donzellini saw medicine as a practical discipline 'whose purpose is operational' ('il cui fine è l'opera'). He was therefore confident in the effectiveness of treatment. Indeed, thanks to the reason and experience of the good physician, it could even wipe out an aggressive disease like the plague. This humanist optimism about the huge potential and capability of human ingenuity – a key concept in his cultural and religious visions – was not only applied to medical practitioners. Indeed, he wrote the tract in the vernacular, hoping to encourage people to implement his 'preservative and curative [system] against the plague' ('preservativo e curativo della peste'). Once the inhabitants of the city were able to recognise the symptoms of the disease, identify its contagious nature, and observe its 'growth' ('accrescimento'), they would take suitable precautions immediately to limit its spread. He also suggested a series of practical measures for securing the collaboration of the townspeople and curbing the epidemic. These included employing honest, qualified physicians in hospitals; purifying the air and contaminated items with bonfires; encouraging evacuation from infected cities for those who could afford to leave; and using town criers to help promote a series of medicines (purgatives, oils, and sudorific powders that were simple to prepare, with recipes provided), which the sick would be able to obtain easily or even make themselves, thereby gaining valuable time.

Donzellini's practical attitude towards care of the body and his willingness to embrace the latest developments in sixteenth-century medical and naturalistic knowledge can also be seen in his correspondence. In addition to the above observations on his publishing collaboration with Zwinger, it is worth examining his epistolary exchange with Camerarius. In 1586, Donzellini was waiting for the physician from Nuremberg to send his 'Botanicon,' which was probably the *De plantis epitome utilissima* (*Most Useful Synopsis of Plants*, Frankfurt, 1586, later translated into German as the *Kreutterbuch*, literally *Plant Book*). This text was a reworking of Mattioli's *Discorsi* (*Discourses*, Venice, 1550) on the six books of Dioscorides's *De materia medica* (*On Medical Material*), the most famous and valued systematic pharmaceutical-botanical study of the time. The year before, in 1585, Girolamo had edited a critical edition of the *Consilia* (*Medical Advice*, Lyon, 1586) and *Epistolae* (*Letters*, Lyon, 1586) by Vittore Trincavelli, a Venetian professor of practical medicine at Padua University (where he had taken Da Monte's place). Trincavelli was a key player in the relaunch of Hippocratic and Galenic culture to counter its Scholastic and

Arabic counterpart. Donzellini played an active role in the distribution of these two texts and sent copies to Camerarius, who in turn was supposed to share them with the imperial physician Johannes Crato von Krafftheim and the Protestant jurist Johann Baptist Fischart.[75]

Donzellini was also involved in publishing projects aimed at reforming medicine during his time in Venice. In 1579, he collaborated with the printer Vincenzo Valgrisi on a plan to publish the eighth part of the *Curationum medicinalium centuriae* (*Centuries of Medical Healing*) by Amatus Lusitanus. This was a collection of clinical cases, which were described with great attention to the specific context in which the diseases had appeared and analysed through the author's extensive theoretical, anatomical, and pharmacological expertise. A Jew of Portuguese origin, Lusitanus lived variously in Venice, Ferrara, Ancona, and Rome in the second half of the century. He mixed in medical humanist circles until Pope Paul IV's new policy on Jews led to attacks against him as a *marrano* (crypto-Jew). He then decided to return to Judaism and joined the Jewish community in Thessalonica in the last decade of his life. He continued working on the epic *Centuriae* until his death in 1568. Around ten years later, his son delivered the manuscript of the eighth book of the *Centuriae* directly to Valgrisi, who brought in Donzellini. Among other things, Girolamo was supposed to rework certain controversial statements made by Lusitanus against Mattioli's *Discorsi*, probably concerning the identification of some medicinal plants (the rivalry between Lusitanus and the imperial physician is well known).[76] The project never came to fruition, but Donzellini's involvement in the attempt to publish a work by Lusitanus is interesting. Not only was the Portuguese author familiar with the direct observation of natural and clinical phenomena, but he also valued Neoplatonic thought. Indeed, when he was in Thessalonica in 1559, he read, enjoyed, and set out to issue an edition of the *De harmonia mundi* (*On the Harmony of the World*) by the Neoplatonic philosopher Judah Abravanel (Leone Ebreo), which still remains unpublished. Significantly, the *Centuriae* was placed on the Index in the 1590 s for its discussion of the dietary excesses and abnormal sexual practices of members of the regular clergy, along with the resulting diseases.[77]

Donzellini's correspondence not only highlights his medical and publishing interests but also casts light on his medical practices, confirming elements discussed above. First of all, it demonstrates his involvement in the preparation of medicaments and above all his fascination with theriac. He was part of a production chain for this potent antidote in which he collaborated with the Veronese apothecary Bellicocco and Camerarius. From Italy, he sent Bellicocco's sometimes secret recipes for theriac and other remedies created in Verona to Camerarius, as well as seeds that were impossible to find in Germany but widely available in the Republic (although he also procured them from friends in Cyprus, Crete, Constantinople, and Alexandria).[78] In exchange, Camerarius provided Donzellini with potash alum. This essential ingredient for the production of theriac was ordered from Hieronymus Herold, an archiater from Leipzig, and delivered to Bellicocco's shop, where it was collected by Donzellini.[79]

Donzellini's letters also shed light on his penchant for experimentation, confirming among other things the above observations on his interest in the 'spagyric miracle.' He frequently studied and discussed the potential of new remedies and techniques in the medical world, adding them to his professional skill set without abandoning the teachings of the humanist tradition. Some of his letters written in 1577, just after his release from prison, reveal that he discovered tobacco (known at the time as *erba regina* or *santa croce*) through Melchiorre Guilandino, a botanist in Padua who was already using the name *tabacus* for the prodigious plant. Various physicians and naturalists in Rome also sent him a tobacco juice palliative. In one letter to Camerarius, Girolamo enclosed the recipe for this medication together with the required tobacco in order to sound him out on the new substance that had recently arrived from the Americas.[80] His curiosity about the properties of natural remedies from distant worlds is also apparent in his interaction at more or less the same time with a merchant of African origin, whom he asked about the properties of *nux vomica* (the "vomiting nut," widespread in the forests of South-East Asia). We do not know how this traveller ended up in Venice and came into contact with Donzellini, but his description of *nux vomica* was then referred to Camerarius. Donzellini was therefore eager to consolidate his international network after leaving prison and update his medical and naturalistic knowledge through reading, correspondence, and personal encounters.

Donzellini's research interests did not distract him from his everyday medical practice, which extended to all levels of society including marginal figures like prisoners of the Inquisition. While in 1578 he tended to the health of his former cellmate Nascimbene Nascimbeni, in 1584 he treated Laura Malpiero, a woman accused of witchcraft and imprisoned in Venice. He wrote a letter supporting her cause on 15 December that year, a document included in the records of her trial. Handwritten by 'Girolamo Donzellini, physical medical physician' ('Hieronimo Donzellini dottor medico fisico'), it attests to the woman's poor state of health and recommends her release. Given that she was 'riddled with pain, with extremely troublesome fever and colic ache that make her cry out day and night' ('carica di male con febbri e dolori colici molestissimi, che la sforza a gridare dì et notte'), the physician concluded that she would not benefit from any 'appropriate help or assistance' ('aiuto et soccorso conveniente') as long as she remained in prison.[81] The regrettable episode of Nascimbeni's escape while in Donzellini's custody had clearly not compromised the latter's professional ethics or charitable nature. Whether his patients were wealthy patricians or forlorn prisoners of the Inquisition, his work was still guided by their needs, even if defending a heretic or a witch could further jeopardise his already marred reputation.

The repercussions of Donzellini's intellectual research were therefore extremely practical. His quest for knowledge, conducted on the basis of an animated vision of the cosmos in which humankind and nature were connected by mysterious correspondences, was expressed first and foremost in practical science. This enabled Donzellini to adopt a hands-on approach towards the body and indeed creation. In this way, he not only implemented the teachings of the ancients, which were revived through encounters with texts and scholars in the *Repubblica medica*, but also incorporated innovative doctrines and experimented with new natural products and "miraculous" alchemy techniques. At the same time, his research also featured a highly practical and moral religiosity with Latitudinarian, spiritual, and mystical influences; through these religious beliefs, the acquisition of knowledge became a vehicle for action based on dialogue, tolerance, and the imitation of Christ.

Notes

1 Many studies in historiography have focused on the figure of Paracelsus. The first to analyse his life and thought was Walter Pagel, whose studies are still a valuable resource: see Walter Pagel, *An Introduction to Philosophical Medicine* (Basel: Kerger, 1958). Today, one of the greatest experts is Charles Webster: see in particular Charles Webster, *From Paracelsus to Newton. Magic and the Making of Modern Science* (New York: Cambridge University Press, 1982); idem, *Paracelsus: Medicine as a Popular Protest,* in Grell, Cunningham (eds.), *Medicine and the Reformation*, 57–77; idem, *Paracelsus. Medicine, Magic and the Mission at the End of Time* (New Haven: Yale University Press, 2008). Other important works are: Ole Peter Grell (ed.), *Paracelsus: The Man and His Reputation, His Ideas and Their Transformation* (Leiden – Boston: Brill, 1998); Gerhild Sholz Williams, Charles D. Gunnoe jr (eds.), *Paracelsian Moments: Science, Medicine and Astrology in Early Modern Europe* (Kirksville: Truman State University Press, 2002); for an English translation of the works written by Paracelsus between 1529 and 1532, see Andrew Weeks (ed.), *Paracelsus (Theophrastus Bombastus von Hohenheim, 1493–1541). Essential Theoretical Writings* (Leiden – Boston: Brill, 2008).

2 Tommaso Zefiriele Bovio, *Melampigo, overo confusione de medici sofisti che s'intitolano rationali* (Verona: Girolamo Discepoli et Fratelli), 1585, 44–46.

3 There is an in-depth analysis of the issues discussed below in Celati, *Medicine*.

4 See Lorenz Scholtz von Rosenau, *Epistolarum philosophicarum, medicinalium, ac chymicarum a summis nostrae aetatis philosophis ac medicis exaratarum volumen* (Frankfurt: And. Wecheli haeredes, Claudium di Marni, & Ioh. Aubrium, 1598), 155. The letter is also cited in Giancarlo Zanier, 'La medicina paracelsiana in Italia, aspetti di un'accoglienza particolare,' *Rivista di Storia della filosofia*, 4 (1985), 635, and in Ingegno, *Il medico*,169.

5 See Marco Ferrari, 'Alcune vie di diffusione in Italia di idee e di testi di Paracelso,' in *Scienze, credenze occulte, livelli di cultura. Convegno internazionale di studi, Firenze, 26–30 giugno 1980* (Florence: Olschki, 1982), 23–24; Antonio Clericuzio, 'Chemical Medicine and Paracelsianism in Italy 1550–1650,' in Margaret Pelling, Scott Mandelbrote (eds.), *The Practice of Reform in Health, Medicine and Science, 1500–2000: Essays for Charles Webster* (Aldershot: Ashgate, 2005, 59–79).

6 See Zanier, *La medicina*, 628, 635; Paolo Galluzzi, 'Motivi paracelsiani nella Toscana di Cosimo I e di don Antonio dei Medici: alchimia, medicina "chimica' e riforma del sapere,' in *Scienze, credenze occulte,* 56–62.

7 See the interesting overview in Mammola, *La ragione*, 195–99.

8 David Gentilcore, *Medical Charlatanism in Early Modern Italy* (Oxford: Oxford University Press, 2006), 227.

9 Ibidem.

10 'I used to own all books by Paracelsus, but since I could not learn anything from them, I exchanged them with some others and did not want to keep them in my library as they did not teach anything' ('Ego aliquando libros omnes Paracelsi apud me habui, sed cum ex eorum lectione nihil proficerem, pro aliis permutavi, nec in mea Bibliotheca tales libros haerere volui, qui nihil docerent.' Scholtz von Rosenau, *Epistolarum*, 155. On the imperial court and the role that Crato covered there see Louthan, *The Quest for Compromise*.

11 'But learn about another spagyric miracle' ('Sed accipe aliud spagiricum miraculum'); Scholtz von Rosenau, Epistolarum, 155.

12 'And I think that if anything worthwhile was said or written by him [Paracelsus], it would have been reported by Andernach in his books' ('Ac puto, si quid dignum unquam ab eo dictum aut scriptum est, id ab Andernaco in suos libros fuisse traslatum.'); ibidem. On the spread of Paracelsianism in Europe and the first attempts to compromise between Galen and Paracelsus, see Michaela Valente, *Johann Wier. Agli albori della critica razionale dell'occulto e del demoniaco nell'Europa del Cinquecento* (Florence: Olschki, 118–20); Didier Kahn, *Alchimie et paracelsisme en France à la fin de la Renaissance (1567–1625)* (Geneva: Librairie Droz, 2007), 200–07.

13 Thomas Erastus, *Disputationes de medicina nova Philippi Paracelsi pars prima. In qua, quae de remediis superstitiosis & magicis curationibus ille prodidit, praecipue examinantur* (*First Part of the Disputations on the New Medicine of Philip Paracelsus, which examines above all his accounts of remedies of superstitious and magical treatments*, Basel, 1571); *Disputationes de medicina nova Philippi Paracelsi pars altera. In qua philosophiae Paracelsicae principia & elementa explorantur* (*Second Part of the Disputations on the New Medicine of Philip Paracelsus, which explores the principles and elements of Paracelsian philosophy*, Basel, 1572); *Disputationes de medicina nova Philippi Paracelsi pars tertia* (*Third Part of the Disputations on the New Medicine of Philip Paracelsus*, Basel, 1572); *Disputationes de medicina nova Philippi Paracelsi pars quarta et ultima* (*Fourth and Final Part of the Disputations on the New Medicine of Philip Paracelsus*, Basel, 1573); See Charles D. Gunnoe jr., 'Erastus and Paracelsianism. Theological Motifs in Thomas Erastus' Rejection of Paracelsian Natural Philosophy,' in Allen G. Debus, Michael Thomson Walton (eds.), *Reading the Book of Nature: The Other Side of the Scientific Revolution* (Kirksville: Truman State University Press, 1998), 45–66; Charles D. Gunnoe, *Thomas Erastus and the Palatinate. A Renaissance Physician in the Second Reformation* (Leiden – Boston: Brill, 2011), especially pp. 242–47.

14 Emanuele D. Vitali, entry 'Algarotti, Vittorio,' in *Dizionario Biografico degli Italiani*, 2 (1960).

15 Between 1590 and 1593 there was a predominantly negative view of Paracelsus's works; nevertheless, this opinion was not shared by all members of the Congregation of the Index. After a long discussion, Paracelsus was included among the authors in the first class; despite this officially definitive decision, further attempts were made to place him in the class of authors whose texts were prohibited *donec corrigatur* (until corrected); Baldini, Spruit, *Catholic Church*, vol. 3, 2166–70.

16 Charles Webster, 'Conrad Gessner and the Infidelity of Paracelsus,' in John Henry, Sarah Hutton (eds.), *New Perspectives on Renaissance Thought: Essays in the History of Science, Education and Philosophy in Memory of Charles B. Schmitt* (London: Duckworth, 1990), 13–23.

17 Girolamo Donzellini, *Remedium ferendarum iniuriarum, sive de compescenda ira* (Venice: Francesco Ziletti, 1586), on which see Alessandro Arcangeli, 'Girolamo Donzellini on Anger: Managing Emotions Between Inquisition Trials,' in Federico Barbierato, Alessandra Veronese (eds.), *Late Medieval and Early Modern Religious Dissents: Conflicts and Plurality in Renaissance Europe* (Pisa: Edizioni Il Campano Arnus University Books, 2012), 58–77. Arcangeli is one of the few scholars that have analysed the Remedium ferendarum iniuriarum, also offering a brief reconstruction of the most widespread philosophical interpretations of the question of anger in classical, Christian, and Renaissance culture. See also Redmond, *Girolamo Donzellino*: according to the author, Donzellini's thought is reminiscent of that of Boethius in the *De consolatione philosophiae* (Consolation of Philosophy). There are also references to Donzellini's work in Ingegno, 'Il medico' 169–70.

18 On Ziletti, see Grendler, *The Roman Inquisition*, 191, 111.

19 For a general discussion of the notion of anger in the early modern period and an analysis of how it was developed in philosophical, theological, moral, medical, literary, and artistic terms, see Karl A.E. Enenkel, Anita Traninger (eds.), *Discourses of Anger in the Early Modern Period* (Leiden – Boston: Brill, 2015).

20 See Arcangeli, 'Girolamo Donzellini on Anger,' 75.

21 Donzellini, *Remedium*, 8 (dedication to Sisto Visdomini).

22 'La religiosità viva e mistica della Riforma,' Cantimori, *Eretici italiani*, 121.

23 Basel, Universitätsbibliothek, Abteilung Frey-Gryn Mscr GII 37, letter of 3 November 1586. Donzellini agreed with Aristotle that anger was a natural element, a constituent part of every man's temperament. However, he rebuked the Greek philosopher for being too gentle in his criticism of the passion. Specifically, Donzellini did not subscribe to the Aristotelian theory of the "golden mean" with regard to vices of the soul; see Arcangeli, 'Girolamo Donzellini on Anger,' 73.

24 Donzellini, *Remedium*, 24v.

25 'Arbitramur enim unam solam, ac veram philosophiam esse, cum vera ac germana religione penitus consentientem, cuius finis sit veritas sincera Dei cognitio et cultus'; ibidem.

26 On Ficino's contribution to the renewal of medicine and above all his idea of medicine strongly influenced by Florentine Neoplatonism – 'a physical and medical version of Platonism' ('una versione fisica e medica del platonismo') – see Teodoro Katinis, *Medicina e filosofia in Marsilio Ficino: il Consilio contro la pestilenza* (Rome: Edizioni di Storia e Letteratura, 2007), 68–83. Ficino assigned the good physician with the role of 'minister' ('ministro') of nature and instrument of God, comparing the figure to a sorceror or sage, capable of assisting the action of nature and controlling its occult forces. The Florentine praised medicine as a point of intersection with other fields of knowledge, given that it was closely linked to astrology, magic, and philosophy. Similar ideas can also be found in the thinking of Italian heterodox physicians like Guglielmo Grataroli and Girolamo Donzellini. On the concept of *religio* (religion) in Ficino, closely connected to the notion of *sapiential* (wisdom), and a clear point of reference in Donzellini's philosophical output, see Cesare Vasoli, 'Il *De christiana religione* di Marsilio Ficino,' *Bruniana & Campanelliana*, 13, no. 2 (2007), 403–28. On the Neoplatonic framework that pervaded Florentine humanism, see idem, 'Prisca theologia.' Donzellini refers to Ficino as the 'illustrator' ('illustratore') of Platonism in Donzellini, *Remedium*, 47v.

27 Ibidem.

28 Si Deus Sol est incorporeus, infinitus, omnia permeans, omnia occupans, omnibus praesens: si Deus lux est iucundissima, atque aeterna: si ex eius luminis communione, homo non tantum Angelis Dei, sed Deo ipsi similis efficitur: quin immo Dei filius, ac in Deo alter veluti Deus: & in beatissimo beatus, si haec beatitudo omnes voluptetes, & gaudia comprahendit, aut potius immenso superat intervallo, quae habuit, ac habiturum est genus humanum a Mundi exordio ad eius usque exitum, ac finem: si denique Deus erit omnia in omnibus: idest, ita aderit singulis, ut illis seipsum communicando, omne simul bonum comunicet: quid superest, nisi ut unusquisque alia omni cogitatione semota, in illud unum incumbat, ut ad tantae felicitatis possessionem possit pervenire?'; Ibid., 49r.

29 Antonio Rotondò, 'La censura ecclesiastica e la cultura,' in *Storia d'Italia*, vol. 5, *I documenti* (Turin: Einaudi, 1973), 1454–60.

30 On Patricius and his thought, see Maria Muccillo, 'La filosofia antica nelle Discussiones peripateticae di Francesco Patrizi da Cherso,' in eadem, *Platonismo ermetismo e "Prisca theologia". Ricerche di storiografia filosofica rinascimentale* (Florence: Olschki, 1996), 73–193; Margherita Palumbo, entry 'Patrizi, Francesco,' in *Dizionario Biografico degli Italiani*, 81 (2014); Baldini, Spruit, *Catholic Church*, vol. 1, 2197–264.

31 Delio Cantimori, *Anabattismo e neoplatonismo nel XVI secolo in Italia* (Rome: Aseq, 2009, first edition 1936), 24.

32 Idem., *Eretici italiani*, 18. For the humanist solution to the religious problems inherited by 'Italian heretics' in the following century and often tackled using similar models, see ibid., 15–22.

33 See the well-known sentence in the Hermetic text *Asclepius*: 'Mankind is a great miracle' ('Magnum miraculum est homo'); there is a similar statement in Donzellini, *Remedium*, 18r: 'Man, namely the divine miracle, is the outstanding and superior work of God' ('Hominem scilicet divinum miraculum, optimumque, ac praestantissimum Dei opificium esse').

34 'Una sostanza corruttibile,' Rotondò, 'Pietro Perna,' 388–89.

35 God is defined as αόρατον και άρρετον, Donzellini, *Remedium*, 47v. With these expressions, Donzellini was referring to the *priscus philosophus* (ancient sage) Philo of Alexandria, a source also used by Servetus along with Lactantius, Origen, and the Neoplatonic philosophers. Philo is defined as a supreme master of wisdom, together with Hermes Trismegistus, in Donzellini, *Themistii Euphradae*, 11. The *Remedium* also contains multiple references to the work and thinking of Lactantius. Considered one of the Fathers of the Church most indebted to the Hermetic tradition, Lactantius supported its spread in Christian culture and was committed to encouraging conciliation between pagan cults and Christianity; see Francis Yates, *Giordano Bruno e la tradizione ermetica* (Rome – Bari: Laterza, 2006, first edition 1964); Paolo Scarpi, 'La divina auctoritas di Ermete Trismegisto: per una nuova religione di tolleranza,' in Salvatore Gaspa (ed.), *From Source to History: Studies on Ancient Near Eastern Worlds and Beyond: Dedicated to Giovanni Battista Lanfranchi on the Occasion of His 65th Birthday on June 23, 2014* (Münster: Ugarit-Verlat, 2014), 650–52. With regard to Servetus and his reception of the thought of Lactantius, see Manzoni, *Umanesimo ed eresia*, 98. On Origen and his importance in the theology of Servetus, see ibid., ad indicem. As mentioned above, Donzellini displayed a strong interest in Origen's thinking, offering Zwinger an edition of the *Origines in Ioannem volumina 4*; see Basel, Universitätsbibliothek, Abteilung Frey-Gryn Mscr II 2, letter of 20 August 1583.

36 Manzoni, *Umanesimo ed eresia*, 126.

37 I Cor 15:28.

38 'Deum esse sphaeram cuius centrum est ubique'; Donzellini, *Remedium ferendarum iniuriarum*, 48r. The expression became well known through the *Liber XXIV philosophorum* (*Book of the Twenty-Four Philosophers*), where it was included in statement number 2: this anonymous pseudo-Hermetic work, an anthology of Christianised Neoplatonic doctrine, was conceived as an account of a symposium between twenty-four theologians meeting to find a suitable definition for describing the nature of God; see Paolo Lucentini (ed.), *Il libro dei ventiquattro filosofi* (Milan: Adelphi, 1999). The text was first cited in the *Regulae coelestis iuris* (*Rules of Celestial Law*) by Alain de Lille (1125–1203) and became extremely popular during the Renaissance through the work of Cusano and Ficino.

39 Donzellini, *Remedium*, 47r–47v.

40 Ibid., 47v.

41 'La Parola era eterna. Il figlio di Dio non era eterno,' Bainton, *Vita e morte*, 934.

42 Addante, *Valentino Gentile*, 189. The Christ-Word is defined in the dedication as 'that eternal Son of God generated by the Father since time immemorial ('aeternus ille dei filius, ab infinitis seculorum aetatibus ex patre genitus'); Donzellini, *Remedium*, 8.

43 One exemplary case concerns Antonio Francesco Pigafetta, a heterodox physician from Vicenza who, while in exile in Heidelberg, stated that he supported the opinion of a 'certain Spaniard who is an expert in surgery' ('Hispanus quidam sectionis peritus') with regard to blood circulation in the heart. Giuseppe Ongaro demonstrated that he must have been referring to Servetus and identified the open-endedness of the statement as 'a vague memory and chance reading' ('una vaga reminescenza e una lettura accidentale') by the physician years before during his time in Padua; see Ongaro, 'La scoperta della circolazione,' 37.

44 See, moreover, the way in which the *Cento e dieci divine considerazioni* (*One Hundred and Ten Divine Considerations*), a text known to Donzellini, discouraged the true Christian from struggling to understand such a complex and mysterious theological matter: see consideration number 95: 'Men are incapable of the divine generation of the son of God and of the spiritual regeneration of the sons of God' ('Che gli uomini sono incapaci della divina generazione del figliuolo di Dio e della spirituale rigenerazione delli figliuoli di Dio'); Valdés, *Le cento e dieci divine considerazioni*, 345–49.

45 There are also lexical and content-based similarities between the *Remedium* and the *Explicatio* by Fausto Sozzini, but the evidence is too fragmentary to suggest that Donzellini had read the text by the Italian anti-Trinitarian theologian. It is worth remembering, though, that Sozzini had been in close contact with Castellio while writing the *Explicatio* (1562–1563) and that the latter, like his companions in Basel Martin Borrhaus and Celio Secondo Curione, had accepted Erasmus's teaching that interpreted the Logos in its literal sense of *sermo* or *oratio*. It cannot be excluded that Donzellini developed these ideas in his long-term contact with the more innovative cultural circles in the Swiss city, which, as we know, continued after he returned to his homeland. Furthermore, between the late 1570s and the 1580s Donzellini was in contact with the heterodox alchemist Claudio Textor, who was a close friend of Cornelio, Fausto Sozzini's uncle, in Venice: the physician might also have become acquainted with the Sienese theologian's thinking through these friendships. On Fausto Sozzini, the *Explicatio* and Socinianism see Sergio Carletto, Graziano Lingua, *Logos o uomo? Testi antitrinitari di Michele Serveto e Fausto Sozzini* (Dronero: L'Arciere, 2009); Mario Biagioni, 'Fausto Socini e i sociniani', in *Il contributo italiano alla storia del pensiero*, Michele Ciliberto (ed.) (Rome: Istituto dell'Enciclopedia italiana, 2012), 221–29; Biagioni, Felici, *La Riforma radicale*, 124–42.

46 Donzellini, *Remedium*, 50r.
47 Ibid., 8v.
48 Ibid., 9r–9v.
49 Ibid., 9r.
50 Ibid., 44r.
51 Ibidem.
52 In the light of the analysis of the theological and philosophical content of the *Remedium*, in addition to what was highlighted in the previous chapter when reviewing Donzellini's publishing work, I feel there is little basis for Quaranta's suggestion that the physician was influenced by the Calvinist doctrine and supported the dogma of predestination, made on the basis of his references to the concept of providence in his correspondence. In fact, this notion had a different meaning for him, which did not exclude individual freedom, the key element of his humanist religion. See Quaranta, *Medici italiani*, 79–80; 103–06.
53 Donzellini, *Remedium*, 10–11, dedication to Bishop Sisto Visdomini (the numbering is mine, as the pages of the dedication are unnumbered).
54 Ronald Breugelmans, *Fac et spera, Joannes Maire Publisher, Printer and Bookseller in Leiden, 1603–1657. A Bibliography of His Publications* (Leiden – Boston: Brill, 2003).
55 'For one thing, spiritualism's reliance on the working of the inner spirit accorded with the research on the invisible forces at work within the human body [...]; for another, with its deprecation of traditional written authorities, spiritualism helped "physicians" to dispute the heretofore invincible medical treatises of the ancients.' Waite advanced this suggestive hypothesis in reference to David Joris and his circle of friends and medical correspondents, in particular Johannes Wier, a physician with spiritual tendencies; Waite, 'Radical Religion,' 167–85.
56 Donzellini, *Remedium*, 40r.
57 The most malignant was dry or 'hot' ('torrida') bile, which was denser than other forms. Although those affected by it were slow to anger, they were also less likely to calm down and forgive. Their rage tended to escalate into resentment, developing into hatred that could only be quelled through revenge. At the opposite extreme were subjects with a 'hot temperament' ('temperamento caldo'), whose anger flared up more easily (which, as Donzellini pointed out, had also been observed by Lucretius in *De rerum natura*); 40v.
58 Ibidem.
59 Ibid., 40v–41r.
60 Ibidem. On the subject of using music as a healing remedy, see Concetta Pennuto, 'Curare con la musica,' in Antonio Clericuzio, Germana Ernst (eds.), *Il Rinascimento Italiano e l'Europa,* vol. 5, *Le scienze* (Treviso: Angelo Colla editore, 2008), 297–306.
61 'As it indeed appears evident from this, there is truth to the definition which says that medicine is the philosophy of the body and inversely philosophy is the medicine of the soul, where the physician heals not only bodies but also souls and is a master at indicating good behaviour. It follows from this that the medical art will be increasingly glorious in the future and will be used exceptionally for a long time to come. Because it can improve not only bodies but also souls, especially for lovers of virtue and honesty.' ('Ut ex eo facile appareat minime veram esse definitionem illa quae dicit Medicinam esse philosophiam corporis, Philosophiam vero animi Medicinam, cum Medicus non tantum corporum, sed etiam animorum sit curator, et morum magister. Ex quo sit, ut Ars medica longe gloriosior futura sit, ac eius usus longe optimus. Quae non tantum corpora meliora, sed animos etiam virtutis, ac honestatis magis amantes, ac studiosos possit efficere.'); ibid., 32r.

62 Ibid., 40r.
63 Hiro Hirai, 'Alter Galenus: Jean Fernel et son interprétation plantonico-chrétienne de Galien,' *Early Science and Medicine*, 10, no. 1 (2005), 1–35.
64 'France has also provided Budé, Lefevre, Fernel, Castellio' ('Gallia etiam tulit Budaeu, Fabrum, Fernellium, Castalionem'); Donzellini, *Themistii Euphradae*, 25. See also the references to the quality of 'tota substantia' in the treatise written under the name of Claudio Gelli in 1584, on which see Mammola, *La ragione*, 201.
65 Ibid., 201–08, in particular 204.
66 Ibidem.
67 Ibid., 207.
68 Donzellini, *Remedium*, 51r–51v.
69 I focused on this treatise in more detail in Celati, 'The Experience of The Physician Girolamo Donzellini,' 197–202. For analysis of the treatise, see also Samuel Cohn, *Cultures of Plague: Medical Thinking at the End of the Renaissance* (Oxford: Oxford University Press, 2010), 274–76.
70 On this matter, see Nancy Siraisi, *History, Medicine, and the Traditions of Renaissance Learning* (Ann Arbor: University of Michigan Press, 2007), 102–05; Richard Palmer, 'Girolamo Mercuriale and the Plague of Venice,' in Arcangeli, Nutton, *Girolamo Mercuriale*, 51–65; Vivian Nutton, 'With Benefit of Hindsight: Girolamo Mercuriale and Simone Simoni on Plague,' *Medicina e Storia*, 11 (2006), 5–19.
71 Donzellini defines plague as a 'popular epidemic that is shared by the majority of people where it prevails. This is not part of the essence of the plague but is an element of chance, extrinsic to its nature. It follows on from the effect of the plague, namely infection, which is also the cause of the plague shared by the whole population. If there were just one person in the world with this poisoned quality, which is the true essence of plague together with its characteristic effects and random manifestations, there is no doubt it would be plague [...]. It is certainly true that it spreads quickly where multitudes are found.' ('epidemia popolare e comune al più di quella gente dove regna, il che non pertiene a quell'essenza della peste ma è accidente estrinseco alla natura sua, e segue l'effetto della peste, che è il contagio, e anche la causa di essa peste che è comune a tutto il popolo. Ma posto caso che nel mondo fosse uno solo che avesse quella venenata qualità che è la vera essenza della peste insieme col caratterismo de suoi effetti e accidenti non vi è dubbio che saria peste [...]. Egli è ben vero che dove si trova moltitudine presto si diffonde.'); Girolamo Donzellini, *Discorso nobilissimo e dottissimo preservativo e curativo della peste* (Venice: Orazio Gobi da Salò, 1577), 1r.
72 In the thought of Fracastoro, a versatile intellectual who was active in the fields of astronomy and literature as well as philosophy and medicine, the theories of ancient authors are reworked on the basis of observation and direct experience of natural phenomena, with the complete convergence of the philosophy of nature and medical doctrine. On him, see Vivian Nutton, 'The Reception of Fracastoro's Theory of Contagion: The Seed that Fell Among Thorns?,' *Osiris*, 6 (1990), 196–34; Enrico Peruzzi, entry 'Fracastoro, Girolamo,' in *Dizionario Biografico degli Italiani*, 49 (1997); Alessandro Pastore, Enrico Peruzzi (eds.), *Girolamo Fracastoro: tra medicina, filosofia e scienze della natura. Atti del Convegno (Verona-Padova, 9–11 ottobre 2003)* (Florence: Olschki, 2006); Concetta Pennuto, *Simpatia, fantasia e contagio. Il pensiero medico* **e** *il pensiero filosofico di Girolamo Fracastoro* (Rome: Edizioni di Storia e Letteratura, 2008).
73 'Il vitalismo onnipresente dell'*anima mundi*,' Peruzzi, 'Fracastoro, Girolamo.'
74 Donzellini, *Discorso nobilissimo*, 2r.

75 On these exchanges, see Quaranta, *Medici italiani*, 201, 202, 214, 215.
76 On this publishing venture, see ibid., 198–99. On Donzellini's role as a mediator in another controversy in the *Respublica medica* that again involved Mattioli, this time against the naturalist Gessner, about how to depict the plant *aconitum primum* correctly (a polemic which continued for about a decade), see Candice Delisle, 'The Letter: Private Text or Public Place? The Mattioli-Gesner Controversy about the *Aconitum Primum*,' *Gesnerus*, 61, no. 3–4 (2004), 161–76.
77 Quaranta, *Medici italiani*, 199. The physician and censor Girolamo Rossi was responsible for the expurgation (after he had intervened in the works of Guglielmo Grataroli, the Italian physician in exile in Basel); see Baldini-Spruit, Catholic Church, vol. 1, 1689. On Rossi, see Hannah Marcus, 'Girolamo Rossi, a Physician and Censor for the Congregation of the Index,' *Early Science and Medicine*, 23 no. 1–2 (2018), 14–33; eadem, *Forbidden Knowledge,* ad indicem.uaq
78 On Donzellini's friendships in the Orient, see Quaranta, *Medici italiani*, 190.
79 Eadem, *Exile Experiences*, 88–90.
80 Eadem, *Medici italiani*, 269–70.
81 'I, Girolamo Donzellini, physical medical physician, attest that I examined an old woman, Laura Malipiero, in the prisons of the Holy Office. I found her riddled with pain, with extremely troublesome fever and colic ache that make her cry out day and night. I cannot provide appropriate help or assistance in that place. My conscience prompted me to testify to this on oath, signing it by hand' ('Faccio fede io Hieronimo Donzellini dottor medico fisico haver visitato nelle prigioni del s.to uffizio una madonna Laura Malipiero vecchia et trovatala carica di male con febbri e dolori colici molestissimi, che la sforza a gridare dì et notte, ne in tal loco posso io farli aiuto et soccorso conveniente, di che per propria coscienza con giuramento ho voluto farve testimonio sottoscrivendo di mia mano propria.'); ASV, Sant'Uffizio, *Processi, Contro Laura Malipiero*, Bu. 52, Fide di Girolamo Donzellini.

Conclusions

Beyond the frontiers of knowledge: Networks and practices of dissent between science and faith

Donzellini always maintained a *heterodox* profile in the deepest sense of the term, refusing to conform to any single confession. The combined analysis of his network, his intellectual output, and his correspondence has highlighted a life that blended irenic ideas with elements of the most radical movements of the Italian and European Reformation, giving rise to eclectic personal religious proclivities in which cultural and spiritual rebirth were inseparable elements. Girolamo Donzellini's religious sensibilities were the product of his effusive intellectual curiosity and his dogged adherence to the values of humanist culture. These traits were heavily influenced by the themes of the Reformation, which he absorbed in different ways and environments ranging from the religious debates organised by his father in Orzi Nuovi in the 1520s to the teachings of an exceptional tutor like Michelangelo Florio. Other influences included Padua University with its widespread heretical ideas, the Spiritual groups in Rome with ties to Di Capua, and the situations in Venice and beyond the Alps. Girolamo then reworked these principles beyond any form of dogmatism, moving in different, potentially subversive directions whose sole common denominator was the struggle for tolerance and freedom of research. Against this backdrop, for around forty years (between the 1540s and the 1580s) Donzellini played an essential role in the international network for the production and distribution – as well as smuggling – of books and knowledge that were incompatible with traditional scholastic teaching.

A connection can be drawn between Donzellini's interest in mnemonics, his attachment to *prisca theologia*, his curiosity about the thinking of Paracelsus, and his religious spiritualism. More generally, he entertained ideas and associated with groups and individuals that embraced an esoteric conception of religion and philosophy and also engaged in medical practices based on a sympathetic understanding of nature (in this respect, his fascination with theriac also extended beyond reasons of practicality and pharmacological effectiveness). It is also significant that Donzellini forged friendships with men like Giuseppe Valdagno and Tommaso Bovio, who were not in circles openly involved in religious dissent but were interested in Neoplatonism and alchemy. This reinforces the impression that he was a

DOI: 10.4324/9781003218852-8

prime mover in a network of scholars who were drawn to the secrets of nature and published humanist editions of ancient Neoplatonic texts.

The cultural and religious climate that Donzellini experienced was fraught with tension and open to new definitions drawing an increasingly close association between religious and philosophical 'heterodoxy' – the latter term is used in reference to ways of thinking that were far removed from both Catholic and Reformed orthodoxies and Scholastic Aristotelianism. Girolamo Donzellini was by no means a lone figure within this framework. As this final chapter shows, many physicians (and humanists) involved in the Italian Reformed movement acted as intermediaries between religious spiritualism and a form of naturalistic philosophy that was open to Hermetic ideas and practices of alchemy and magic. The next pages will corroborate this picture by reconstructing the broader network that included Girolamo Donzellini and his Venetian colleagues Teofilo Panarelli and Decio Bellebuono.[1] Regardless of whether these three physicians knew each other personally (which is not supported by the sources but cannot be excluded), the reconstruction shows that they were part of the same 'social movement,' frequenting the same places and sharing practices, readings, ideas, and contacts. More extensive than their individual networks, this group had specific common cultural, scientific, and religious features. The movement was active in Venice, Padua, Basel, and the Kingdom of Naples for around forty years before it was destroyed by death and repression.

This reconstruction can be used to detail the specific role played by physicians like Donzellini, Panarelli, and Bellebuono (along with their cohorts) in the sixteenth century religious crisis and to connect it to coeval complex developments in medical and philosophical culture. Driven by the belief that research could only be advanced through total intellectual and religious freedom, Donzellini and his companions combined a desire for cultural and religious renewal with experimentation in the field of nature. In this way, they developed unprecedented interest in practical forms of knowledge and in direct inquiry into natural secrets. The examination of this 'network of networks' also enriches our current understanding of early modern Italian society and culture. On the one hand, it helps to contextualise the impact of the repressive action of the Inquisition on Italian culture and society, as well as shedding light on the strategies of intellectual and religious resistance adopted by its opponents. On the other hand, it underlines the interaction between elite knowledge and so-called popular culture at the junction between healing the body and curing the soul. The following pages demonstrate that the connection between fledgling modern science – above all medicine – and religious and philosophical heresies went far beyond the recurrence of certain themes in the reading and output of figures in the heterodox movement. There was also a relational dimension encompassing friendships, complicity, competition, correspondence, verbal exchanges, and various types of collaborations within the Venetian medical community (and between the latter and humanists, philosophers, booksellers, polygraphs, technicians, empirics, and alchemists). Indeed, the inextricable link between religious dissent and the desire for cultural renewal took shape in everyday life in the alleys, bridges, and houses of the city.

This network was founded on an ideal agenda that was essentially unachievable in the late sixteenth century as it attempted to use spiritual, scientific, and societal renewal to overcome dogmatic barriers, fiercely opposing any form of religious violence. The project aimed to further investigate the occult forces of nature, which was seen as animated by the spirit of God. Indeed, only humans, as privileged beings, were capable of unveiling its most hidden dynamics by acting on the 'sympathies' between natural elements and between creation and creator. The agenda also included promoting cultural discourses and publishing projects with profound spiritual influences in the fields of philosophy and religion, sometimes straying into pantheism with an intrinsic rejection of all forms of confessionalisation and intolerance.[2] In a century of theological wars and fanaticism, this community of dissidents was thus connected by shared minority positions, which prompted significant developments in intellectual history. At the height of the Counter-Reformation, they kept alive the values of humanism through their commitment to the free circulation of books and knowledge, and their endorsement of pantheist and irenic doctrines.

As we have seen, Donzellini included his thoughts on the continuous nature of wisdom in the preface to the orations of the rhetorician Themistius, who had defended religious tolerance in the Late Roman Empire. It is probably no coincidence that Themistius's work was included in the *Somma*, a summary of past and future publications by the Accademia della Fama (Academy of Fame) in Venice, founded by the aristocrat Federico Badoer in 1556. The publications and general cultural programme of this institution – defined by Lina Bolzoni as an 'encyclopaedic utopia' ('utopia enciclopedica') – were inspired in more than one respect by the notion of *prisca theologia* or the *docta religio*. The works scheduled to be published and/or translated into the vernacular included texts by Giulio Camillo Delminio, Francesco Zorzi, and Rodolphus Agricola, as well as ancient texts in the Hermetic, Pythagorean, and (Neo)Platonic tradition.[3] Members of the Academy included Decio Bellebuono from at least 1559 onwards[4] and a young Franciscus Patricius, who soon became one of the best known critics of Aristotle and advocated a form of Platonism with a naturalistic tinge – he was duly placed in charge of the Academy library. For his part, Badoer was in close contact with Donzellini's friend Alessandro Citolini, who also collaborated with the Academy.

The Accademia della Fama was notable for its wide range of interests: law and humanity, theology and music, mathematics and physics, and, naturally, philosophy. The approach to the latter was clearly concordist, with the subject divided into five parts: supernatural philosophy, natural philosophy, logic, medicine, and moral philosophy. The institution was also involved in popularising the thinking of Petrus Ramus (Theodor Zwinger's former master) in the Italian peninsula; this school of thought featured a method for summarising and memorising all forms and fields of knowledge which also drew on Hermetic and Lullian paradigms. The mission of the Academy was to publish texts: both original works (which required the unanimous approval of members) and editions or vernacular versions of ancient and recent works.

The Academy dissolved in 1561 when its founder went bankrupt. It is possible, though, that there were other underlying reasons. For instance, the institution was viewed with suspicion in religious terms as its members had ties with well-known Italian heterodox figures, most notably those connected to spiritual movements.[5] Furthermore, it was founded at the same time (the late 1550s) that there was an increase in censorship and repression in Venice, aiming to combat such restrictions by circulating knowledge more widely and making it accessible to everyone through vernacular publications. In pursuing this goal, members maintained communication channels with the German book market in an attempt to overcome the religious divide. While Pietro Perna stocked publications by the Academy in his Frankfurt warehouse, more than thirty years after the closure of the institution Gian Vincenzo Pinelli sent Jacob, Theodor Zwinger's son, a 'brief index' of its published works that were no longer available (which was probably the list of texts that academicians had previously sent to the Frankfurt fairs).[6]

Nevertheless, there was no room for the utopian syncretism and cosmopolitanism of the Academy in confessional Europe. The academicians even failed when they strove to establish working partnerships with Italian Protestant refugees (like Pier Paolo Vergerio) in order to extend the reach of their publishing programme: such projects were perceived as 'paganesque humanism,' which was outlawed both on Reformed soil and in Catholic Italy.[7] For its part, the Counter-Reformation Church perceived Platonic spiritualism as no less pernicious than Aristotelian materialism. Indeed, as Cardinal Bellarmine explained, the similarities between Platonism and Christianity made it more dangerous to the stability of the Holy Mother Church than unrelated philosophies, just as Christian heresies constituted a greater threat than pagan worship.[8] The new Tridentine orthodoxy could not tolerate the essentially non-confessional content of the Hermetic and Neoplatonic tradition. Moreover, the emanationist understanding of the cosmos could potentially lead to pantheistic visions and endorse heretical notions of the Trinitarian dogma. It is therefore no surprise that the first Neoplatonic text systematically subjected to censorship in 1578 was one of the most important in the Academy's publishing programme: the *De harmonia mundi*, by Francesco Zorzi.

The polygraph, editor, and alchemist Girolamo Ruscelli also had contact with the Academy. It is not known whether Donzellini knew him personally, but both were habitués of the Platonist and Erasmian circles in Brescia.

Ruscelli's anthology *Rime di diversi eccellenti autori bresciani* (*Lyric Poems by Various Excellent Brescian Authors*) served as a showcase for these groups (containing, among other works, poetry by Giovanni Andrea Ugoni and Fortunato Martinengo).[9] Girolamo was certainly familiar with Ruscelli's work, citing it in his *Discorso nobilissimo* (*Very Noble Discourse*) in 1577 in relation to preparing 'do-it-yourself' remedies for the plague. It is known that Ruscelli and Bellebuono were part of the same alchemical and academic networks in Venice (where Franciscus Patricius edited Ruscelli's *Imprese illustri* [*Emblems of Illustrious Men*]). As we have already seen, it is also documented that Teofilo Panarelli was Ruscelli's housemate and brother-in-law. Ruscelli, in turn, had been a pupil of Giulio Camillo Delminio. He saw the universe as the result of a complex system of aggregation and repulsion between different natural elements and studied the most hidden parts of nature throughout his life. According to his preface to the *Segreti nuovi* (*New Secrets*), he founded and headed the Accademia Segreta (Secret Academy) in Naples between 1543 and 1552; unlike many sixteenth-century academies, which were characterised by literary and rhetorical interests, it was notable for its alchemical and Hermetic elements, and for its pronounced experimentalism.[10] Ruscelli explained that the members personally tested recipes and 'secrets' learned by word of mouth or contained in books and manuscripts on magic and alchemy. They were assisted in their work by eleven artisans, who provided the necessary materials. This undertaking combined practical-technical knowledge with alchemical secrets in a proto-scientific method based on direct observation of physical phenomena and repetition of tests (which had to be carried out three times in order to be considered valid).[11] The *Secreti nuovi* only contained vague information about precisely where and when the Academy was active, probably because, as seen above with regard to the Venetian Academy, such institutions were viewed with great suspicion in political and religious terms. According to Eamon, the Accademia Segreta ceased to exist (either voluntarily or by force) at more or less the same time as the 1547 uprising against the Holy Office, despite the support that Ruscelli had received from Prince Sanseverino (after an introduction had been arranged by the former's patron Alfonso D'Avalois, one of the prince's political allies).[12] After his time in Naples, Ruscelli moved to Venice, where he became famous in the 1550s and 1560s as a writer of 'books of secrets' and worked as a proof-reader at Vincenzo Valgrisi's printing house.[13]

Ruscelli and Panarelli lived together in Venice until the former died in 1566. Another member of the household was their housekeeper Dionora Calia, also tried by the Holy Office, who can be seen as a bridge between Panarelli's and Decio Bellebuono's respective circles. She lived with Ruscelli and Panarelli in San Luca until the polygraph's demise. At some unknown point she was also in the service of Lodovico Dolce, another polygraph who was an acquaintance and rival of Ruscelli. Dolce also authored a *Dialogo nel quale si ragiona del modo di accrescere et conservar la memoria* (*Dialogue in which the Method for Enhancing and Retaining Memory is Discussed*, Venice, 1552, a translated reworking of the anthology *Congestorium artificiosae memoriae* [*Congestion of Artificial Memory*, Venice, 1520] by Johann Host von Romberch). Although Calia came from a modest social background, she is depicted in the sources as a charismatic figure who could mobilise and nurture heretical relations just as effectively – or even more so – as a man, blending religious ideas with personal and even sentimental reasons. As has already been noted, the role of women in heterodox networks in sixteenth-century Venice was more significant than historiography has thus far demonstrated.[14] This was not only in their roles as sisters and wives but also in their own right; they helped to establish connections in the heretical network as cohorts, friends, patients, employers, and workers.

Aged about sixty, Calia had a powerful voice and an especially pugnacious temperament for a working-class woman; she was esteemed by her friends, who not without reason called her *madama.* Her heterodoxy was expressed first and foremost through her behaviour. For example, she ate meat 'indifferently and on Fridays, Saturdays, and all the other forbidden days' ('indifferentemente et venerdi et sabato et gli altri giorni proibiti'), although she swiftly threw it into the fire if she received a visit from anyone outside her heretical circle. She also denied the value of confession and communion and rarely went to Mass, seeing the Catholic service as the equivalent of 'going to see a bit of dough' ('andare a vedere un poco de pasta').[15] Panarelli confirmed the suspicions against her at the 1566 trial, probably in an attempt to divert the attention of the Holy Office by accusing a member of his network who was weaker in terms of gender and social status.[16] This first trial failed to induce more orthodox behaviour, and another complaint followed in 1578, partly in reference to past events. After Ruscelli died, she left San Luca and moved to a house in San Samuele where she welcomed heterodox radicals for discussions and forbidden meals. She associated in particular with the empiric and alchemist Antonino Volpe, Bellebuono's rival, who was a frequent house guest. She liaised between Volpe and Camilla, the Paduan woman he had fallen in love with, and defended him during the 1567 trial in which he was involved, thereby helping to generate suspicion about her.[17]

Marziale Clemente, originally from Padua, was another heterodox attendee at Calia's meetings who also lived in her house. After studying in his hometown in the first half of the 1540s, he moved to the School of Salerno to further his knowledge of medicine (without actually practising).[18] In a similar way to Ruscelli, Clemente provides a link between Venice and the Kingdom of Naples, throwing into relief a peninsula-wide network that blended ideas of religious reform with experimental scientific and medical practices. The existence of this network, which deserves to be studied in its own right, is not surprising. After all, Naples was a cultural centre just as vibrant and refined as Venice, with a celebrated heritage of philosophy, astrology, and alchemy.[19] The tradition of Neapolitan studies, which also benefitted from the famous medical school in Salerno, led scholars down highly innovative scientific and naturalistic paths during the sixteenth century. Examples of these include the research led by Vincenzo Pontano, whose naturalism was suffused with astrological-Hermetic readings of the cosmos; the studies conducted by the apothecary and collector Ferrante Imperato, an essential node in the scientific *Respublica* in the second half of the sixteenth century; and the work of Gian Battista Della Porta, which blended ideas of alchemy and magic.[20] Naples was also the centre where Valdesianism first developed. A circle of religious discussion and experimentation formed around Valdés between the 1530s and 1541 (when the master died in the city), also producing radical results in some cases. The movement spread over the following years as members relocated. While it grew above all in Central Italy (Viterbo and Rome, where Donzellini also first encountered Valdesian ideas) and the Venetian Republic (especially Padua and Venice), it remained alive and strong in Salerno in the 1540s. Indeed, it was here where Marziale Clemente became part of the social circle of Prince Ferrante Sanseverino, who was influenced by Valdesian thought (and probably converted to Calvinism in the following years).

The prince's entourage included men of culture who combined natural and religious forms of inquiry (with a spiritual orientation) like the philosopher Scipione Capece, the physician Donato Antonio Altomare, and the alchemist Cesare Mafei.[21] Sanseverino also 'showed great admiration' ('faceva molte carezze') for students from Padua like Clemente who came to Salerno.[22] Indeed, one of the main accusations against Clemente during his trial in 1567 regarded his contact with the court in Salerno. The judges also focused on the prohibited books in his possession: works by Aretino, an unspecified text (in Italian) that questioned the legitimacy of prosecuting heretics, and the *Clavicula Salomonis* (*Key of Solomon*).[23] The latter was one of the most important books of ritual magic in the Renaissance esoteric tradition. Full of Hermetic and Neoplatonic nuances, the text featured '*subversive* magic, based on reason and memory as divine gifts that made man similar to God.'[24] The fact that a text of Hermetic magic sat alongside a work in defence of tolerance on the library shelves of a heterodox member of the network seems to confirm the overlap between religious heresy, philosophical and scientific experimentation, and anti-authoritarian militancy. As the trial records end at the point where the defendant was tortured, the outcome is unknown. It is worth noting, however, that Clemente stressed in his depositions that he was under the protection of Bernardo Tasso, an important member of the Accademia della Fama. The former secretary to Prince Sanseverino, Tasso had embraced Neapolitan Valdesianism and had many friends in the movement.[25] Developing along constantly changing paths, this network of collusion and solidarity was fuelled by personal, political, cultural, and religious relations that extended well beyond the confines of Venice.

With regard to the fates of these protagonists, Ruscelli died in 1566, Panarelli was executed in 1572, Bellebuono died of the plague in 1575, and Volpe disappeared from Venice after his trial, as did Clemente and Calia, the last trace of whom is found in the second trial against the latter. As for the Academy, it had been closed since 1561. However, this was not the end of the story. Despite the spread of an increasingly stifling cultural climate, the ideals shared by members of the network were revived on several occasions (and opposed by the political and religious authorities) during the century.

For example, as we know, Donzellini continued to play an active role in the book smuggling network that extended from Basel to the Po Plain until his execution in 1587. Indeed, his demise was a direct result of this involvement and the forbidden books he possessed. The works that he wanted to print, import into Italy, or distribute on Protestant soil included the manuscript *Philosophiae thesaurus* (*Thesaurus of Philosophy*) by the former member of the Venetian Academy Franciscus Patricius. Girolamo did his best to find a publishing channel for this text but to no avail. Furthermore, as already mentioned, Pietro Perna published another work by Patricius, *Discussiones peripateticae*, in 1581.[26] In the same year, the inquisitor of Como intercepted a shipment containing suspicious books that Swiss printers, including Perna, had sent to a group of Venetian booksellers; the bale was supposed to reach Italy through clandestine channels with Donzellini's help.[27] The works in question were by Paracelsus, Ficino, and Ramon Llull, as well as Pico della Mirandola, Cardano, and indeed Patricius. Damiano Zennari was one of the booksellers involved in this operation. In 1588, he also helped to publish an anonymous Hermetic tract with Grazioso Percacino, another printer with heterodox ties whose involvement attracted the attention of the Holy Office. When Percacino was summoned on 8 May 1588, he was accused of publishing a suspect text without applying for the necessary licence or specifying the name of his printing house, a legal requirement. In his defence, he claimed that he had printed the text on the assumption that Zennari had obtained the necessary permits before sending him the manuscript text.[28] This version of events would not explain, however, why there was no printer's stamp unless the omission had been a strategic choice.

Percacino had been a member of the network since at least the 1550s. As we know, he was a good friend of Teofilo Panarelli, providing him with practical support when he fell victim to the Inquisition. It is also probable that he married Panarelli's sister, Virginia, after the death of her husband, Ruscelli; the main beneficiary of her second will, drafted in 1587, is her niece Marina, whom Teofilo had placed in her care before his execution. In the document, the girl is referred to as 'Marina Percacino.' Besides his personal ties to the movement, Percacino was involved in publishing openly Protestant books by authors like Matthias Flacius Illyricus and Pier Paolo Vergerio. He was still active in the production and distribution of forbidden texts when he secretly printed the manuscript sent by Zennari; he used a single large sheet folded into four, probably so that it could be easily transported, exchanged, and hidden. The tract addressed the highly delicate matter of the 'making' ('factura') of the world and the correlation between macro- and microcosm. The subject matter of the text was defined by the problematic passage of the Johannine tradition 'that which was created; in him was life' ('Quod factum est: in ipso vita erat'). From this starting point, the text went on to describe the relationship between God, man, and the world in monistic, emanationist, and pantheistic-like terms (in his infinite being, God was 'everywhere and in everything in terms of presence, essence, and power' – 'ubique et in omnibus per prasentiam, essentiam et potentiam').[29] Such terminology was very similar to the phrasing used by Donzellini in 1586 in the *Remedium*, his last work. The tract printed by Percacino recognised the existence of an archetypal world of ideas, divine in nature, that was mirrored in the tangible world and achieved the highest level of perfection in the human being or microcosm. The latter, in turn, was thus comparable to God. This topos, which was first developed by Ficino, can also be found in Donzellini's work and in the tradition of radical heresy such as the thought of Servetus.

Due to the need for certainty, typical of a crisis period like the sixteenth century, it became necessary to attribute the mutability of nature to a single divine principle, to establish a full correlation between divinity, the archetypal world, the tangible world, and humankind, and to confirm 'the existence of stable structures of being' ('l'esistenza di strutture stabili dell'essere').[30] The members of the network therefore all followed the same path, albeit with different levels of awareness and intellectual sharpness, driven by a historical, collective, and personal need for renewal and reconciliation. While fascination with occult doctrines became widespread from the 1580s onwards, reflected in the increasing number of occult Inquisition trials and the rise in the smuggling of occult titles, the members of the movement nurtured such ideas systematically and continuously from the 1550s onwards, combining them with religious views that were incompatible with any of the old or new orthodoxies. Moreover, unlike many aristocrats at the time who adopted a strict, rational faith on an individual basis, they moved together as a group, developing not only ideas but also relationships and common practices.[31] It was a complex militant network, committed to societal renewal through philosophy, science, and faith.

It can be argued that this was an active and conscious form of militancy, given the frequently dramatic consequences of the choices made: Donzellini, Panarelli, and Pietro Longo, the bookseller in Girolamo's smuggling network, were all put to death by the Holy Office. Furthermore, at around the same time that Donzellini was drowned, the network was further weakened by the execution of the French alchemist Claudio Textor, who had previously been tried and forced to recant in 1579. Donzellini and Textor were acquainted and shared an interest in alchemy and Hermeticism. They also both adopted the same critical stance towards Catholicism and orthodoxies in general, championing an inclusive Latitudinarian religion. As we saw in Chapter 4, Textor also associated with alchemy enthusiasts Decio and Lelio Bellebuono and was an especially close friend and collaborator of Cornelio Sozzini, the brother of Lelio Sozzini, the famous anti-Trinitarian rationalist theologian.[32] Through him, the network extended to radicals in exile in Poland and Transylvania. As they stated during their trials, Sozzini and Textor sought refuge in Venice because they thought it was a 'free land where everyone could live on his own terms' ('libera patria di poter vivere ciascuno a suo modo'). Indeed, despite the law of 1488 that prohibited all practices of alchemy and divination, it seemed the ideal place to realise the dream of societal and spiritual renewal through advanced alchemical research into the secrets of nature – alchemy was seen as the 'true philosophical science' ('vera scienza filosofica'). Textor started searching for a 'stone beneficial to the soul' ('*lapis* utile per l'anima') while still in France and continued his quest in Rome, Naples, Florence, Genoa, Padua, Treviso, Belluno, and Cividale. On his travels, he also made contact with many alchemists, distillers, apothecaries, and aristocrats, with whom he debated 'philosophy, namely alchemy, which is its form par excellence' ('philosophia cioè della archimia [sic] la quale per eccellenza si chiama così').[33] Textor's book collection (seized and inventoried in 1587 at the time of his second trial) included works by Ramon Llull, Paracelsus, Cardano, and the Calvinist physician Guglielmo Grataroli, himself an iatrochemistry enthusiast.[34]

Sozzini and Textor both encountered groups of religious dissenters in Venice. Fluctuating between Calvinism, Anabaptism, and anti-Trinitarianism, their form of spirituality was totally devoid of any dogmatic asperity. Textor was the son of a heterodox physician and had moved between Catholic and Protestant territories, including Geneva, from an early age, observing first-hand the multiple confessions into which Christianity had split. His doubts started as a result of these experiences and his contact with numerous German students and scholars who 'did not believe anything that the Catholic Church teaches and some believed one side, some the other' ('non credevano cosa alcuna quanto insegna la Chiesa cattolica e altri credevano chi una parte e chi l'altra').[35] After many years of 'serious doubting' ('grande dubitazione'), he settled on the thought that it was enough to 'worship a single God divided into three people' ('adorare un solo Dio distinto in tre persone') and that 'it sufficed just to believe that the sacrament was spiritual nourishment for the soul' ('bastasse solamente credere chel sacramento fosse un nutrimento spirituale dell'anima'). As with Cornelio Sozzini, his religious and intellectual restlessness led him to question orthodox doctrines and develop a spiritualist and rationalist approach. He clearly bonded with others (like Donzellini and Bellebuono) who shared this attitude in the Venetian Republic, thereby sidestepping the confessional issue, which might have led to his false sense of security. In late sixteenth-century Venice, under the rule of Doge Pasquale Cicogna, directives from Rome were implemented with unusual emphasis and the city stopped being a 'free land'; the executions of Textor and Donzellini were accompanied by obsequious reports to the Church authorities.

When the final offensive was launched at the end of the century, more famous defendants like Giordano Bruno and Tommaso Campanella appeared in the Inquisition dock. These figures in turn had ties with members of the Venetian network and other heretical physicians. For example, Bruno and Campanella shared their Roman prison with the physician, architect, and astronomer Nicola Antonio Stigliola, a former pupil of Bartolomeo Maranta, who had associated with Valdesian circles in Naples and had been tried in the 1560s. It is perhaps no coincidence that Maranta was also involved in scientific experimentation with his colleague, compatriot, and fellow habitué of Spiritual circles in Naples Ortensio Abbaticchio, conducting further research into the secret properties of nature, the practice of alchemy, and the mysterious subject of poisons and their antidotes. There was a tragic link between Abbaticchio's interest in the latter and the outcome of his trial: after accusing inquisitor Santoro of engaging him to prepare a potent poison to assassinate Pope Pius IV, he was tortured and hanged on 15 June 1566.[36] Under the influence of the Hermetic teachings and experimental suggestions received from his master, Stigliola also came into contact with Theodor Zwinger and was one of the first to read Giordano Bruno. He was also a personal friend of Campanella. As is known, Bruno and Campanella shared utopian and pantheistic philosophical ideas. Moreover, like many others in the network, they distanced themselves from the confessional disputes to embrace a tolerant and inclusive form of religion.

The links between Bruno, Campanella, and members of the heretical movement in Venice and the rest of the peninsula suggest that there was a connection between religious heresy and philosophical experimentation which deserves further exploration.[37] Besides his contact with Stigliola, Giordano Bruno also associated with Alessandro Citolini after they met in London (where, as we have seen, Citolini had taken refuge) and cited him in his *Cena delle Ceneri* (*The Ash Wednesday Supper*).[38] For his part, Campanella was also in contact with Gian Battista Clario, a young physician from a family of dissidents: his uncle was tried in 1568, his father, also a physician, went into exile in Ljubljana for religious reasons, and his sister, Aurora, married Giambattista Gemma and emigrated to Poland with him before eventually going on trial in Venice in 1620.[39] Gian Battista Clario had a keen interest in Platonic and Pythagorean philosophy and was arrested in Padua in 1592 with his friend Campanella. He published a series of *Dialoghi* (*Dialogues*) in 1608, in which he debated the question of the transmigration of the soul after death, drawing on his conversations with Campanella in prison.[40] In strictly religious terms, Bruno's thought revisited a recurring element in the radical experience of many heretics, above all physicians (from Servetus onwards), namely the rejection of the dogma of the Holy Trinity and the idea that the Son and the Holy Spirit were 'manifestations' of the only God, infinite and present throughout nature. The frequently underground community of heretical physicians and their cohorts therefore seems to have exerted both direct and indirect influence on late Renaissance thinking.

This matrix of connections reveals the presence of a movement with uniform cultural features and varied social characteristics.[41] Extending from the South of Italy to Basel via Padua and Venice, it brought together a variety of figures: physicians, philosophers, empirics, alchemists, engineers, free thinkers with an interest in religious and scientific debate, aristocrats, and housekeepers. Unsurprisingly, the most represented professions in the network were physicians – the starting point of the research for this book – and humanists/philosophers, their natural interlocutors. Nevertheless, booksellers and alchemists also had a strong presence; although they lacked the same level of education and humanist formation as physicians, they contributed to the production and circulation of knowledge. Despite the important patronage that patricians provided to physicians, not without heretical complicity, they constituted a smaller group (which does not mean that the class factor did not guide strategic choices, especially in relation to repression). The existence of such a community proves that elite knowledge did not move in parallel with its popular counterpart. Instead, one fuelled the other in a kind of continual osmosis between the practices, information, and theories provided by the different individuals in the network. The printing industry also made a valuable contribution, enabling various magical, alchemical, and Hermetic texts to be distributed at every level of society, as shown by the broadside printed by Percacino. Although medical and philosophical humanism cannot be equated with the empirical practices conducted in apothecary shops and workshops, the two dimensions can and must be interpreted as intrinsically interconnected. The magical, Hermetic, and occult world did not exist separately in an academic ivory tower or a remote laboratory but formed a part of everyday life in households and families, playing a role in both personal and professional relations.[42]

From the 1570s onwards, network connections were based more on the production and distribution of books than heretical practices like communal readings of heterodox works or celebrating Communion (which were the distinctive features of Panarelli's circle in the 1560s, for example). However, this new focus was not unconnected to the theological debate. In fact, it was a product of it. Attempts to propose a philosophical religion or a religious philosophy, a monistic cosmic vision, and a holistic notion of knowledge and the spiritual dimension were intended to offer an inclusive and reassuring solution to the confessional crisis. Many heterodox physicians in particular seem to have played a pivotal role between the spiritual religious tradition and the philosophical heritage. For practitioners who took care of souls as well as bodies, an interest in the widespread sixteenth-century theological debate was probably used to rework the characteristic spiritualism of the Italian Reformation into a functional, rational, and militant approach imbued with irenicism, Hermeticism, and natural inquiry.

The story of the network also demonstrates that there was still opposition to the disciplinary measures of the Catholic Church (and institutional Churches in general) at the height of the Counter-Reformation. In this respect, the experiences of Donzellini and his companions suggest that the Counter-Reformation was not a monolithic and reductionist process, a form of blanket repression that prevented any form of religious or intellectual creativity in Italy through trials and torture. Instead, it appears more like a complex, multifaceted process in which attempts at standardisation and regulation were countered more or less overtly by resistance, conflict, and alternative world views and lifestyles. Once the religious field had become unworkable, channels of expression were sought and sometimes found in science and philosophy.

By focusing on the biography of Donzellini, which constantly intersected with and was influenced by the male and female members of his contact network, this book has attempted to demonstrate that medicine, philosophy, religion, and society were not separate environments. The story which has been narrated derives from the distinctive actions of the individuals who created, experienced, and reconstructed these religious, cultural, and social dimensions. I hope that the experiences of Donzellini and the others in the social movement to which he adhered will cast light on the meanings attributed to categories like religious dissent, humanist medicine, Renaissance esotericism, and Counter-Reformation by men and women in the sixteenth century, as they conducted their everyday lives and relationships.

Notes

1 An initial survey of this type was included in my methodological article Celati, 'A Digital Exploration,' of which this chapter offers an extended version.

2 On the philosophical concept of 'spirit,' see Eugenio Garin, 'Il termine "spiritus" in alcune discussioni fra Quattrocento e Cinquecento,' in idem, *Umanisti, artisti, scienziati. Studi sul Rinascimento Italiano* (Rome: Editori Riuniti, 1989), 295–303. 'The terms spirit and spiritual were extremely widespread in both learned and vernacular contexts. This usage was rife with ancient but also medieval meanings; even though the usage was full of ambiguity, it was historically and culturally significant. Spirit and spiritual became terminologically speaking [...] the meeting point – with an equivocalness that seems to have served the different parties – of the new [...] philosophical trends influenced by Neoplatonism, Pythagoreanism, Hermeticism, and so on [...] not without the presence of the medical and philosophical-medical traditions, with which astrology was associated' ('I termini spirito e spirituale avevano un'enorme diffusione, sia dotta che volgare. In tale uso rifluivano significati antichi, ma anche medievali, e in un modo tutt'altro che privo di equivoci, eppure storicamente e culturalmente significativo. Spirito e spirituale divengono terminologicamente [...] il luogo di incontro – con una equivocità che sembra servire alle varie parti – delle nuove [...] tendenze filosofiche neoplatoniche,

pitagorizzanti, ermetizzanti ecc [...] non senza la presenza delle tradizioni mediche e medico-filosofiche, a cui si collegava l'astrologia'); ibid., 297.

3 On this Academy, see Lina Bolzoni, 'Rendere visibile il sapere. L'Accademia veneziana tra modernità e utopia,' in David Chambers, Francois Quivigier (eds.), *Italian Academies of the Sixteenth Century* (London: The Warburg Institute University of London, 1995), 61–75; eadem, 'L'Accademia veneziana. Splendore e decadenza di un'utopia enciclopedica,' in Laetitia Boehm, Ezio Raimondi (eds.), *Università, Accademie e Società scientifiche, in Italia e in Germania dal Cinquecento al Settecento* (Bologna: Il Mulino, 1981), 117–67; Simone Testa, *Italian Academies and their Networks, 1525–1700. From Local to Global* (New York: Palgrave Macmillan, 2015), especially 96–122; Valeria Guarna, *L'Accademia veneziana della fama (1557–1561). Storia, cultura e editoria* (Manziana: Vecchiarelli editore, 2018).

4 Giuseppe Luigi Fossati, *Memoria sopra due celebri accademie veneziane* (Venice: Perlini, 1806), 47: see the list of members who promised to observe the rules of the Academy in August 1559. The list is taken from the *Capitoli dell'Accademia* (*Chapters of the Academy*), found in a manuscript held at the Biblioteca Albani entitled *Istruzioni diverse* (*Various Instructions*) and published by Perlini. See also the signatures in the *Capitoli e convenzioni fatte e sottoscritte di propria mano dai signori Accademici a di 13 agosto 1559* (*Chapters and conventions written and signed by the members of the Academy on 13 August 1559*), published in Paul Lawrence Rose, 'The Academia Venetiana. Science and culture in Renaissance Venice,' *Studi Veneziani*, 2, (1969), 222–24.

5 See the contact between Paolo Manuzio, head of the Academy's printing house, and Giovanni Morone, Reginald Pole, and Pietro Carnesecchi. Furthermore, Federico Badoer appears in a dialogue by Antonio Brucioli; see Bolzoni, 'Rendere visibile,' 74. See also the figure of Luca Contile, who was 'head of the Council of Sciences' ('reggente del consiglio delle scienze') at the Academy and was in contact with Mino Celsi and Vittoria Colonna. Among other things, Contile expressed radical ideas in his *Dialogi spirituali* (*Spiritual Dialogues*) by hoping for reconciliation between Muslims, Jews, and Christians through common reference to the figure of Christ and drawing on the thought of Michael Servetus; see Simonetta Adorni Braccesi, 'Tra ermetismo ed eresia: Luca Contile, Alessandro Farra e la "filosofia simbolica,"' *Bruniana & Campanelliana* 17, no. 2 (2011), 545–54.

6 Perini, *La vita e i tempi,* 124–25; Anna Laura Puliafito, 'Due lettere del Pinelli e l'Accademia della Fama,' *Studi Veneziani*, 18 (1989), 285–398.

7 'Umanesimo paganeggiante'; Bolzoni, 'Rendere visibile,' 74.

8 'Plato was far more dangerous to be studied than Aristotle as he was closer to our dogma, in the same way that more damage derives from reading heretical books than those by Gentiles' ('Assai più pericoloso era su le scuole Platone di quello che fosse Aristotele per essere quello più vicino ai nostri dogmi, in quella guisa che tutto dì s'esperimenta maggior danno dalla letione de libri eretici che di quelli de' Gentili.'); Giacomo Fuligatti, *Vita del cardinale Roberto Bellarmino* (Rome: Herede di Bartolomeo Zannetti, 1624), 116–17, cited in Rotondò, *La censura ecclesiastica*, 1455.

9 Valeria Di Iasio, 'Le Rime di diversi eccellenti autori bresciani di Girolamo Ruscelli. Le ragioni (varie) di un'antologia,' in Marco Bizzarini, Elisabetta Selmi (eds.), *Fortunato Martinengo. Un gentiluomo del Rinascimento fra arti, lettere e musica. Annali di Storia bresciana*, no. 6 (Brescia: Morcelliana: 2018), 123–314; Marco Faini, 'Fortunato Martinengo, Girolamo Ruscelli e l'Accademia dei Dubbiosi tra Brescia e Venezia,' in Paolo Marini, Paolo Procaccioli (eds.), *Girolamo Ruscelli. Dall'Accademia, alla corte alla tipografia, Atti del Convegno*

internazionale di studi (Viterbo, 6–8 ottobre 2011) (Manziana: Vecchiarelli editore, 2012), 455–19.

10 On the Accademia Segreta, see William Eamon, Francoise Paheau, 'The Accademia Segreta of Girolamo Ruscelli: A Sixteenth-Century Italian Scientific Society,' *Isis* 75, no. 2 (1984), 327–442.

11 Ibid., 333.

12 Ibid., 330. According to Paolo Procaccioli, the Accademia Segreta was no more than a literary invention; see Procaccioli, 'Ruscelli, Girolamo.' Even if this were the case, it seems significant to me that Ruscelli imagined an academy with the aforementioned characteristics to demonstrate his scientific expertise.

13 On the literature of secrets, an astonishly popular genre in the sixteenth century, see Sabrina Minuzzi, *Sul filo dei segreti, Farmacopea, libri e pratiche terapeutiche a Venezia in età moderna* (Milan: Unicopli, 2016); Laura Balbiani, 'Tra gli scaffali della biblioteca di Don Ferrante, Segreti della natura, magia popolare e scienza,' in Germana Ernst, Guido Giglioni (eds.), *I vincoli della natura. Magia e stregoneria nel Rinascimento* (Rome: Carocci, 2012), 99–115.

14 This historiographic gap, regarding above all women who were not members of the aristocracy, has now been partially bridged by the volume edited by Marina Caffiero and Alessia Lirosi, *Donne e Inquisizione*. See in particular the first two essays by Michaela Valente, 'Tra i silenzi della storia. Primi appunti su donne e Inquisizione romana nella prima età moderna,' pages 1–25, and Susanna Peyronel Rambaldi, 'Inquisizione e donne accusate di luteranesimo,' pages 27–54, which provide a more extensive bibliography.

15 ASV, Sant'Uffizio, *Processi, Contro Dionora Calia*, Busta 21, complaint against Dionora Calia (anonymous and undated) and passim.

16 Ibid., testimony by Teofilo Panarelli of 30 June 1566.

17 '[Dionora] persists in her bad habits both directly and indirectly by abetting heretics with testimonies, as she did by testifying in favour of a friar from Apulia, Antonino Volpe, an oil distiller at the Order of St Augustine in Padua, a defrocked friar from Mantua named Francesco, and Marziale Clemente from Mantua, all three Lutheran prisoners' ('continua nelle sue cattive operationi si intrinsiehi come extrinsiechi favoreggiando eretici con examini, come si examinò in favor de un frate Antonino Volpe puliese distillatore di ogli del ordine di S.to Agostino di Padova e un Francesco Mantuano sfratato un Martial Clementi di Padova tutti e tre pregionati per Luterani'); ibid., complaint against Dionora Calia.

18 Ibidem; ivi, *Contro Marziale Clemente*, Bu. 25.

19 On the scientific and philosophical context and the study of the secrets of nature in sixteenth-century Naples, see Donato Verardi, *La scienza e i segreti della natura a Napoli nel Rinascimento. La magia naturale di Giovan Battista Della Porta* (Florence: Florence University Press), 2018.

20 There is an extensive bibliography on these figures. As a starting point see Patrizia Calenda, 'I trattati astrologici di Giovanni Pontano,' in AA.VV., *Le terre della Sibilla appenninica, antico crocevia di idee, scienza e cultura* (Montemonaco: Miriamica, 1999), 135–44; on Imperato, for an initial bibliography see Cesare Preti, entry 'Imperato, Ferrante,' in *Dizionario Biografico degli Italiani*, 62 (2004); on Della Porta, Michaela Valente, 'Della Porta e l'Inquisizione. Nuovi documenti dell'archivio del Sant'Uffizio,' *Bruniana & Campanelliana*, 5 (1999), 415–35; eadem, 'Della Porta inquisito, censurato e proibito,' in Marco Santoro (ed.), *La "Mirabile" natura. Magia e scienza in Giovan Battista Della Porta (1615–2015). Atti del convegno internazionale Napoli · Vico Equense, 13–17 ottobre 2015* (Pisa – Rome: Fabrizio Serra Editore, 2016), 233–40; Verardi, *La scienza e i segreti.*

21 Addante, *Eretici e libertini,* ad indicem, and on Capece in particular pp. 61–76. See this text also for the radical consequences of Valdesianism between the Kingdom of Naples and Venice. See also idem, entry 'Sanseverino, Ferrante,' in *Dizionario Biografico degli Italiani*, 90 (2017).
22 ASV, Sant'Uffizio, *Processi, Contro Marziale Clemente*, Bu. 25, interrogation of Clemente on 19 August 1568.
23 Ibid., 12r: Clemente was accused of having a 'work in which it is claimed that heretics must not be prosecuted, which begins "if from God on high"' ('scrittura in cui si sostiene che gli eretici non devono essere perseguitati che inizia "se da l'alto Iddio"'). On the *Clavicula Salomonis*, see Federico Barbierato, *Nella stanza dei circoli. Clavicula Salomonis e libri di magia a Venezia nei secoli XVII e XVIII* (Milan: Sylvestre Bonnard, 2002).
24 'Una magia *sovversiva*, fondata sulla ragione e la memoria come doni divini che rendevano l'uomo simile a Dio,' Vittoria Perrone Compagni, 'Ermete nel Medioevo cristiano,' in Gian Maria Cazzaniga, *Esoterismo* (Turin: Einaudi, 194–73), cited in Ernst, Giglioni, *I vincoli della natura*, 20.
25 Rosanna Morace, entry 'Tasso, Bernardo,' in *Dizionario Biografico degli Italiani*, 95 (2019).
26 On the publication and circulation of the *Discussiones peripateticae*, see Margherita Palumbo, 'Books on The Run. The Case of Francesco Patrizi,' in *Fruits of Migration*, 45–71, especially 48–49.
27 Perini, *La vita e i tempi*, 238; Baldini-Spruit, *Catholic Church*, vol. 1, 683–704.
28 ASV, Sant'Uffizio, *Processi, Contro Gratioso Percacino*, Busta 61.
29 Ibid., see the enclosed sheet.
30 Ernst, Giglioni, *I vincoli della natura*, 20–21. See in general the introduction of the editors at the pages 1–25.
31 Ulvioni, 'Cultura politica,' 630–31.
32 There is a description of Cornelio Sozzini's scientific and religious profile, and his dealings with the Inquisition, with many references to Textor, in Stella, *Dall'anabattismo al socinianesimo,* in particular see 144–63; 169–73. On Textor, see ASV, Sant'Uffizio, *Processi, Contro Socini Cornelio, Textor Claudio*, Bu. 42; ivi, *Contro Claudio francese*, Bu. 59.
33 Ivi, *Contro Socini Cornelio, Textor Claudio*, Bu. 42, 11r.
34 Ivi, *Contro Claudio francese*, Bu. 59, 11r–11v.
35 Ivi, *Contro Socini Cornelio, Textor Claudio*, Bu. 42, 20v, 21r.
36 Ortensio Abbaticchio was physician to the heterodox Neapolitan Pompeo Delli Monti, for whom he prepared distillates that could soothe and treat kidney pain. See Delio Cantimori, entry 'Abbaticchio, Ortensio' in *Dizionario Biografico degli Italiani*, 1 (1960); Saverio Ricci, *Il sommo inquisitore: Giulio Antonio Santori tra autobiografia e storia (1532–1602)* (Salerno – Rome: 2002), ad indicem.
37 To this end, there are interesting avenues of research in the studies of Luca Addante, who also highlights the connections between Telesio and the Valdesian world in Luca Addante, entry 'Telesio, Bernardino,' in *Dizionario Biografico degli Italiani*, 95 (2019).
38 On Bruno's English stay see Michele Ciliberto, *Il sapiente furore. Vita di Giordano Bruno* (Milan: Adelphi, 2020), 209 and following.
39 ASV, Sant'Uffizio, *Processi, Contro De Domo Marco, Gemma Aurora*, Bu. 80.
40 On which, see Giacomo Moro, 'Tracce dell'incontro con Campanella nelle opere di Giovan Battista Clario,' in *Bruniana & Campanelliana* 21, no. 1 (2015), 55–65.
41 See a digital visualisation of this 'network of networks,' with percentage of the professions of the nodes within it in the appendix of this book (figures A3 and A.4).
42 The notion of a connection between learned and popular magic was put forward in the field of the history of ideas in Ernst, Giglioni, *I vincoli della natura*.

Dramatis personae

To guide the reader through the web of stories told in this book, here follows a list of characters with a brief description of their professions, places of work, religious orientations, and ties to the main protagonists. It includes physicians and other figures who play a significant role in the analysis of networks conducted herein.

Abioso, Agostino:	Friend and cohort of G. Donzellini; physician and heterodox dissenter; active in Venice and Romagna.
Abioso, Ludovico:	Friend and cohort of the physician T. Panarelli; son of Agostino Abioso; heterodox merchant; active in Venice.
Altieri, Baldassarre:	Friend and cohort of G. Donzellini; secretary to the English ambassador in Venice; heterodox dissenter.
Arrivabene, Andrea:	Bookseller in Venice; involved in the publication and distribution of prohibited books; friend and cohort of G. Donzellini and T. Panarelli.
Badoer, Federico:	Venetian aristocrat; founder of the Accademia della Fama; in contact with the heterodox physician D. Bellebuono.
Bellebuono, Decio:	Heterodox physician from Campania; active in Venice; collaborator and rival of the empiric A. Volpe.
Bellebuono, Lelio:	Son of D. Bellebuono; alchemy aficionado; friend of C. Sozzini and C. Textor in Venice.
Bellebuono, Properzio:	Brother of D. Bellebuono; debtor to the empiric A. Volpe in Venice.
Biandrata, Giorgio:	Heterodox physician; archiater in Poland and Transylvania; protector of exiles and theologian.

Bovio, Tommaso Zefiriele:	Empirical physician; friend and rival of G. Donzellini; active in Verona.
Buccella, Niccolò:	Physician and surgeon from Padua; later an exile in Poland, where he is court physician; friend of G. Biandrata; rival of S. Simoni.
Cagnon, Marietta:	Venetian commoner; cohort turned accuser of G. Donzellini.
Calia, Dionora:	Heterodox housekeeper; active in Venice in household of G. Ruscelli and T. Panarelli; friend of A. Volpe and M. Clemente.
Camerarius, Joaquim:	Physician and humanist; active in Nuremberg; correspondent of G. Donzellini.
Canova, Giambattista:	Heterodox physician; friend and cohort of G. Donzellini in Venice.
Capua di, Pietro Antonio:	Archbishop; driving force behind heterodox circles in Rome; frequented by G. Donzellini.
Castellio, Sebastian:	Anti-Calvinist theologian and humanist; active in Basel; probably in contact with G. Donzellini.
Caterina, known by two surnames, Colbertalda and Sartora:	Housekeeper of L. Maggi and G. Donzellini in Venice; accuser of G. Donzellini in the 1550s; in turn tried by the Holy Office in the 1570s.
Cipolla, Zanetto:	Barber surgeon at the *Ospedale degli Incurabili*; heterodox dissenter.
Citolini, Alessandro:	Humanist active in Venice; later an exile; friend and cohort of G. Donzellini; pupil of Giulio Camillo Delminio and mnemotechnics aficionado.
Clario, Gian Battista:	Heterodox physician; active in Padua; friend of T. Campanella, with whom he is imprisoned by the Holy Office.
Clario, Aurora:	Sister of G.B. Clario; married to G.B Gemma; heterodox dissenter.
Clemente, Marziale:	Humanist active in the Kingdom of Naples and the Republic of Venice; tried in 1568; magic aficionado; friend of A. Volpe and D. Calia.
Curione, Celio Secondo:	Humanist; an exile in Basel; in contact with G. Donzellini; author of *Pasquino in estasi.*
Da Canal, Marcantonio:	Venetian patrician; pupil of C. Donzellini; later active in T. Panarelli's heterodox group.
Dandolo, Andrea:	Venetian patrician; active in T. Panarelli's heterodox group; close friend of G.B. Gemma.
De Megis, Pietro:	Alchemist, empirical physician, and heterodox dissenter; active in Venice; first husband of C. Colbertalda.

De Freschi Olivi, Giovan Battista:	Converted Jew and physician; friend of P. De Megis; active in Venice.
De Neri, Andrea:	Heterodox physician; friend and cohort of G. Donzellini and P. Perna in Venice.
Donzellini, Buonamonte:	Father of G. and C. Donzellini; active in Orzi Nuovi; heterodox dissenter.
Donzellini, Cornelio:	Brother of G. Donzellini; defrocked friar; heterodox dissenter; active in the Republic of Venice, Ferrara, and Florence.
Donzellini, Girolamo:	Heterodox physician; active in the Republic of Venice; an exile in Protestant Europe for seven years; "citizen" of the *Respublica medicorum.*
Donzellini, Lucrezia:	Veronese wife of G. Donzellini.
Emo, Francesco:	Venetian patrician; active in T. Panarelli's heterodox group.
Fabbri, Matteo:	Heterodox physician; friend and cohort of G. Donzellini in Venice; later active in Ferrara as physician to Duchess Renée of France.
Fano da, Guido Giannetti:	Politician; secretary to P.A. di Capua in Rome; later active at the English embassy in Venice; friend and cohort of G. Donzellini.
Fenari, brothers (Marco and Ippolito):	Apothecaries active in Venice; collaborators of G. Donzellini.
Florio, Michelangelo:	Preacher and tutor of G. Donzellini; heterodox dissenter.
Fonzio, Bartolomeo:	Preacher and tutor of T. Panarelli; heterodox dissenter.
Gadaldino, Agostino:	Physician from Modena; friend and cohort of G. Donzellini in Venice.
Gallo, Nicola:	Sardinian physician; an exile in Geneva; tried for anti-Trinitarianism by Calvin.
Gatta, Giovanni:	Heterodox physician, active in Venice in T. Panarelli's heterodox group.
Gemma, Giambattista:	Apothecary at the *Due Colombine* and heterodox physician; son of S. Gemma and active in T. Panarelli's group in Venice; later an exile in Poland.
Gemma, Silvestro:	Head of the Gemma family, the owners of the *Due Colombine* apothecary shop in Venice; heterodox dissenter.
Gemma, Marcantonio Jr:	Son of S. Gemma and brother of G.B. Gemma; apothecary at the *Due Colombine* in Venice; heterodox dissenter.

Gemma, Marcantonio Sr:	Brother of S. Gemma; apothecary at the *Gatta* in Venice, where various heterodox dissenters are welcomed.
Gemma, Marita:	Wife of M.A Gemma Jr.; cousin of Caterina Colbertalda.
Grataroli, Guglielmo:	Physician from Bergamo; an exile in Basel, where he opposes S. Castellio's circle to defend Calvin; probably in contact with G. Donzellini; alchemy and Hermeticism aficionado.
Goineo, Giovanni Battista:	Heterodox physician in Pirano; later a religious exile.
Guarniera, Caterina:	Partner of T. Panarelli and mother of his children; involved in the trial against him.
Harvel, Edmund:	English ambassador in Venice until 1550; patient and protector of Donzellini.
Lando, Ortensio:	Heterodox physician active in Venice; friend and cohort of G. Donzellini.
Longo, Pietro:	Intermediary in book smuggling operation between Venice and Basel; in contact with Donzellini; heterodox dissenter.
Maggi, Vincenzo:	Philosopher; acquaintance of G. Donzellini, whom he hosts in Padua at the beginning of his escape.
Maggi, Vincenzo:	Diplomat; friend and cohort of G. Donzellini in Venice; the physician acts as witness at his wedding; heterodox dissenter.
Maggi, Lucrezia:	Wife of the diplomat V. Maggi; patient, friend, and cohort of G. Donzellini; heterodox dissenter.
Manna, Ludovico:	Defrocked friar; heterodox physician; friend and cohort of G. Donzellini in Venice.
Marcello, Paola:	Aristocrat; nun at the convent of Santa Lucia in Venice, from which she escapes with Donzellini's help.
Massari, Girolamo:	Heterodox physician from Vicenza; an exile in Strasbourg.
Michiel, Gian Battista:	Diplomat; friend, and cohort of C. Colbertalda and L. Maggi; active in the heterodox network in Venice from the 1550s to the 1570s.
Morosini, Cecilia:	Aristocrat; nun at the convent of Santa Lucia in Venice, from which she escapes with the help of Donzellini, her physician.
Moscardo, Paolo:	Attorney; heterodox dissenter; friend and cohort of T. Panarelli in Venice.

Moscardo, Giuseppe:	Physician and heterodox dissenter; friend and cohort of T. Panarelli in Venice; later an exile; brother of P. Moscardo.
Nascimbeni, Nascimbene:	Cellmate of G. Donzellini and later his patient; heterodox dissenter.
Negron, Giacomo:	Musician and heterodox dissenter; active in Venice in T. Panarelli's group.
Negroni, Vincenzo:	Physician and heterodox dissenter; active in the heterodox network in Venice in the 1560s.
Noise, Angelo:	German; active in Venice in T. Panarelli's heterodox group; provides the group with access to the Fondaco dei Tedeschi.
Panarelli, Nicola Antonio:	Physician and heterodox dissenter from Monopoli; later active in the Republic of Venice; father of T. Panarelli and V. Panarelli.
Panarelli, Teofilo:	Heterodox physician; key driving force behind a heretical circle in Venice in the 1560s.
Panarelli, Virginia:	Sister of T. Panarelli; wife of G. Ruscelli; heterodox dissenter; involved in the trial of her brother in Venice.
Panvinio, Paolo:	Veronese; brother of the papal historian Onofrio Panvinio; attempts to publish some of his brother's books with the involvement of G. Donzellini.
Parma, Gasparo:	Accountant from Modena; friend and cohort of G. Donzellini in Venice; heterodox dissenter.
Parma, Pantasilea:	Wife of G. Parma; patient of G. Donzellini; heterodox dissenter; Donzellini's accomplice when the nuns escape from Santa Lucia.
Parto, Girolamo:	Notary and heterodox dissenter; half-brother of G.B Michiel.
Passeri, Marcantonio:	Professor of philosopher at Padua University; master of G. Donzellini; still associates with the latter in the early 1550s in Venice, where he is involved with heretical circles and ideas.
Patricius, Franciscus:	Neoplatonic philosopher; member of the Accademia della Fama; author of texts that Donzellini attempts to publish at P. Perna's printing house in Basel.
Pegolotto, Francesco:	Physician from Reggio Emilia; heterodox dissenter; active in Venice in T. Panarelli's heterodox group.
Percacino, Grazioso:	Printer and bookseller; friend and cohort of T. Panarelli first in Padua and then in Venice, where he remains active in the production and

	distribution of suspect publications until the 1580s.
Perna, Pietro:	An exile from Lucca; printer in Basel; friend and cohort of G. Donzellini, with whose help he introduces his publications secretly into the Republic of Venice.
Renée, Duchess of Ferrara:	French Calvinist; wife of Duke Ercole II d'Este; protector of various heterodox dissenters including C. and G. Donzellini in Ferrara.
Ruscelli, Girolamo:	Polygraph, printer, and alchemist; member of academies; husband of V. Panarelli; lives with T. Panarelli in the 1560s in Venice, where his housekeeper is D. Calia.
Rustici, Filippo:	Physician from Lucca; an exile in Geneva; asks fellow radical G. Biandrata to be godfather to his child; brother-in-law of his colleague S. Simoni.
Sauli, Caterina:	Noblewoman from Genoa; plays host to a heterodox circle in her house in Padua; protects friends and cohorts of G. Donzellini like A. Citolini, O. Lando, and G. Parma.
Sanseverino, Ferrante:	Prince of Salerno; close to heretical environments and protector of heterodox dissenters; has M. Clemente as a house guest in Salerno.
Schiavona, Marchetta:	From Zara; known for her learning; friend and cohort of G. Donzellini and the Parma spouses; involved in the escape of the nuns from the convent of Santa Lucia in Venice.
Simoni, Simone:	Physician from Lucca; heterodox dissenter turned atheist; an exile in various European countries; rival of N. Buccella at the court in Kraków.
Sozzini, Cornelio:	Alchemist active in Venice; heterodox dissenter; brother of L. Sozzini; friend of L. Bellebuono and C. Textor.
Sozzini, Fausto:	Theologian from Siena; founder of Socinianism with his uncle Lelio; collaborates with Biandrata to establish the Unitarian Church, friend of N. Buccella.
Sozzini, Lelio:	From Siena; active in Padua and Bologna; travels at length in Reformed Europe; theologian and founder of Socinianism with his nephew Fausto.

Spinola, Publio Francesco: Humanist from Milan; friend and cohort of G. Donzellini; responsible for the conversion of C. Colbertalda to the Reformation.

Squarcialupi, Marcello: From Piombino; physician and heterodox dissenter; an exile in various European countries; interested in astronomical matters; antagonist of S. Simoni, whom he accuses of atheism.

Stella, Francesco: Physician from Treviso; heterodox dissenter; active in the Republic of Venice in the distribution of heterodox books; in contact with G. Donzellini.

Strozza, Caterina: Partner of Francesco Strozzi; later in contact with G. Donzellini, to whom she rents a room in her house in Venice; involved in the trial against the physician.

Strozzi, Francesco: Florentine; translator of the *Pasquillus extaticus* by C.S. Curione; heterodox dissenter; active in Tuscany, Rome, and Venice, where he is a friend and cohort of G. Donzellini.

Susio, Giambattista: Heterodox physician; friend and cohort of G. Donzellini in Venice; personal physician of C. Sauli.

Tasso, Bernardo: Secretary to F. Sanseverino; later a member of the Accademia della Fama; protector of M. Clemente.

Textor, Claudio: French alchemist; friend, collaborator, and cohort of C. Sozzini; in contact with D. Bellebuono and G. Donzellini.

Ugoni, Andrea Giovanni: Friend of G. Donzellini and in contact with other members of his network in Brescia and Venice.

Valgrisi, Giorgio: Printer and bookseller; son of V. Valgrisi; friend and cohort of G. Donzellini in Venice; heterodox dissenter.

Valgrisi, Vincenzo: Founder of a printing house that publishes and sells prohibited texts in Venice; in contact with various heterodox physicians.

Vanni, Pietro: From Lucca; English ambassador in Venice; successor to E. Harvel; patient and protector of G. Donzellini.

Volpe, Antonino: Empirical physician and alchemist from Lucania; friend of D. Calia and M. Clemente in Venice and Padua; collaborator and rival of D. Bellebuono; heterodox dissenter.

Zennari, Damiano:	Bookseller; active in Donzellini's book network.
Ziletti, Giordano:	Printer and bookseller; friend of Donzellini since childhood turned accuser.
Ziletti, Francesco:	Son of Giordano; printer of Donzellini's *Remedium Ferendarum Iniuriarum.*
Zwinger, Theodor:	Swiss physician and humanist; friend, correspondent, and collaborator of Donzellini; plays an active role in the latter's book network.

Appendix: Visualisations

1. Places

Figures A.1 and A.2.

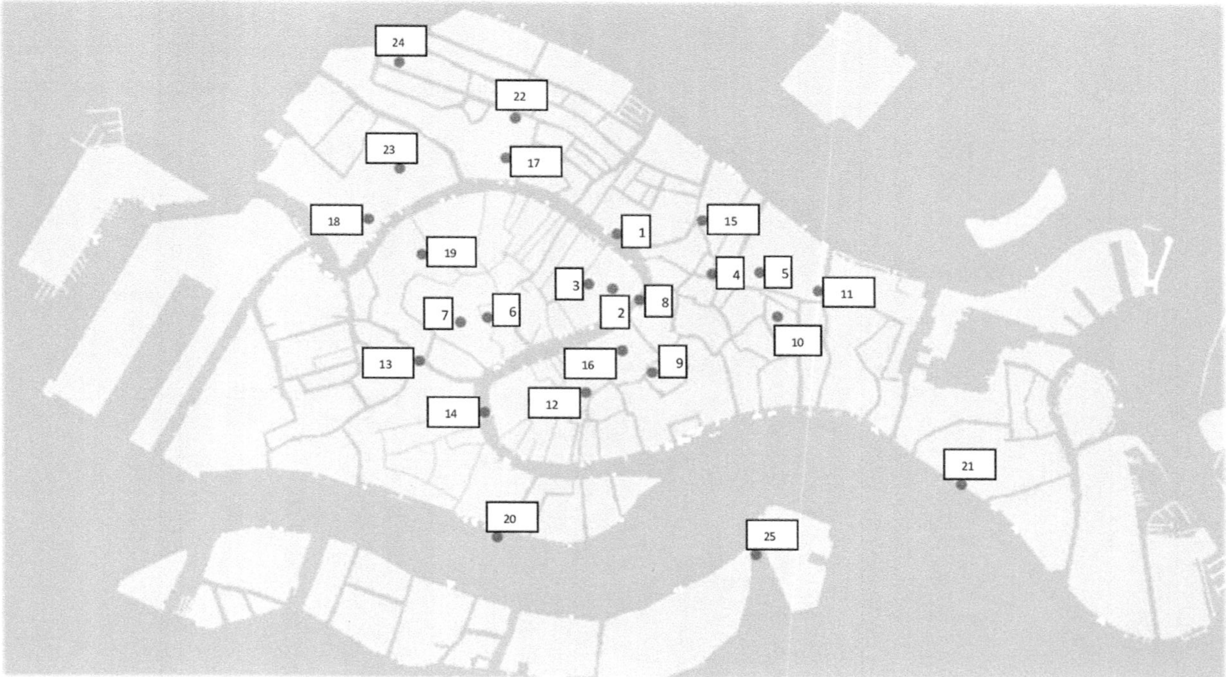

Figure A.1 Map of the main Venetian places mentioned in the book.
1 = Church of Santi Apostoli; 2 = Fondaco dei Tedeschi; 3 = Ruga dei Oresi; 4 = Church of Santi Giovanni e Paolo; 5 = Ospedale dei Derelitti; 6 = Church of San Polo; 7 = Basilica dei Frari; 8 = Campo San Bartolomeo; 9 = Merceria; 10 = Campo San Lorenzo; 11 = Church of San Francesco della Vigna; 12 = Frezzaria; 13 = Campo San Pantalon; 14 = Campo San Samuele; 15 = Campo San Canzian; 16 = Campo San Luca; 17 = Spezieria delle Due Colombine; 18 = Santa Lucia Convent; 19 = Rio Marin; 20 = Ospedale degli Incurabili; 21 = Fondamenta San Domenico; 22 = Spezieria della Gatta; 23 = Church of San Geremia; 24 = Campo San Girolamo; 25 = Island of San Giorgio.

Source: Venice State Archive.

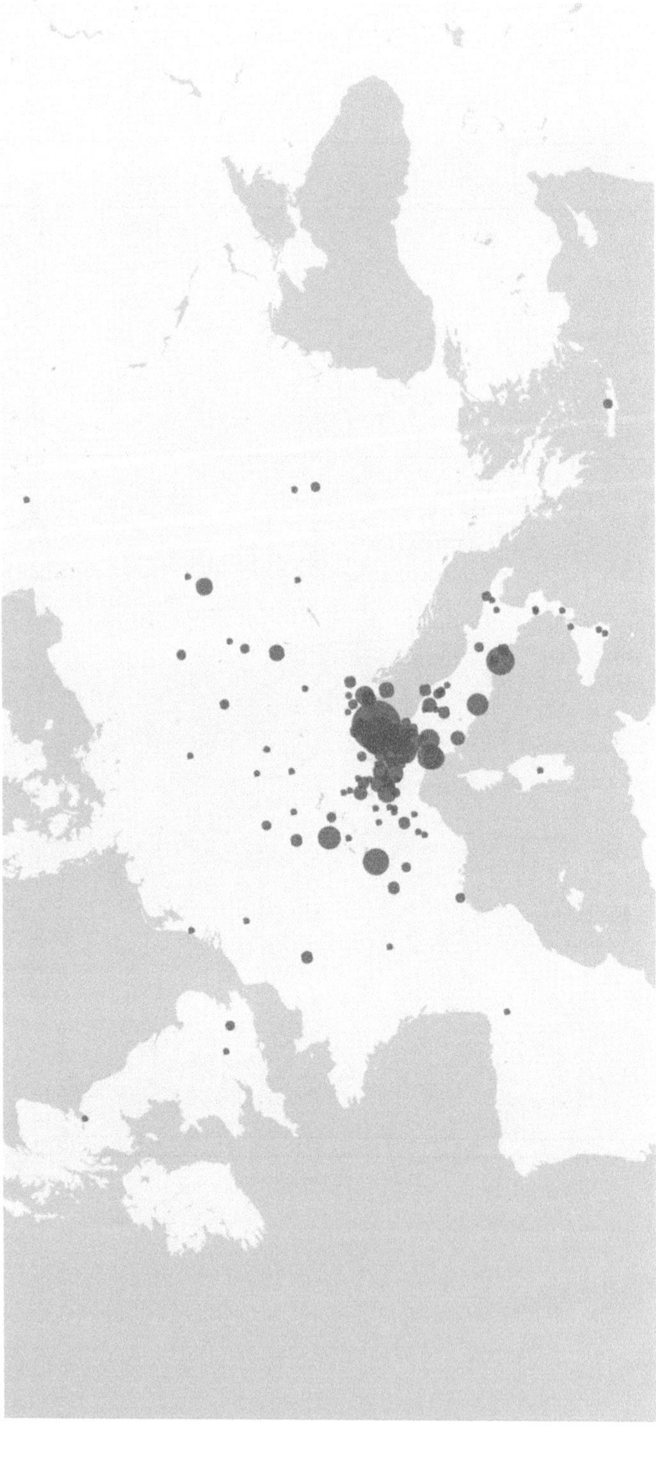

Figure A.2 European distribution of Italian heterodox physicians.

Sources: Figures A.1 and A.2 produced by Palladio.

2. Networks

In the following network visualisations (figures A.3 and A.4) nodes and edges provide information about the network described in the conclusion of the book, and the relationships that bonded together the people within it. In figure A.3 the colours of the nodes indicate people's professions (A.3a), while in figure A.4 they are set with respect to repression (A.4a). The size of the nodes represents their centrality (that is the number of links held by each node). In figure A.3 edges are set by the 'category' of the relationship (that is the kind of bond which linked the people who interacted in the network: A.3b); in figure A.4 they are set by the place where the interaction took place (A.4b). The arrowed edges indicate a 'direct' relationship: the protection offered to Clemente by Tasso and the one given by Ferrante Sanseverino to several nodes (including his contribution to Ruscelli's Secret Academy); a teacher-pupil relationship like in the case of Maranta and Stigliola/Delminio and Citolini; Zwinger and Donzellini's attempts to publish Patricius' texts; employment relationships like in the case of Ruscelli and Calia/Perna and Longo; Longo's shipping of books to Donzellini; accusation against Calia by Panarelli. Various "categories" of relationship can often overlap, linking people in different ways; in these cases, in order to set the edges' colours (figure A.3), I have chosen those which were more relevant for the themes of the book (for instance, the edge between Perna and Longo is arrowed, but it is coloured as to represent "books", rather than "employment").

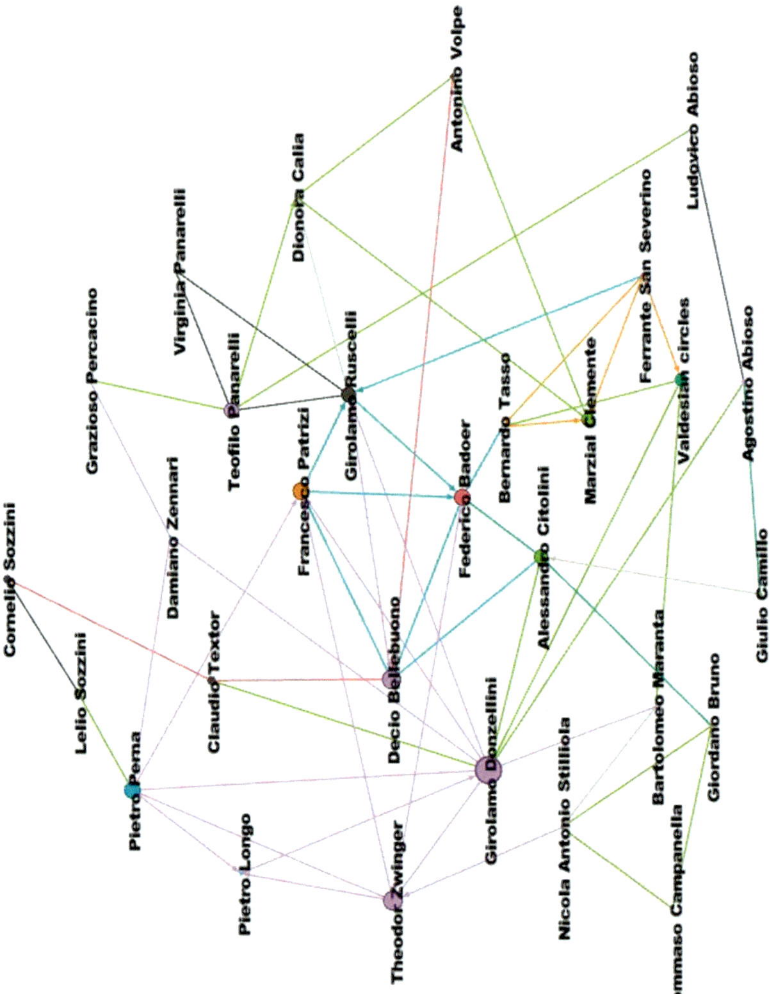

Figure A.3 Network described in the conclusions of the book.

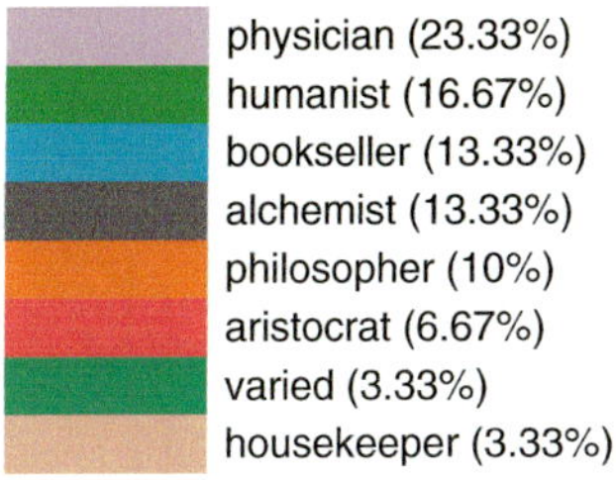

Figure A.3a Nodes legend (indexed according to profession).

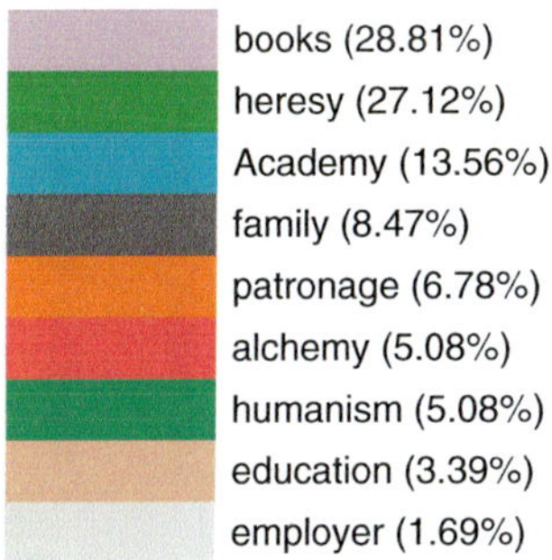

Figure A.3b Edges legend (indexed according to type of relationship).

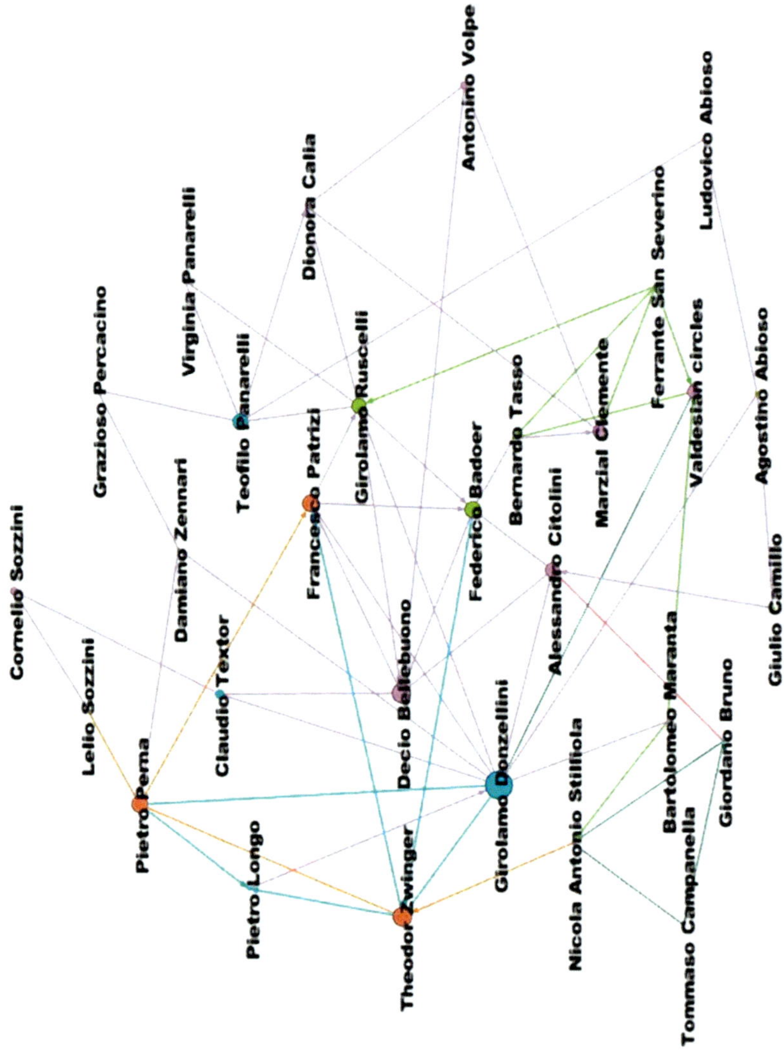

Figure A.4 Network described in the conclusions of the book.

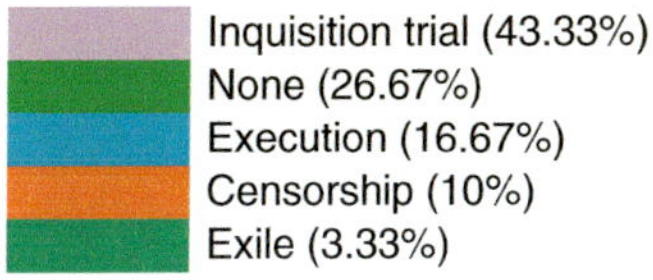
Inquisition trial (43.33%)
None (26.67%)
Execution (16.67%)
Censorship (10%)
Exile (3.33%)

Figure A.4a Nodes legend (indexed according to Inquisition/Censorship repression).

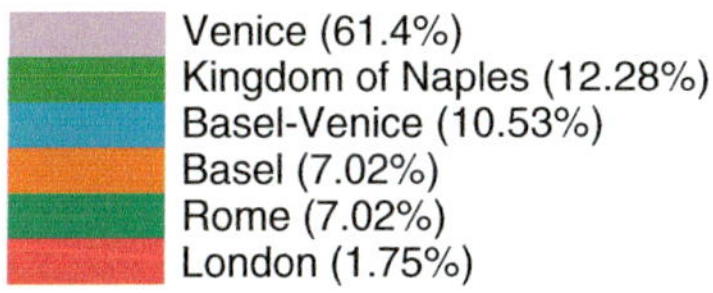

Figure A.4b Edges legend (indexed according to the place where the relationship developed).

Source: Venice State Archive. Figures A.3 and A.4 produced by Gephi.

Index

Note: Page numbers in *italics* refer to figures.

For Product Safety Concerns and Information please contact our EU representative GPSR@taylorandfrancis.com Taylor & Francis Verlag GmbH, Kaufingerstraße 24, 80331 München, Germany